AT WHAT COST
Modern Capitalism and the Future of Health

Nicholas Freudenberg

OXFORD
UNIVERSITY PRESS

OXFORD
UNIVERSITY PRESS

Oxford University Press is a department of the University of Oxford. It furthers
the University's objective of excellence in research, scholarship, and education
by publishing worldwide. Oxford is a registered trade mark of Oxford University
Press in the UK and certain other countries.

Published in the United States of America by Oxford University Press
198 Madison Avenue, New York, NY 10016, United States of America.

© Oxford University Press 2021

Library of Congress Cataloging-in-Publication Data
Names: Freudenberg, Nicholas, author.
Title: At what cost : modern capitalism and the future of health / by Nicholas Freudenberg.
Description: New York, NY : Oxford University Press, [2021] |
Includes bibliographical references and index.
Identifiers: LCCN 2020044862 (print) | LCCN 2020044863 (ebook) |
ISBN 9780190078621 (hardcover) | ISBN 9780190078645 (epub)
 Subjects: MESH: Public Health Administration | Industry | Socioeconomic Factors |
Capitalism| History, 21st Century | United States
Classification: LCC RA418 (print) | LCC RA418 (ebook) | NLM WA 540 AA1 |
DDC 362.1—dc23
LC record available at https://lccn.loc.gov/2020044862
LC ebook record available at https://lccn.loc.gov/2020044863

9 8 7 6 5 4 3 2 1

Printed by LSC Communications, United States of America

CONTENTS

PREFACE

2020 was a banner year for followers of the apocalypse. Massive fires, often aggravated by heat waves and droughts, burned forests and houses in California, Washington, Oregon, Nevada, and Colorado as well as in Indonesia, Brazil, and Australia. A record-breaking 30 tropical storms or hurricanes hit states on the Gulf and Atlantic coasts as well as in the Caribbean, killing almost 400 people, destroying homes and communities, and imposing costs of more than $33 billion. And of course there was the COVID-19 pandemic, estimated by the end of 2020 to have infected at least 60 million people and killed at least 1.5 million around the world. In the United States alone, the pandemic put 30 million people out of work temporarily or permanently, pushing many into hunger and food insecurity, homelessness, and misery.

Political apocalypses also proliferated. Around the world, authoritarian, nationalist, anti-democratic or corrupt governments undermined democracy in Brazil, Turkey, Poland, Saudi Arabia, and the United States, leading to predictions of the collapse of liberal Western civilization. Racial and economic inequality, already at record levels globally and in the United States, further widened, precipitating the largest mass mobilizations in U.S history. The election defeat of President Donald Trump in November raised hope for a restoration of democracy in the U.S. but the almost 74 million votes he received signaled the continuing support for his brand of denigrating science, challenging norms of decency and compassion, and supporting the ultra-rich.

The catastrophes of 2020 amplified a cascade of other long-brewing health and social crises—human-induced climate change, a persistent crisis of affordable housing, growing burdens of chronic diseases, rising "deaths of despair" from drug overdoses, alcoholism and suicide in many wealthy countries, increased surveillance and interference with people's private lives through digital technologies, and a level of political polarization and disrespect for truth that jeopardized rational discourse as a strategy for solving problems.

While the spectacular disasters of 2020 attracted public and media attention, less noticed were the daily tribulations that ordinary Americans faced in their pursuit of health, life, liberty, and happiness. For the 34 million

Americans with diabetes and the 88 million at risk of the disease, every meal can be a battle to find tasty, healthy food they can afford. For the 10 million Americans estimated to have lost their homes in the Great Recession of 2008 or the 500,000 Americans who now sleep on the street every night, safe, stable housing remains an elusive goal. For the 44 million Americans who have outstanding student loan debts totaling more than $1.7 trillion, the American dream of supporting a family, buying a house, and having a better life than your parents often seems out of reach. About two in five American workers—53 million men and women—earn low wages, with many lacking benefits, health and safety protections, or the right to unionize. The synergistic impact of these experiences disproportionately affect Blacks, Latinx, recent immigrants, and women. Their constant struggles can make day-to-day living an ordeal and undermine self-esteem, dignity, and hope for the future, key foundations of health.

Will the human and environmental costs inflicted by the disasters of 2020 and before create new openings for imagining a different, more sustainable world? Or, as we saw in the national response to the 2008 financial crisis, will the nation's commitment to business-as-usual whatever the cost predominate? Will the power that has been concentrated in the hands of corporations and the wealthiest Americans over the last few decades again enable them to resist meaningful changes that improve the well-being of humanity and our planet? These are the questions I explore in *At What Cost*.

My explorations are shaped by my experiences as a public health researcher, practitioner, and activist. For the past four decades, I have studied and taught how social, economic, and political forces shape the health of communities and the opportunities for improving health and reducing health inequalities. With community organizations, schools, youth organizations, local government officials, my students, and other health workers, I have contributed to planning, launching, and evaluating health programs and policies created to reduce the health and social problems that threaten well-being in the United States and elsewhere. As an activist, I have had the privilege of participating in and studying many of the social movements that have struggled to create alternatives to health damaging policies and social structures. Two centuries of public health history have convinced me that it is the mix of science, public health practice, and social mobilization that leads to improvements in the health of populations. My goal here is to discover the magic blend of these three in these times that can reverse the damage to health and the cost to society of recent political and economic changes in the American economy.

For many years, those of us who came of age during the Cold War avoided using the word *capitalism*, fearful of its old-fashioned resonance or its risk of precipitating McCarthyite retaliation. Many chose more anodyne terms—free markets, neoliberalism, private sector—hoping perhaps to engage rather than alienate defenders of the status quo. More recently, in public health scholarship, the term "commercial determinants of health" has been used to describe how markets and the quest for profits shape health and disease, a term that may further obscure the roots of global threats to health.

In *At What Cost*, I choose to use the word capitalism, focusing on the variant that has emerged in the last few decades, what I call modern capitalism or 21ˢᵗ-century capitalism. I argue that recent changes in capitalism have precipitated or aggravated both the apocalypses of 2020 and the slower-motion disasters of the last two decades. In this view, modern capitalism has become the fundamental influence on individual and global health and disease, shaping the spread of pandemics, the impact of human-induced climate change, and the growing burden of chronic diseases like cardiovascular conditions, diabetes, and cancers. Capitalism also creates the actual options ordinary people face in their daily pursuit of what I call the pillars of health: food, education, health care, work, transport, and connections to others.

For these reasons, I have come to believe that understanding the economic system called capitalism, its influences on well-being, and its variants and alternatives are essential tasks not only for public health researchers, practitioners, and activists, but also for concerned citizens, reformers, and social movements. For those who seek improvements in global and individual health, avoiding the word and idea of capitalism is like physicians avoiding the mention of bodies for fear of embarrassing others. By describing the pathways by which recent changes in capitalism have disrupted or complicated people's quest for those pillars essential for health, I hope to spark conversation, debate, and strategizing about alternatives.

In a hopeful sign, public opinion polls show that many, especially young people, now question whether capitalism as practiced can safeguard our present and future and a new generation of scholars are subjecting this system to the intensive scrutiny that may suggest alternative paths.

As I discuss in the last chapters of the book, charting ways to reduce the costs to human and planetary health of the current configuration of capitalism does not require readers to agree on the specifics of what comes next or on what brand of the many varieties of capitalism and socialism now on offer around the world will follow.

But making progress in resolving the grand challenges to well-being facing the world in the opening decades of the 21st century does require some new commitments. Above all, it requires rejection of the dogma that there is no alternative to the world the way it is. It also requires a commitment to collecting and analyzing the evidence that documents the true costs and benefits of the current system, not a faith-based adherence to market fundamentalism whatever capitalism's costs to current and future generations and our planet. It requires those seeking both incremental and transformative change and those committed to racial justice, gender justice, environmental justice, food justice, and health justice to search for common ground, shared agendas, and collective strategies rather than pursuing moral purity, siloed goals, or exclusionary principles.

Throughout the book, I profile a few of the many organizations and individuals who are showing the way to forge such unity and highlight the obstacles they encounter. In the United States, as President-Elect Joe Biden and Vice President-Elect Kamala Harris chart their directions for their administration and then begin to implement these plans, these organizations and individuals have the opportunity to, as President Franklin D. Roosevelt once famously put it, make these leaders do the right thing.

In 2020 what became clear is that our future could be far worse than our present. But the events of the year also showed but by acting together, we might muster the vision, power, and strategies for a far better world. As in every prior period in human history, when crises disrupt normal life, they also precipitate new social and political tidal waves that in turn open possibilities and hope in the United States and around the world. In *At What Cost*, I invite readers to define a role for themselves in riding these waves to a better, healthier, and more sustainable world.

ACKNOWLEDGMENTS

No single discipline, source, research method, or point of view can provide the knowledge needed to take on the task of mapping modern capitalism and its impact on human and planetary well-being. Therefore, my quest to understand the future of health in the current era has depended on many generous scholars, scientists, activists, journalists, students, friends, and other informants.

Several colleagues were kind enough to read one or more draft chapters and give me constructive advice. These include Sherry Baron, Wendy Chavkin, Nevin Cohen, Lori Dorfman, Michelle Fine, Sasha Freudenberg Chavkin, David Himmelstein, Rositsa Ilieva, Jennifer Lacy-Nichols, Kelley Lee, Jerry Markowitz, Chris Palmedo, Jan Poppendieck, Barbara Reisman, Eric Scherzer, Gyorgy Scrinis, Emilia Vignola, Craig Willingham, and Steffie Woolhandler. Their insights helped to make this a better, more accurate account.

I am especially indebted to Jerry Markowitz, who read all the chapters and with whom I have several times taught a public health and history graduate course on corporations, health, and democracy at City University of New York. The students in this course have also helped me to deepen my understanding of how corporations influence health. Special thanks to the students in the Spring 2020 semester who were especially helpful in giving feedback on book chapters and the ideas in this book.

In addition to those listed above, a larger group of scholars and activists, some also friends, have produced a body of work that built the foundation of this book. These include Mary Bassett, Fran Baum, Fred Block, Sharon Friel, Sandro Galea, Corinna Hawkes, Ibram X. Kendi, Naomi Klein, Nancy Krieger, Ron La Bonte, Carlos Monteiro, Marion Nestle, David Rosner, Arundhati Roy, David Sanders, Harriet Washington, David Williams, Timothy Wu, Shoshana Zuboff, and many others cited in the references. I am grateful for the information and inspiration they have provided over the years. Of course, all errors in judgment and fact are my responsibility.

Although my work has been mostly in the United States, over the last several years I have had the opportunity to participate in several international gatherings to learn more about the ways that corporations and markets influence health in other places. The 2015 Bellagio meeting on Health Impact Assessment of Transnational Corporations; the sessions on media representations of the alcohol, tobacco and food industries at the 2015 meeting of the European Public Health Association in Milan; the sessions on the political economy of public health nutrition at the Cape Town World Nutrition Conference in 2016; my meetings and presentations to El Poder del Consumadores in Mexico City in 2017; the Pan American Health Organization meeting on corporate influences on health promotion in Brasilia in 2018; and the discussions with the People's Health Movement at the 2019 Prince Mahidol Award Conference meeting in Bangkok, Thailand, and my collaboration with Kelley Lee and others to explore the commercial determinants of health introduced me to activists, professionals, and scholars working on this topic in other countries. These gatherings also gave me a chance to get feedback on the concepts presented in this book and deepen my understanding of the global dynamics of 21st-century capitalism. My thanks to all the participants in these sessions.

I have been privileged to spend most of my academic career at CUNY, the last five years at our School of Public Health and Health Policy. CUNY exemplifies the best of this nation's public sector—and the ongoing challenges it faces. Several academic leaders including Marilyn Auerbach, Ayman El-Mohandes, Felo Matos-Rodriquez, Susan Klitzman, Vita Rabinowitz, and Diana Romero have made me feel welcome at CUNY over the years, defended its traditions of student access, affordability, critical inquiry, and academic freedom, and encouraged my colleagues and me to journey on the road of public scholarship.

At Oxford University Press, I have had the pleasure of two talented and engaged editors, first Chad Zimmerman, then Sarah Humphreville. My deep thanks to each for their help in moving this book along and making it better. Also thanks to Emma Hodgdon, Sarah Payne, Amy Whitmer, and several others at Oxford who helped to bring this book to press. Big thanks also to Angela Baggetta my publicist who helped to get the word out about the book, an essential task for achieving its goals.

This book was completed during the pandemic quarantine, so I am especially grateful to my colleagues, friends, my partner Wendy, and my son Sasha who now and always keep me entertained, engaged, and hopeful about the future.

December 2020, New York City

PART I

Introduction

Part 1

CHAPTER 1
The Changing Face of US and Global Capitalism

Well, capitalism is a big problem, because with capitalism you're just going to keep buying and selling things until there's nothing else to buy and sell, which means gobbling up the planet.

—Alice Walker

PESSIMISM AT DAVOS

Despite the snow-covered peaks, the crisp mountain air, and the strains of Yo-Yo Ma himself playing Bach's sixth Cello Suite in the mountain camp, a mood of gloom and uncertainty hung over the 2020 World Economic Forum meeting in Davos, Switzerland. Why the ambiance of pessimism among the individuals who lead the world's most powerful corporations and financial institutions?

One reason, perhaps, is that a significant number of people around the world were again asking whether the reigning form of capitalism was capable of meeting the world's greatest challenges—climate change, growing inequality, rising nationalism and authoritarianism, continuing financial volatility, epidemics of mental health, chronic and infectious diseases, and increasing deaths of despair.

Were the emerging questions about the future of capitalism a real threat, jeopardizing the global economic and political order that had emerged since the 1970s? Or did they promise new opportunities for a healthier, more equitable future? After all, in the late nineteenth century, the early twentieth century, after the Great Depression, and again in the 1960s and 1970s, reformers and activists had organized movements that shook the established order.

Was this emerging criticism another blip, like the 2008 financial crisis, a disaster that capitalism ended up using to strengthen its control of the world economy?

At the Davos meeting, some participants, like Marc Benioff, chair and co-CEO of Salesforce, a global tech company with 2019 revenues of more than $13 billion, put it bluntly. "Capitalism as we have known it is dead," he said. "This obsession we have with maximizing profits for shareholders alone has led to an incredible inequality and a planetary emergency."[1]

Other business leaders tried to put a happier face on the situation. Feike Sybesma, the chief executive officer and chair of Royal DSM NV, a Dutch transnational food and health corporation, observed:

> Business leaders now have an incredible opportunity. By giving stakeholder capitalism concrete meaning, they can move beyond their legal obligations and uphold their duty to society. They can bring the world closer to achieving shared goals, such as those outlined in the Paris climate agreement and the United Nations Sustainable Development Agenda. If they really want to leave their mark on the world, there is no alternative.[2]

Stakeholder capitalism, according to the Davos 2020 Manifesto, released shortly before the forum, sought to engage "all its stakeholders in shared and sustained value creation." Among those to be included as stakeholders were "employees, customers, suppliers, local communities and society at large." However, to keep all eyes firmly focused on the bottom line, the manifesto went on to observe that "the best way to understand and harmonize the divergent interests of all stakeholders is through a shared commitment to policies and decisions that strengthen the long-term prosperity of a company."[3]

Tim Wu, the Columbia University legal scholar who writes about the perils of tech company monopolies, observed that, "walking around [Davos], I thought at first I had mistakenly wandered into a business-casual Bernie Sanders rally: unrestrained capitalism has gone too far; corporate greed has endangered the planet; the time has come for radical change."[4]

Klaus Schwab, the founder and longtime CEO of the World Economic Forum, optimistically added to the happy face spin: "If you aggregate our goodwill and action," Schwab told the Davos participants, "we can say to the next generation: 'You can rely on us.'"[5]

But at least one next generation participant, Greta Thunberg, the teenage Swedish climate activist attending her second Davos forum, seemed unwilling to rely on Schwab and his peers. "I've been warned that telling people to panic about the climate crisis is a very dangerous thing to do," Thunberg told the attendees. "But don't worry, it's fine. Trust me, I've done this before, and I can assure you: It doesn't lead to anything."[6]

Beneath the competing efforts to frame a global debate, however, the 2020 Davos meeting crystallized the uncertainty among many "stakeholders" about whether or not the variant of capitalism that emerged in the late twentieth century could solve the problems now facing the world.

A survey of 1,581 CEOs of global corporations conducted for the 2020 Davos forum by PwC, a global accounting company, found that more than a third of the corporate leaders were "extremely worried" about over-regulation, trade conflicts, and uncertain economic growth.[7] United States CEOs were more pessimistic than their global peers, with 62 percent projecting a decline in the pace of their business's growth in the next year, compared to 53 percent for all CEOs. In the United States, 83 percent of CEOs were planning "operational efficiencies" such as cuts in staffing, selling off businesses, or deferring investments to help drive growth. What impact will these efficiencies have on workers, consumers, and the public at large? And what voices will participate in making these decisions? And don't such decisions belie their statements about using the crisis to improve the world?

Corporate leaders' concerns about the economy's future are amplified by other economic trends. Although the global economy has expanded for years, productivity has barely budged, suggesting that the previous relationships between growth and increasing productivity might be broken. Broken as well is the long-term relationship between an expanding economy and rising wages. The wealthiest are of course earning much more but incomes are stagnant or declining for the bottom 90 percent of wage earners. These trends make it impossible to follow the model set up by Henry Ford in the early twentieth century, where paying workers more enabled them to buy the Model Ts they were making, fueling consumption and economic growth.

Finally, business leaders were worried that the tried and true tricks that governments have used to fight off economic downturns in the past may have reached their limits. Between 2008 and 2017, four central banks injected $10 trillion into the global economy but productivity growth continued to stagnate.[8]

If corporate leaders' record on improving productivity is poor, their progress on climate change is dismal. True, the proportion of CEOs extremely concerned about climate change had increased by more than 25 percent since the 2019 survey. In a letter to CEOs sent shortly before the Davos meeting, BlackRock chief executive Larry Fink showed that some executives now believe that climate change is a salient threat to their business. This provides a rationale for acting in the interests of that largest of shared stakeholders, the planet itself. "Climate change has become a defining factor in companies' long-term prospects," wrote Fink, "but awareness is rapidly changing, and I believe we are on the edge of a fundamental reshaping of finance." He pledged to begin moving those parts of BlackRock's almost $7 trillion of assets it managed out of fossil fuels.[9]

However, in 2020, climate change ranked only eleventh in the list of the top 15 CEO concerns, despite the International Climate Change Panel's warning that climate change was the gravest existential threat facing the world's land, oceans, economy, health, and social cohesion today.[10] In fact, a report from Greenpeace, the global activist environmental organization, released at the Davos forum, found that banks and pension funds with CEOs attending Davos have collectively made loans or investments in fossil fuel companies to the tune of $1.4 trillion.[11] Illustrating the lack of consensus among global elites, US Treasury Secretary Steven Mnuchin used the Davos meeting to ridicule Greta Thunberg and the calls for fossil fuel divestment (See Figures 1.1a and 1.1b). "We don't believe there should be carbon taxes," he said. "We want to cut taxes. We think that industry can deal with this issue on its own."[12] Even extreme perils to the planet's future have not overcome differences among capitalism's leaders, jeopardizing the prospects for meaningful action.

Another report released at the 2020 Davos forum, this one by Oxfam International, found that the world's 2,153 billionaires now have more wealth than the 4.6 billion people who make up 60 percent of the planet's population.[13] To address this problem of growing income and wealth inequality, Davos participants would need to make significant changes in tax, trade, wage, education, childcare, healthcare, gender, and economic development policies, an appetite that seemed lacking at Davos.

Some participants in Davos did voice support for new thinking. One of the highlights of the meeting was an appearance by will.i.am, described as a creative innovator, futurist, entertainer, technology investor, and founder and chief executive officer of I.AM+. He told the Davos participants, "It's a brand new decade, y'all. This decade is going to define the rest of freaking humanity."[14]

If CEOs left Davos with worries, their fears exploded only a few weeks later as the COVID-19 pandemic infected the world's populations. Not only did COVID-19 kill or sicken millions of people in low-, middle-, and high-income countries, it also triggered a global economic crisis that rivaled the Great Depression of 1929.

Against this backdrop, *At What Cost* examines what role capitalism plays in shaping the future of the "rest of freaking humanity." The book explores how the transformations of twenty-first century capitalism have changed people's search for well-being and happiness and for the basic necessities of life—food, healthcare, education, and work. Far from the glitz of Davos, I investigate ordinary people's encounters with corporations as these individuals pursue their daily tasks and seek health and life satisfaction for themselves, their families and their communities. I ask whether out of these daily quests, those who seek a healthier, more just, and sustainable world can create new alliances, that can, over time, forge another world where human need takes precedence over profit. I focus on the United States, the country I know best, but since the

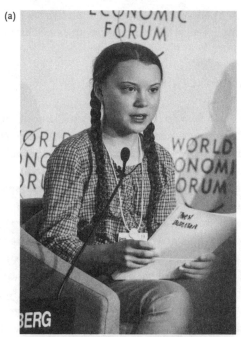

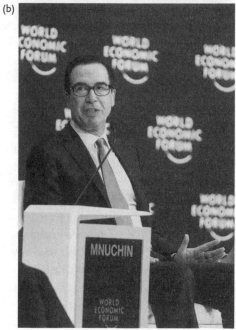

Figs. 1.1a and 1.1b At the 2020 World Economic Forum in Davos, Greta Thunberg, the Swedish climate activist, and Steven Mnuchin, the US Secretary of the Treasury, expressed conflicting ideas on how to address climate change.

daily experiences of people in the United States are shaped by and shape the experiences of people everywhere, my perspective is inevitably global.

SIGNS OF DISSATISFACTION

It is not only the CEOs who go to Davos who worry about the future. Evidence suggests that most Americans are not happier, healthier, enjoying more freedom, and more confident about their own and their family and friends' future than in the past. Nearly 250 years after the Declaration of Independence proclaimed inalienable rights to life, liberty, and the pursuit of happiness, all three are still elusive goals in the United States.

Public opinion polls, media reporting, and academic research show that many in the United States are dissatisfied with the current state of our society. Exploring the ways that changes in modern capitalism have contributed to this "dis-ease"—a growing sense of distrust, disappointed dreams, and social exclusion—can set the stage for considering alternatives. One such 2019 survey of more than 34,000 people in twenty-eight countries conducted by Edelman, a global communications company, found that only 43 percent of the US general population believed that they and their families will be better off in five years' time, a decline of 7 percent in just one year. More than half the US respondents worried that "people like me" will lose "the respect and dignity I once enjoyed in this country." About half the Americans feared they might lose their job as a result of the gig economy, their lack of training or skills, the looming recession, immigration, or automation, the defining characteristics of this period.[15] Only a few months later, the COVID-19 pandemic turned these fears into reality for millions of people.

Americans' willingness to support capitalism has long depended on the belief that it was the system that best offered them the chance to achieve the American dream: a better life than their parents and opportunities for their children to realize their aspirations. Yet today, 47 percent of the people in the US Edelman sample agreed with the statement that capitalism as it exists today does more harm than good in the world.[16] Among young people, support for capitalism is even lower. A 2016 Harvard University survey found that 51 percent of American youth aged eighteen to twenty-nine no longer support capitalism. Only 42 percent said they back it, while just 19 percent were willing to call themselves "capitalists."[17] As support for capitalism declines, will more Americans seek alternatives to the arrangements that the current order offers?

Trust and confidence in social institutions are also key indicators of social well-being. Annual public opinion polls by Pew Research Center show that the proportion of US residents who trust the government in Washington to do what is right "just about always" or "most of the time" fell from a high of

77 percent in 1964 to 17 percent in 2019.[18] A 2018 Edelman poll showed that people in the United States were more distrustful of the media than in fourteen other nations, of business than in fifteen other nations, of non-governmental organizations than in nineteen other nations, and of government than in twenty other nations. Further, these low levels of trust in mainstream institutions fell sharply between 2017 and 2018. Overall, the United States had the biggest drop in trust across the four institutions assessed by Edelman, a total one-year decline of 37 percent in the proportion trusting.[19]

Many Americans report that part of their worries about our social order arise from its impact on their psychological and physical well-being. A recent Gallup Poll found that 55 percent of Americans felt stressed about their lives in 2018. That was a record high for this country and higher than global averages regarding stress and worrying. Levels of anger are also high—22 percent of Americans said they were angry, almost 40 percent higher than just a decade previously.[20]

Stress and anger are well documented contributors to more serious psychological problems. Rising rates of mental health problems such as depression, anxiety, and psychological distress provide another cause for concern that all is not well in the United States. A 2018 study by Blue Cross Blue Shield found that diagnoses of major depression have risen by 33 percent since 2013. This rate is rising even faster among millennials (up 47 percent) and adolescents (up 47 percent for boys and 65 percent for girls).[21] The COVID-19 pandemic and the police killing of George Floyd significantly worsened these already high levels of depression and anxiety.

In the United States, comparison studies of adults in the mid-1990s and early 2010s show increasing psychological distress and declining well-being concentrated among low-socioeconomic-status individuals of all ages from the young to older adults.[22] Other surveys show that money problems are the major cause of psychological distress for most Americans and that loss of housing and employment precipitated by the 2008 financial crisis contributed to higher levels of distress.[23]

Rising debt also influences well-being. Approximately three out of every four millennials in the US have some form of debt, according to an NBC News/GenForward survey, and they are putting off major milestones because they cannot pay up. The most common form of debt is for credit card payments with college loan debts a close second. Forty-nine percent of African American millennials have student loan debt — more than any other racial subgroup.[24] In the first four months of the COVID-19 pandemic more than 20 million Americans lost their jobs, further worsening debt, especially among those with the least resources.

In the decade since investment bank Lehman Brothers collapsed and the economy spiraled into the Great Recession, about 10 million Americans lost their homes.[25] In many cities, the financial practices that triggered the housing crisis of 2008 led to a slow-burn increase in homelessness. In Los Angeles, for example, homelessness surged by 75 percent in six years.[26] By 2013, the number of homeless children in the United States was three times higher than in 1983, the previous peak.[27] These increases in homeless and housing instability disproportionately affect Blacks and Latinos, further widening health inequalities.

Other health problems are also worsening. In an influential series of studies, Princeton University researchers Anna Case and Angus Deaton document increases since 2000 in death and illness rates among middle-aged non-Hispanic whites without a college degree. They call this excess mortality "deaths of despair," attributing the increases on one level to drug overdoses, suicide, and alcohol-related diseases but on a deeper level to the economic insecurity of contemporary capitalism.[28]

Premature deaths and preventable illnesses from chronic conditions such as cardiovascular diseases, diabetes, and cancer constitute a rising portion of the US health burden and also contribute to persistent class and racial/ethnic inequities in health and disability.[29] The World Health Organization identifies tobacco and alcohol use, unhealthy diets, and physical inactivity as the primary drivers of these chronic conditions.[30] In the United States, dietary factors are associated with a substantial and growing proportion of deaths from heart disease, stroke, type 2 diabetes,[31] and now COVID-19.

Modern capitalism contributes to this burden by aggressive marketing of sickening products; encouraging consumers to cope with stress and anxiety with the use of tobacco, alcohol, unhealthy food, and prescription drugs; and by making these unhealthy products ubiquitous and inexpensive. In these ways, our current economic and political system directly contradicts the public health advice that healthy choices should be easy choices.

In the last five years, in the United States and other high-income countries, longevity has declined for the first time in decades, wide gaps in health between different social groups persist or even widen, income inequality has skyrocketed, and urban air pollution has worsened in many cities. For the most part, however, the US government has been unable or unwilling to enact the measures known to mitigate or reverse these trends, an incapacity starkly illustrated by the inept federal response to COVID-19.

Public opinion polls suggest that these changes in health influence how Americans feel about their most basic choices in their daily lives. For example, in a Gallup Poll from 2019 only 26 percent of Americans believe they are eating a very healthy diet.[32] A 2018 Pew Poll showed that 51 percent of US adults say the average person is exposed to additives in the food they eat every day that pose a serious risk to their health.[33] Another poll showed that many Americans are confused about information they receive on food from advertisers and the media. Half of respondents say that conflicting information causes them to doubt the choices they make. Among millennials 60 percent doubt their food choices.[34]

Similar doubts characterize healthcare users. In 2018, reports a Gallup Poll, 48 percent of adults said that their overall view of the US healthcare industry was somewhat or very negative; only 34 percent reported a positive view. Almost four in five said they were generally dissatisfied with the total cost of healthcare in this country.[35]

In the last two decades, scholars and policy makers have become dissatisfied with the exclusive use of economic indicators such as the Gross Domestic Product (GDP), the standard indicator of economic growth. Instead they have proposed new measures of well-being that include subjective perceptions of happiness, life purpose, as well as cognitive assessments of individuals' status compared to others.[36]

One such indicator, the Happy Planet Index, measures how nations are doing at achieving long, happy, sustainable lives for their residents. It compares how efficiently residents of different countries are using natural resources to achieve long, healthy, satisfying lives.[37] On this index, the United States ranks 108th out of 140 countries, with lower life expectancy than 30 countries, higher levels of economic inequality than 33, and a more damaging environmental impact on the world than 136 other nations. Evidence from many cross-national studies shows that higher happiness scores lead to better health and better educational and social outcomes.[38] While any indicator of a concept as subjective as happiness is subject to uncertainty, a team of internationally recognized researchers aptly note that in measuring key social outcomes it is "better to be approximately right than precisely wrong."[39]

If so many Americans are dissatisfied or having trouble negotiating the basic tasks of daily living—getting food, healthcare, and education—then the United States has an obligation to consider alternatives. Moreover, comparative data suggests that current social and economic arrangements make Americans less happy, healthy, educated, and fulfilled at work and in relationships than they do people in other high-income nations, a clear indictor that the United States can do better.

In every era, people confront serious challenges and strive to better their lives. What distinguishes the current period is the prevalent belief that there are no palatable alternatives to the current economic and political arrangements, to the system of modern capitalism that has emerged in the years since World War II. The old alternatives—the Soviet Union and China—collapsed and were reborn with some of the same capitalist features that trouble Americans now. The new alternative—the authoritarian, nationalist, sometimes populist, often-corrupt governments that have emerged in Brazil, Russia, Turkey, India, Poland, the Philippines, the UK, and the United States—seem equally unappealing.

The 2008 financial crisis could have been a turning point. It could have led the people and the government of the United States to examine more closely whether the market economy's growing influence on people's daily lives needed to change. But these changes did not occur. Instead, for the last decade we have seen deteriorating health for many Americans, growing debt, persistent inequality, the rise of low-wage labor, distrust of most social institutions, seemingly irreconcilable political conflicts, and worsening global warming. Will the global economic decline triggered by the COVID-19 pandemic provide another opportunity to construct meaningful alternatives?

To assess the prospects for change requires a deeper analysis of the shifts in capitalism in the last fifty years.

THE ROLE OF CORPORATIONS IN MODERN CAPITALISM

Until recently, talking about capitalism in the United States made the speaker seem naive or perhaps was an indicator of the person being trapped in an antiquated nineteenth-century ideology. Some business leaders claimed the label—the business magazine *Forbes* proudly adopted the slogan "the capitalist tool." But for the most part more anodyne terms like the "free market system" were favored by business leaders, politicians, the public, scholars, and the media.

The 2008 fiscal crisis brought the word back into mainstream discourse. The economist Thomas Piketty's 2013 book, *Capital in the Twenty-First Century*, became an unlikely bestseller. In the following years, more than three dozen new books and untold numbers of magazine articles were published on the topic. Like rare birds in the rainforest, new species of capitalism were identified and dissected including surveillance capitalism, neoliberal capitalism, casino capitalism, disaster capitalism, carceral capitalism, supercapitalism, crony capitalism, predatory capitalism, philanthrocapitalism, and more.[40] In 2020, *Foreign Affairs*, the voice of the nation's international and economic policy establishment, published a series of articles on "The Future of Capitalism," with several articles by Nobel Prize–winning economists and a sober assessment of its prospects.[41] The COVID-19 pandemic sparked further questions about whether capitalism and well-being were compatible.

At What Cost focuses on the variant of capitalism that emerged in the United States in the last decades of the twentieth century and into the twenty-first century. American capitalism, a global system that influences and is influenced by every other nation, is a complex structure that changes over time and place. As the political economist Fred Block observed, proponents of modern capitalism often claim that it is a natural arrangement that follows fixed laws and is therefore the inevitable global social and economic system of the twenty-first century.[42] Even a cursory scan of the variation in capitalist forms in the last century in Europe, the United States, China, Russia, and emerging middle-income countries contradicts this simplistic myth.

As a public health researcher, my primary motivations for studying modern capitalism are to understand its impact on human well-being and planetary health, identify features that magnify or mitigate harm, and discover strategies that reduce such harms.[43]

For these reasons, I am especially interested in understanding the actors—individuals and organizations—whose behaviors, practices, and decisions influence well-being. Thus, corporations are central characters in this story.

Why the focus on corporations? Isn't the problem simply greedy or unscrupulous individuals—the bad acts of people like Martin Shkreli, the founder and former CEO of Turing Pharmaceuticals who bought the license for a life-saving drug and then raised its price from $13.50 to $750 per pill? Or Elizabeth Holmes, CEO of Theranos, who raised more than $700 million from venture capitalists and private investors based on false claims that she had devised new breakthroughs on blood-testing technologies? And aren't other institutions also to blame for the declines in Americans' satisfaction with their lives—inefficient or corrupt government bureaucracies; faith organizations more concerned with protecting their own or promulgating ideology than promoting moral values; or parents who have abdicated responsibility for raising healthy, well-behaved children?

Of course, many individuals and organizations share responsibility for the world's most serious problems. But since World War II, there is wide consensus that corporations have become the most powerful economic, political, and social force in the world. In 1959, reflecting the views of corporate executives, Ford Company vice president William Gossett wrote that the modern corporation is the dominant institution in our society.[44] As he left office in 1961, President Dwight Eisenhower warned of the rise of the military-industrial complex, an alliance between defense corporations and the US military that, in Eisenhower's views endangered our liberties and democratic processes.[45]

In 1977, John Kenneth Galbraith, the economist who studied corporate power, wrote that the modern corporation was "the institution that most changes our lives we least understand or, more correctly, seek most elaborately to misunderstand. . . . Week by week, month by month, year by year, it exercises a greater influence on our livelihood and the way we live than unions, universities, politicians and government."[46]

To understand how modern capitalism influences our "livelihood and the way we live" requires investigation not of an abstract system, but of the specific institutions that make decisions that determine what people eat, how they get educated, and where and how they work.

The increasing power of corporations to shape lives is the result of their changing role in our society. As a result of the trends that have shaped modern capitalism, no other modern organization has amassed so much technology, capital, and political power. No other organization has the capacity to penetrate so many aspects of so many people's daily lives. No other organization has the global reach or the ability to act with so few structural constraints. Unlike governments, which are unable to move to another country if they incur the disfavor of their voters, corporations can move capital, workers, and markets to other nations when upstart political leaders seek to constrict their autonomy.

Of course, neither capitalism nor corporations are homogenous. They can and do disagree and their conflicts can promote well-being or intensify the harm they do. But compared to governments, voters, or civil society groups, the shared values and practices of corporations have more in common and enable the largest transnational corporations to speak on many global issues with a common voice.

For those concerned with improving global well-being, corporations make a particularly suitable focus of inquiry. Compared to changing the behavior of the world's 7.7 billion people, the environments of hundreds of thousands of communities, or the thousands of cultures that influence people, changing the business and political practices of the two thousand corporations that dominate the world's economy is conceptually, if not politically, simple.

How important are these top corporations to the world's economy? The top two thousand public corporations on the 2018 Forbes Global 2000 List included companies from sixty countries that account for $39.1 trillion in sales, $3.2 trillion in profit, and $189 trillion in assets. The 288 largest private companies on Forbes 2019 List added another $1.7 trillion in revenues.[47]

Between 2003—when Forbes compiled its first Global 2000 list—and 2018, the value of the assets of these corporations almost doubled in inflation-adjusted dollars.[48] In 2011, corporations made up 5 percent of all businesses but earned 62 percent of annual revenues.[49] Of the 200 organizations in the world with the highest annual revenues, 157 are corporations and only 43 are governments.[50]

Since the 1970s, changes in capitalism triggered a transformation of the United States from the consumption-oriented welfare economy and politics that emerged after World War II. As a result, global corporations, the public face and executive agents of twenty-first-century capitalism, now interact with governments, civil society, and social movements in new ways. Today, the decisions of corporations, banks, and other businesses shape how individuals encounter six pillars of health—food, education, healthcare, work, transportation, and social connections. In turn, the choices people make among the options corporations offer determine the health of individuals, families, communities, and the planet itself.

Modern capitalism has brought amazing benefits to many people in the United States and around the world. Its creativity and innovation offer the hope that problems that have confronted humanity since its inception could be solved. Big global corporations employ millions, pay taxes, and produce vital goods such as essential medicines and food and also products and services that entertain, allow people to communicate easily across what used to be boundaries, and reduce burdensome and monotonous work.

In the twentieth century, capitalism showed its remarkable capacity to promote economic growth and generate wealth, even if it left inequality mostly unaddressed. However, for hundreds of millions of Americans and billions more in other parts of the world, how capitalism has evolved now undermines health, widens inequality, worsens climate change, and erodes democracy. Food, education, healthcare, labor, transportation, and social relationships constitute the most basic necessities of life. Converting them into commodities that must bring profits to their producers if they are to be offered imposes a cost on human and planetary well-being. A conversation about the benefits and costs of contemporary capitalism can set the stage for a deeper consideration of adjustments and alternatives.

In the 1970s, the brand of capitalism that had dominated America since the end of World War II, an arrangement forged in a struggle that reflected a compromise between corporations and some sectors of working people, began to erode. Mapping the changing landscape of contemporary corporate influences on daily lives shows how companies now design lifestyles and living conditions that enable corporate America to achieve its objectives of raising revenues, profits, and shareholder value while maintaining their influence on politics and the economy.

THE RISE OF MASS CONSUMPTION

Following the Great Depression and World War II, the United States forged an economic and political system that promoted mass consumption as the motor of economic growth. Henry Ford's innovation of paying his workers enough to afford the cars they produced created a system of production and consumption that spurred economic growth for decades. It also led to the creation of a middle class that provided political and moral support for sustaining this system. The labor movement won important concessions from ruling elites that expanded workers' share of this growth.

The parallel development of a welfare state that, over time, provided Social Security, Medicare, Medicaid, food stamps, public housing, and other social benefits protected vulnerable populations against market swings and also contained dissent from those bypassed by the growing economy. In the 1960s and 1970s, new federal environmental, health, consumer protection, and business regulations provided additional protection against corporate harms.

Of course, this consumption-oriented economy shielded by a welfare state did not emerge without conflict. Significant sectors of the population—Blacks, immigrants, poor people, women, together a majority—were inadequately protected or unprotected. The civil rights, labor, environmental, women's, and other social movements played an important role in strengthening these protections and monitoring enforcement.

By the 1970s, however, social, economic, and political developments, operating at the local, national, and global levels, challenged this model of growth. Several of these trends warrant further exploration.

In the last seventy-five years, the consumer economy in the United States has grown remarkably. At the end of World War II, consumer spending replaced wartime production to propel the growth of the American economy. Between 1945 and 1949, Americans purchased 20 million refrigerators, 21.4 million cars, and 5.5 million stoves, a trend that continued into the 1950s.[51] By 2016, consumer spending accounted for 68 percent of the GDP, making it the driving force of the economy.[52] Between 1945 and 2017, the unadjusted annual personal consumption expenditures of the average American increased almost fiftyfold.[53]

As more Americans acquired refrigerators, cars, and televisions, and later computers and mobile phones, consumer spending increased its share of the economy and big corporations became ever more dependent on what Americans spend. Finding new ways to increase consumer spending became the path of choice for both CEOs and political leaders. For CEOs, increasing consumer spending was the way to continue to grow revenues and profits and for both liberal and conservative politicians it was the way to offer a better life to voters. In some ways, many consumers also benefited from increased consumption but since the 1970s, the health, environmental, and social justice costs of the paths that corporations chose to increase their profits through increased consumption grew even faster.

Two threats jeopardized unlimited growth. Economic downturns such as the 2007 to 2009 Great Recession, when the GDP declined 5.1 percent and its predecessors in 1990–91, 1980–82, and 1929–33[54] interrupted consumption and made restoring consumer spending a top corporate and political priority.

To reduce the impact of such economic contractions on profitability, businesses devised several countermeasures. These include reducing labor costs by automating or moving factories to lower-wage states or nations, lowering prices for some products, and targeting more sales to high-income consumers. Credit cards, introduced in the 1960s, enabled even more consumer spending while also sparking a rise in debt, another key strategy for promoting consumption. The rise of home mortgage credit in the run up to the collapse of the housing bubble and the recent ballooning of college and automobile debt illustrate this practice.

A more enduring threat is overproduction, defined as producing more than consumers can purchase, leading to excess inventories and lost profits. Marxists and capitalists agree that profitability requires improving worker productivity while holding down hourly costs. An efficient way to lower costs is to reduce labor costs, either by deploying new technologies to automate or moving jobs to regions where workers can be paid less. Both strategies threaten the Fordist model of increasing consumption by paying workers more.

From 1920 to 1970, productivity of American factories, as measured by output per hour, grew much more rapidly than in the decades before or after, an increase economists attribute to rapid innovation and technological change.[55] By the 1970s, however, American corporations were producing far more than they could sell. To maintain profits in the face of declining sales, businesses decided to cut labor costs, a trigger to outsourcing, automation, and corporate campaigns against unionization. These strategies, however, led to subsequent decades of stagnant wages, which reduced the buying power of workers, and led to further declines in corporate revenues, a vicious downward cycle. Another strategy for increasing consumption, one that became increasingly important, was to develop new markets in other parts of the world.

By the mid-twentieth century, American capitalism had created a system that met many people's needs but increasingly threatened long-term human and planetary well-being. In the last several decades, new economic and social trends have made that system more toxic.

SIX TRENDS THAT CHANGED CAPITALISM IN THE TRANSITION FROM TWENTIETH TO TWENTY-FIRST CENTURIES
Globalization and Global Trade

Globalization describes the movement of capital, goods and services, ideas, and people from one nation to another. Capitalism has always been a global system. In the seventeenth and eighteenth centuries, its growth was fueled by trade among many nations in sugar, tobacco, and slaves. In the nineteenth and twentieth centuries, Western nations extracted the wealth that allowed their continued expansion from the natural resources and labor of their colonies in Africa, Asia, and Latin America.

Today's globalization has made moving capital, goods and services, people, and ideas around the world faster and easier than ever before. The Bank for International Settlements estimates that $220 billion moves across borders every hour.

As national consumer spending grew, globalization brought new opportunities for corporations. In 1970, global trade accounted for 9 percent of the US economy; by 2015, it had more than tripled to 30 percent of GDP.[56] Corporations were the drivers and prime beneficiaries of this new trade, responsible for 80 percent of global trade.[57]

In 2017, the total global trade in goods and services was about $23 trillion, doubling from $12.5 trillion in 2005.[58] This growth in global trade enables US transnational corporations to move capital, factories, and profits to the places where return on investment will be highest, regulations least burdensome, and wages and taxes lowest. Even before President Donald Trump's 2017 trillion-dollar tax break, US companies in 2015 shifted $600 billion in profits to tax havens, where they paid low or no taxes.[59]

Globalization moves people too. According to the United Nations, the number of international migrants, defined as those living outside their country of birth, reached 272 million in 2019, an increase of 51 million since 2010. Currently, international migrants compose 3.5 percent of the global population, an increase of 25 percent since 2000.[60] More than a billion people travel as tourists each year and many people cross borders regularly to work or escape poverty or persecution. This river of people means that ideas, food, pathogens such as the coronavirus or Ebola, and illicit products such as drugs and guns can move around the world at breakneck speed, challenging regulators, autocrats, and public health officials. Anti-immigration policies and the COVID-19 pandemic and the economic collapse it precipitated have for now reduced the flow of people but both economic growth and further contraction each trigger new migrations.

A striking change of this period was the shift in responsibility for setting trade rules from governments to corporations. In 1947, corporate leaders successfully influenced the General Agreement on Tariffs and Trade (GATT), which set the framework for global trade. Subsequently the World Trade Organization (WTO), negotiated between 1986 and 1999, and the North American Free Trade Agreement (NAFTA), a three-country agreement among the governments of Canada, Mexico, and the United States that entered into force in 1994, redefined trade negotiations. Previously, national governments had the strongest voice in ensuring that trade rules protected national interests. Now corporations dominate trade treaty negotiations to protect their interests. It is as if the National Basketball Association had reassigned monitoring and enforcing the rules of the game from referees to players.

Globalization of trade also helped corporations find new markets and expand sales of consumer goods from food, alcohol, and tobacco to cars and social media accounts. As health and other concerns led Americans and residents of other high-income countries to reduce their purchases of unhealthy commodities such as tobacco, alcohol, soda, fast food, and polluting or unsafe automobiles, these industries found new customers in middle- and low-income countries.[61] In Latin America, for example, expanded marketing of credit allowed more Brazilians and Mexicans to purchase automobiles, increasing the demand for US cars as well as the levels of debt and the number of traffic deaths in those countries.[62]

The global trade treaties negotiated in the last few decades also influence health and the environment through their protection of corporate intellectual property rights for essential medicines, the mechanisms they create for resolving disputes between nations and corporations, and rules on labor and environmental standards. They also set the rules for trade in unhealthy commodities such as tobacco or highly processed food.[63]

An example illustrates both the power of corporations to influence trade and the resistance from governments and civil society. Philip Morris International, a leading global tobacco maker, used the International Centre for the Settlement of Investment Disputes (ICSID), an arbitration panel of the World Bank, to bring cases against the governments of Uruguay and Australia, which had proposed stark new health warning labels on every cigarette pack. In 2010, Philip Morris claimed that Uruguay's tobacco control laws violated a treaty with Switzerland, the country in which Philip Morris had its headquarters. The law required graphic health warnings on the front and back of cigarette packets, a policy shown to reduce tobacco use.

Philip Morris asked the trade court to order Uruguay to end these measures and pay the company $25 million.[64] In this case, the court upheld the national rules and required Philip Morris to pay court costs, an important victory that strengthened governments' capacity to protect their citizens from aggressive tobacco industry marketing. Previous threats by Philip Morris to file similar legal actions against Canada and Australia had delayed action on warning labels in these nations for two decades. Uruguay's victory was in part possible because the Bloomberg Foundation contributed millions of dollars toward that nation's legal expenses.[65]

In theory, trade agreements also have the potential to protect labor rights. And yet, of the 580 investor-state dispute settlements (ISDS) on property rights cases concluded by mid-2018, not a single settlement of a dispute on labor rights had been made under trade treaties.[66]

More broadly, the failure of NAFTA and its successors to require enforcement of US labor laws, prohibit investment decisions that result in increased poverty across participating nations, or engage workers in monitoring implementation mean that these agreements often undermine, rather than support, labor rights.[67]

Trade agreements also spell out the rules for investors to increase their stakes in foreign companies to gain profits or increase shareholder value. Investors, often from high-income countries, invest in low- or middle-income ones. Trade and investment treaties set the rules that govern these ventures, often limiting the rights of national governments to monitor and oversee the use and impact of this external investment. In the case of food, transnational companies from high-income nations in the food retail, manufacturing and agricultural sectors have invested in middle- and low-income countries. Corinna Hawkes, who studies the impact of trade agreements on diet, called these investments "a key mechanism in shaping the global market for highly processed foods" that contributed to the shift to a less healthy global diet "by enabling and promoting the consumption of these foods in developing countries."[68]

These foreign investment rules can intrude significantly on the "policy space" of signatory countries, reducing their freedom to choose and implement public policies to fulfill their aims.[69] In Mexico, for example, the combination of increased trade with the United States and increased US and Canadian foreign investment in the Mexican food industry changed the nation's diet in ways that contributed to skyrocketing diabetes and obesity rates, imposing several generations of added healthcare costs onto the Mexican people and healthcare system. The trade and investment agreements embodied in NAFTA precluded the Mexican government from acting effectively to reverse these epidemics of diet-related diseases.[70]

In the last five years, President Trump's trade wars, the British exit from the European Union, and the global resurgence of nationalism have triggered additional conflicts about global trade. In both the United States and United Kingdom, governments, and their backers from industries with strong national roots, such as steel, have urged a more nationalist approach to trade agreements, an approach that favored their interests over those of more globalized corporations. While these new conflicts may have changed which corporate sectors benefit from new trade agreements, they have done little to better protect labor, health, or the environment or to bring voices representing these interests into the trade negotiations.

The pandemic in 2020 showed the gap between the ability of private enterprise to enable customers, goods, and services—and viruses—to travel around the world with minimal interference and the capacity of governments to take effective action when such global journeys threated health. In this case, the diminished capacity of international organizations was exacerbated by the World Health Organization's inability to act swiftly, in part as a result of austerity-induced government cutbacks in funding and in part due to distortion of mission and priorities by governments in wealthy nations like China and the United States and billionaire philanthropists.[71]

The 1999 Seattle protests against the World Trade Organization were the most visible opposition to corporate globalization up to that point. Since then, defenders of corporate managed globalization have sought to portray opponents of globalization as ignorant King Canutes, vainly trying to resist the inevitable rise of globalization's tide.[72] But as Jeremy Brecher and his colleagues noted as early as 2000, the choice was not between globalization or no globalization. The real option is to find the balance between globalization from below (solidarity movements among workers, citizen groups, and governments) and globalization from above (led by corporate and financial elites).[73] This clash will continue to shape the next stage of globalization.

Financialization

As overproduction and falling demand limited opportunities for profit, investors looked for new ways to increase returns on their capital. Financialization, defined as a "pattern of accumulation in which profit making occurs increasingly through financial channels rather than through trade and commodity production"[74] has now become a major influence on individuals and families, governments, and businesses. Encouraging more consumer debt through mortgages, credit cards, and loans started as a way to promote consumer spending. Soon, however, profiting from financial speculation turned into an end in itself, a way to increase return on investment and shareholder value.

Financialization moves money that had been involved in the production and sales of real goods and services into the speculative economy where investors profit by making loans, packaging debts, or trading in future prices of commodities like oil, grains, or beef. Financialization affects interest rates, debt, access to markets, financial stability, and the ups and downs of the economic cycle that have worsened the lives of so many people around the world.

The proportion of all corporate profits that came from the financial industry increased from 20 percent in 1980 to about 40 percent by 2000.[75] Financialization also benefited non-financial corporations by providing new opportunities to profit from financial transactions rather than producing and selling products. But a 2015 report from the International Monetary Fund warned that the financial sector in the US, Japan, and other advanced economies has become too big and grown faster than regulators can keep up with. The study's authors wrote, "Beyond a certain level of financial development, the positive effect on economic growth begins to decline, while costs in terms of economic and financial volatility begin to rise."[76]

Financialization became an important strategy by which corporate managers could respond to the growing demand from investors for increasing shareholder value, defined as management's ability to increase sales, earnings, and cash flow in order to increase dividends and capital gains for shareholders. If making money by making things had become too challenging in the new economic environment, then companies could instead make money by engaging in the many ingenious financial transactions they had created since the 1970s.

In the view of Rana Foroohar, an award-winning business journalist, financialization and the rise of the finance sector has led to the fall of American business by diverting capital from more productive uses, slowing increases in productivity, and rewarding lobbying for policies that favored its interests at the expense of other business sectors.[77]

Each of these strategies increased financial churn and contributed to a less stable economy. Stock buybacks enable investors to buy back corporate shares owned by others to increase their own share of profits. In 1982, President Ronald Reagan's Security and Exchange Commission loosened restrictions on stock buybacks, rules originally set to discourage managers from manipulating the price of stocks without improving operations or profits.[78] By 2016, the value of stock buybacks and dividends that the S & P 500 companies returned to shareholders was greater than their total operating profits.[79] After the 2017 $2.3 billion tax cut, US corporations reported stock buybacks that exceeded $1 trillion, a new record.[80] This windfall could have been spent instead on research, increasing worker pay, building more affordable housing, or reducing carbon emissions, all activities that could have also led to returns on investment, albeit at a lower rate.

Another consequence of financialization was growing debt. Lending money to consumers, then packaging and selling the cash flow of pooled debts to third-party investors as securities, a process known as securitization, became another source of profit. As companies produced more than they could easily sell, loans leading to consumer debt became an important strategy for increasing markets and revenues. Since 2000, rising debts for housing mortgages, college loans, credit cards, medical treatment, and auto payments enriched investors but made the lives of millions of Americans more precarious and stressful.

Financialization often benefited corporations in ways that harmed consumers.[81] Speculation in food futures in commodities markets led to food shortages, increased prices, and perhaps increased malnutrition.[82] In higher education, financialization encouraged financial service firms to lend to the growing number of lower-income students enrolling in college but left millions of students with debt that burdened them for decades. In healthcare, The Carlyle Group, a major private equity fund with more than $200 billion in assets under management, invested in the country's second-largest chain of nursing homes but then cut staff to increase profits, leading to unemployment, deterioration in care, preventable deaths of residents, and, ultimately, the chain's bankruptcy.[83] According to a *Washington Post* investigation, the rise in health-code violations at the chain began after Carlyle and other investors completed a 2011 financial deal that extracted $1.3 billion from the company for investors but burdened the chain with what turned out to be unmeetable financial obligations.

Financialization and the high rates of return it delivered pressured CEOs to achieve similar high returns on their investors' capital—or risk losing it to the many financial schemes that did bring satisfying profit rates. In 1997, the Statement on Corporate Governance of The Business Roundtable, a leading business trade association, asserted that in its view, "the paramount duty of management and of boards of directors is to the corporation's stockholders; the interests of other stakeholders are relevant as a derivative of the duty to stockholders. The notion that the board must somehow balance the interests of stockholders against the interests of other stakeholders fundamentally misconstrues the role of directors."[84]

More than twenty years later, the Business Roundtable changed its position, releasing in 2019 a new Statement on Purpose signed by 181 CEOs who committed to lead their companies for the benefit of all stakeholders— customers, employees, suppliers, communities, and shareholders.[85] But this revision sought to close the barn door on shareholder primacy long after the horses of corporate responsibility had escaped.

As long as that remains true, the Business Roundtable's pledge to put more emphasis on stakeholder value remains mostly rhetorical. This reality was reinforced by the decisions of many CEOs who had taken the pledge to react to the COVID-19 pandemic by furloughing or laying off workers, using cash stockpiles to buy back stocks, giving themselves bonuses, and grabbing government subsidies designed for small businesses.[86]

With its emphasis on speculation, short-term profits, and maximizing quarterly return, financialization encouraged CEOs and other corporate managers to keep their eye on the bottom line, even if that led them to avert their gaze from or cover up ways that their business was harming its workers, consumers, the public at large, or the planet.

Market Concentration and Monopoly

By the start of the twenty-first century, every major industrial sector in the global economy was controlled by no more than five transnational corporations. In about a third of these sectors a single company accounted for more than 40 percent of global sales.[87] Coca Cola, for example, had 51 percent of carbonated soft drink sales, Microsoft has 85 percent of the PC operating systems market, and Merck sold 40 percent of the world's anti-cholesterol statin prescriptions. These global companies were heavily concentrated in high-income countries, and although these nations include only 16 percent of the world's population, they accounted for 95 percent of the Fortune 500 list of companies.[88]

Market concentration and consolidation is both a cause and consequence of the growing political and economic power of the world's largest corporations. While scholars define concentration and monopoly (often used to describe when a single firm controls more than 50 percent of the market) in various ways,[89] highly concentrated industries have a major influence on people's lives.

In general, concentrated industries can charge higher prices because they face less competition. Since corporations in concentrated industries have higher returns and are bigger, they can devote more resources to marketing, enabling them to reach a larger share of the world's population. This contributes to the global rise of premature deaths and preventable illnesses when the products they sell are sickening. For the same reasons, these companies can spend more on lobbying, campaign contributions, and business-sponsored research, giving them a larger voice in shaping policy, politics, labor, and trade agreements than smaller firms. Consolidation reduces companies' need to innovate to stay competitive. In a downward cycle, more concentrated industries can devote more resources to lobbying for public policies that further reinforce concentration and stifle innovation.[90]

As Tim Wu observed, "As a business gets larger, it begins to enjoy a different kind of advantage having less to do with efficiencies of operation, and more to do with its ability to wield economic and political power, by itself or in conjunction with others. In other words, a firm may not actually become more efficient as it gets larger but may become better at raising prices or keeping out competitors."[91]

What caused the recent concentration of global industries across sectors? Peter Nolan, an expert on global economic development, and his colleagues at Cambridge University identified several causes: liberalization of trade and capital flows in the 1980s and 1990s, privatization of many previously public services, the collapse of communism, advances in information technology and computers, and migration as the factors most responsible for increased concentration.[92] In the world created by modern capitalism, bigger is better and those corporations that have the resources to grow and prosper generally get bigger, while those that lack these assets are bought up, stagnate, or fail.

Among the industries that have recently shown increasing consolidation in the United States are hospital care, banking, pharmaceutical companies, transportation and agribusiness—sectors that have a deep influence on the daily experiences of Americans. Between 1985 and 2002, for example, the market share of the top-ten firms in the pharmaceutical industry more than doubled from around 20 percent of global sales to 48 percent.[93] Not surprisingly, profitability in this highly concentrated sector is higher than in less concentrated ones, with pharma companies realizing average operating margins (a measure of profitability) of around 25 percent, compared to 15 percent or less for other consumer goods producers.[94] And as Americans have learned, high profits for drug companies mean big debts, bankruptcies, or foregone treatments for those with serious illnesses.

Other consequences of consolidation are increasing inequality of incomes and wealth. By allowing a small number of firms and investors to capture increasing shares of profits, the process contributes to the new crop of billionaires that has emerged, primarily from the highly concentrated tech industry. Concentration can also discourage innovation and entrepreneurship. If, for example, a national for-profit hospital chain has captured the market in a region, it will be more difficult for small firms or nonprofits to attract the capital, professionals, and patients needed to get started. According to one recent analysis, about 90 percent of hospital markets, 65 percent of specialist physician markets, and 63 percent of insurance markets in the United

States were highly concentrated in 2016[95]—one reason Americans pay more for healthcare than people in any other nation.

Concentration can bring benefits to consumers. The replacement of small, mom-and-pop retail stores by national big-box chains and Internet sales has increased choice and lowered prices for millions of Americans.[96] But even these benefits have their downside: this consolidation has also wrecked Main Streets, increased the number of low-wage workers, and homogenized retail landscapes across the country.

Opposition to monopolization challenges three capitalist myths—that markets are "free," that they operate fairly to allow equal competition, and that they necessarily lead to greater efficiencies. As more Americans have experiences that contradict these myths, the opposition to monopoly control that has erupted periodically throughout American history may again surface. Whether the U.S. Department of Justice's decision to file an antitrust lawsuit against Google in late 2020 serves as an opening salvo or an effort to coopt such a development remains to be seen.

The Neoliberal Agenda: Privatization, Deregulation, Tax Cuts, and Austerity

In response to the economic and political threats to capitalism that emerged in the 1960s and 1970s, a variety of actors including corporations, business and trade associations, right-wing academics, and government officials developed new approaches to allocating government and market responsibilities. Their goal was to create a coherent, defensible and updated alterative to the increasingly threatened model known as Fordism[97] and the welfare capitalist state described by John Maynard Keynes.[98] Scholars have come to use the term "neoliberalism" to describe the new regime that emerged to replace the welfare state.[99] It uses intersecting strategies including privatization, deregulation, tax cuts and austerity to restore the power of markets and capital to guide key economic and political decisions. These strategies have helped to define twenty-first-century capitalism.

As the sociologist Nitsan Chorev observes, neoliberalism is both a set of ideas and a practice.[100] In the United States and the United Kingdom, it was Ronald Reagan and Margaret Thatcher who became the champions for the practice of neoliberalism. For the past forty years, their legacy has been to make the four key planks of neoliberalism the foundation for public social and economic policy. In the United States, the rise of neoliberalism was an effort to restore the ruling class prerogatives under attack by the social movements of the previous decades.[101]

Will the COVID-19 pandemic and the subsequent economic collapse restore the role of government in shaping public policy? Rapid congressional and presidential approval of multi-trillion-dollar stimulus packages, the largest in US history and much more than twice the amount originally requested by the White House; the Federal Reserve's decision to make unlimited purchases of government-backed debt to stabilize financial markets; and President Trump's invocation of the Defense Production Act to compel General Motors, one of the largest corporations in the world, to make medical equipment led some observers to predict the death of neoliberalism.[102] But whether it will be replaced by a genuine revitalization of the public sector or simply give new powers to governments already beholden to markets remains to be seen.

Privatization. Privatization describes the shift of ownership and control of services and facilities from the public into the private sector. Reagan, Thatcher, and other proponents claimed that privatization was more efficient, less expensive, and less intrusive on freedom than maintaining these services or facilities in the public sector.[103] Among the public tasks shifted to the private sector were education, policing and security, sanitation, and healthcare. Also transferred were the ownership and maintenance of bridges, highways, and other infrastructure.

In 1986, President Reagan pronounced that "the nine most terrifying words in the English language are: 'I'm from the Government, and I'm here to help.'"[104] But it turned out that people did still want schooling, healthcare, and garbage pickup, and that on their own, businesses could not deliver these services to all who needed them. So government became the middleman, contracting out and occasionally monitoring performance of a plethora of nonprofit groups, commercial businesses, corporations, and consulting firms.

Each of these enterprises created new opportunities for direct and indirect profits. Private charter schools were often run by churches or other nonprofits but hired for-profit businesses known as educational management companies to rent or lease property, purchase supplies and technology, and provide human resources and legal backup to the schools, each a source for revenues that had previously stayed in the public sector. Similarly, privatization of prisons and jails provided opportunities for profit from running correctional facilities, providing healthcare and food services, and even placing long distance and collect telephone calls.[105]

While some studies have confirmed that privatization can reduce government costs and improve efficiency, there is little evidence that it improves the quality of care or lowers its cost to consumers. In practice, an increase in access appear to be accompanied by increases in price, negating any potential equity-enhancing benefit.[106] In addition, privatization often makes services more available or convenient for the better off than the poor, thus contributing to gaps in access to healthcare, social services, education, sanitation, clean drinking water, and other essential services. Since government is no longer fully responsible for privatized services, accountability is diminished, and democracy compromised.

Privatization can also reduce the wages, benefits, and rights to unionization and worsen the working conditions of workers who move from the public to the private sector. Again, this deterioration most affects already-vulnerable workers—those with a record of underemployment or unemployment, women, people of color and recent immigrants.

In the tech and media sectors, privatizing the digital and mass media public sphere removes public protection from cyberbullying, political manipulation, or net neutrality that a more robust public sector could offer.[107] In past decades, increasing privatization of mass and digital media and the telecommunications industry has turned public space essential for democracy into private hands.

One of the most pernicious effects of privatization is that it shifts the focus of government from ensuring access, quality, equity, and efficiency in the administration of public services to that of a business manager ensuring that contractors are fulfilling the letter of their contracts and remain satisfied so they will continue to provide services.[108] By blurring the lines between government and markets and making meeting the needs of "stakeholders" such as contractors a priority that competes with accountability to the public, privatization undermines government's prime responsibility of protecting the public. Within public health and environmental services, privatization delegates into private hands functions such as vaccine preparation, primary healthcare, or toxic cleanups, leaving the health of the public vulnerable to commercial influences.[109]

Deregulation. An essential element of the neoliberal edifice, deregulation describes the withdrawal, loosening, or non-enforcement of government regulation of capital markets, financial institutions, and public health, consumer, environmental and occupational protections.[110] Deregulation also furthers the ideological agenda of neoliberals. In his book *The War against Regulation*, Philip Cooper described how corporations and their political supporters lobby to slash the budgets of regulatory agencies, then accuse them of being ineffective.[111]

Deregulation also contributes to income inequality. Deregulation of financial services (as well as tax cuts for the wealthy) contributed to massive income redistribution. One study found that President Bill Clinton's deregulation of financial services contributed to rising income inequality, a harm amplified by the relaxation of rules that protected the right for workers to unionize.[112]

"Neoregulation," a term proposed by Gerardo Otero, who studies the global food industry, describes regulations that arise from partnerships between corporations and governments.[113] He observes that neoliberalism not only deregulates but also shifts the focus of government oversight from protecting consumers to protecting corporations. Neoregulation protects the intellectual property rights of agribusinesses and pharmaceutical manufacturers and defends voluntary public-private partnerships as a substitute for mandatory government regulations. According to Otero, neoregulation supports the evolving cooperation between national governments and corporations that characterizes neoliberalism.

The Trump presidency has made deregulation a top priority. In three years, it reversed more than one hundred environmental rules.[114] The administration appointed industry officials to lead the dismantling of regulatory agencies, cut funding for enforcement, and turned over responsibility for writing new regulation to industry insiders.[115] Even after Trump has left office, these actions will leave a long shadow of ill health and environmental degradation resulting from the toxic exposures and harmful business practices enabled by this deregulation.

Together, privatization and deregulation shrink the size and scope of government, making it easier to reduce its influence. As the lobbyist Grover Norquist memorably said in 2001, "I don't want to abolish government. I simply want to reduce it to the size where I can drag it into the bathroom and drown it in the bathtub."[116] While Presidents Reagan, George H. W. Bush, and George W. Bush endorsed this strategy known as "starve the beast" rhetorically, government continued to grow on their watch.

Tax cuts. If privatization and regulation limited the scope of governmental authority, tax cuts served to diminish the resources available for government operations, especially those less essential to business and conservative groups. As a result of their recent successes in modifying democracy and governance, corporations and wealthy elites have dramatically changed the rules on taxes and regulation in ways that have harmed the public good. Neoliberal tax policy reduced tax rates for corporations and the wealthy and shifted more of the tax burden to the poor and middle class through sales, property, and other regressive taxes. For Reagan and his followers, "supply side economics" justified massive tax cuts for the wealthy, a policy they claimed would lead to economic growth for all.[117]

Today, corporations and the wealthy are paying a lower portion of their income in taxes than at any time in recent history. In 1979, corporate taxes constituted 2.6 percent of the gross domestic product; by 2018, this had fallen to 1 percent, a decline of more than 60 percent.[118] Every president from Ronald Reagan to Donald Trump offered some tax cuts for the wealthy and corporations and new rules and enforcement practices that enabled higher tax deductions and easier write-offs. Lax enforcement of tax laws, especially for the wealthy, enabled more tax underreporting and evasion.

A report by the Institute on Taxation and Economic Policy found that in the first year after Trump's 2018 tax cut, the 379 major corporations they studied had paid an average tax rate of 11.3 percent on their US income in 2018, slightly more than half of what is supposed to be the statutory federal tax rate of 21 percent.[119] Many companies paid far less, including ninety-one that had paid nothing in the previous year. Another report found that US corporations hold $2.1 trillion in profits offshore—much in tax havens—in order to avoid being taxed in the US.[120]

How have the reductions in taxes of the recent past influenced well-being, planetary health, equity, and democracy? Tax policy influences health in several ways. It provides revenues for public services that promote well-being and protect health and the environment (fig. 1.2). Progressive taxation redistributes income from the better off to the less well-off, thus contributing to a more equitable society. Some taxes encourage healthier behavior and discourage unhealthy practices on the part of both businesses and individuals. Farmers who grow healthier food can get tax cuts and producers or consumers pay additional taxes on tobacco, alcohol, highly processed food, firearms, and other unhealthy commodities. Finally, a fair tax system increases the credibility, trust, and accountability of government, thus fostering democracy.[121]

As William Wiist points out, insufficient tax revenues harm public health in two ways.[122] First, they deprive local, state, and national governments of the revenues they need to fully protect public health, especially in an era when corporations actively undermine public health and environmental regulations and evade regulations when they can (See Figure 1.2). Second, inadequate public health funding encourages health departments and public health researchers to turn to corporations themselves to establish partnerships that can replace government cuts. But as Wiist notes, "corporations' primary goal

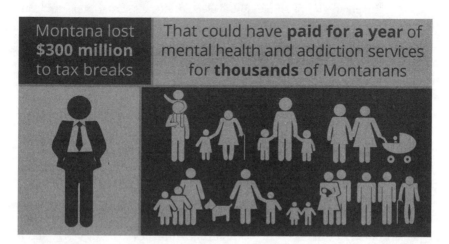

Fig. 1.2 An advocacy group in Montana explained the human costs of tax cuts for businesses.
Photo: Courtesy of the Montana Budget & Policy Center.

is profit and their fiduciary duty is to owners, shareholders, and creditors rather than protecting and promoting the public's health."

Austerity. A final plank of the neoliberal agenda is austerity, policies that aim to reduce government spending through cuts in services and taxes. In the last fifty years, neoliberal governments have used austerity both as a financial tool to cut spending and an ideological lever to discourage citizens from expecting too much of government. The recurrent fiscal crises of modern capitalism provide an opportune justification for the imposition of austerity measures, a tactic Naomi Klein has called the "shock doctrine," the use of natural or economic disasters to enact new policies while people are overwhelmed by deteriorated living conditions and disrupted support systems.[123]

An early field test of austerity occurred in New York City in response to the 1975 fiscal crisis. Rising costs of public services, a decision by banks to end their loans to the city in order to get higher returns elsewhere, and a desire by the newly coalescing Republican right-wing coalition to teach urban liberal policy makers a lesson set the stage for the experiment.[124] In a retrospective assessment of the health impact of the decisions made during the fiscal crisis, my colleagues and I estimated that fiscal-crisis inspired cutbacks in federal, state, and city spending saved about $10 billion in public spending on public health, policing, and other social services in the city. But over the next two decades, just three of the health problems that worsened in significant part as a result of these cuts—the rapid spread of HIV infection, increases in homicide and violence, and the emergence of a tuberculosis epidemic—generated costs of $50 billion to contain and reverse.[125]

These findings suggest that not only do austerity policies impose suffering on the affected populations, they are also a classic example of the penny wise pound foolish strategies of shortsighted elected officials under pressure from the business community.

More recently, scholars in the United Kingdom, Europe, and the United States have assessed the health and social consequences of austerity measures imposed after the 2008 global financial crisis.[126] Stuckler and Basu note that austerity can harm health via two pathways.[127] These policies can increase unemployment, poverty, homelessness and other social risk factors, while cutting effective social protection measures that mitigate their risks to health. In addition, austerity measures can reduce access to or quality of healthcare, thus compromising individuals' capacity to get help for the health problems triggered by worsening living conditions. Another understudied impact of austerity is what some have called "moral distress," a rising prevalence of psychosocial distress, depression, anxiety and fear of the future, unintended consequences of twenty-first-century capitalism that makes so many worry about losing their jobs, homes, or health.[128]

Neoliberalism has also served to reinforce the systemic racism that has long characterized the United States. Privatization removed public services from disenfranchised communities of people of color and often served to reinforce segregation. Deregulation withdrew environmental, occupational, and consumer protections that most benefited African American and Latinx communities. Tax cuts exacerbated the sharp inequalities in income and wealth between Blacks and whites and the austerity cuts in public services harmed people of color most.[129] In these ways, neoliberalism has widened racial gaps in this country and created a space where corporate elites and white nationalists could find common ground.

Together, privatization, deregulation, tax cuts and austerity—the defining characteristics of neoliberalism—have fundamentally altered the relationships between governments, markets, and people, and worsened the living conditions of the vast majority of American people.

New Discoveries in Science and Technology

In the twentieth century, new scientific discoveries, especially in the life sciences, revolutionized the world's potential to solve previously insoluble problems.[130] The discovery of penicillin and other antibiotics allowed medicine and public health to consolidate advances in reducing deaths from infectious diseases, until then the major cause of global mortality. Later, new findings in cellular and genetic biology expanded medicine's formulary for cancer treatment—and in some cases extended the lifespan of those with cancer.[131] Technological advances led to thousands of new medical devices, many of which extended life or buffered the effects of aging.[132]

In the 1950s and 1960s, the so-called Green Revolution promised to end hunger and malnutrition. New discoveries in biology, agriculture, chemistry, and engineering, supported by the Rockefeller and Ford Foundations, led to the development of high-yielding varieties of cereal grains, mechanized irrigation and harvesting infrastructures, modernized agricultural management techniques, and more distribution of hybridized seeds, synthetic fertilizers, and pesticides to farmers to increase food production.[133]

Admirers of the Green Revolution claim that Norman Borlaug, its scientific father, saved a billion people from starvation.[134] Critics, however, point to widespread environmental damage, excessive and inappropriate use of fertilizers and pesticides, increased water pollution, poisoned agricultural workers, and kill-offs of beneficial insects and other wildlife. Together these practices led the eventual abandonment of some of the world's best farming lands. Heavy dependence on a few major cereal varieties has led to loss of biodiversity on farms.[135]

As in other sectors, these adverse impacts are not the inevitable consequences of a particular technology or practice. Rather, as transnational food, chemical, and agricultural supply companies gained control of Green Revolution technologies, they made maximizing profits rather than improving diets or protecting the environment their priority goal, thus losing the opportunity to modify damaging practices based on real-world experience.

Discoveries in computer sciences and the engineering of automation enabled dramatic increases in the speed of communications and the capacity for complex data analysis and reduced the need for dangerous, tedious, and demeaning work.[136] These innovations also increased industrial productivity. Scientists, universities, governments, and businesses sometimes collaborate and sometimes compete to create knowledge, translate such research into practice—and claim the benefits from their application. As historian David Noble has observed, the science and technologies that emerged in the later nineteenth and twentieth centuries were shaped by and inextricably linked with the variant of corporate capitalism of this period.[137] Scientists and engineers may have designed and carried out the research, but corporations and their allies posed the questions that got answered, brought the resulting new products and services to market, and pocketed most of the profit.

Proponents of public ownership of science point to the taxpayer dollars that have supported it. In *Science the Endless Frontier*, an influential 1945 report on US science policy, Vannevar Bush made the case that major investments in research were vital to long-term national interests.[138] Such support, he wrote, speeds the pace of innovation and contributes to national security, medical advances, economic growth, and improved quality of life. Bush argued that by collaborating, government, industry, and academia could accomplish more than by working in isolation. With the creation of the National Science Foundation in 1950; the expansion of the National Institutes of Health; and the establishment of research programs at the Department of Defense, the Department of Agriculture, and other agencies; the federal government translated Bush's report into billions of dollars of annual support for research and development.

In the 1970s, and even more so in the last two decades, transnational corporations responded to the surge of new science and technology by intensifying their efforts to capture the economic rewards of these discoveries for themselves. They sponsored university researchers, but required them to keep research findings secret, withhold evidence that cast doubt on corporate products, or limited their studies to questions that could benefit the company.[139] By deploying science in ways that furthered their business goals—even if the consequence was public harm, these companies challenged the Enlightenment claim that knowledge belongs to humanity.

Recent conflicts over the ownership and use of science illustrate the trend of increasing corporate control. One debate asks who owns the intellectual property developed by scientists. Another asks what role corporations, government, and scientists play in paying for science and setting the rules for scientific integrity.

Intellectual property rights protect the rights of creators of patents and trademarks from appropriation by others. In the United States, the Constitution itself established and defined these rights. Article 1 Section 8 authorizes Congress to "promote the Progress of Science and useful Arts, by securing for limited Times to Authors and inventors the Exclusive Right to their respective Writing and Discoveries." This assertion that ideas as well as tangible goods could be property protected by law was extended to include conflicts over intellectual property rights to concepts, designs, and plans. Previous conflicts had been limited to disputes over ownership of tangible goods such as land, slaves (then shamefully considered property), and machines.

Intellectual property rights are established and protected by governments, but corporations have claimed the right to shape the rules. In the last century, the emergence of a global structure for negotiating trade agreements—first as the General Agreement on Trade and Tariffs (GATT), signed in 1947, and then as its successor, the World Trade Organization (WTO), established in 1995—offered corporations a useful platform for injecting intellectual property rights into trade treaties. High-income countries in Europe, as well as Japan, Canada, and especially the United States wanted to be sure that their transnational corporations could protect their intellectual property in emerging markets in low- and middle-income countries, which had weaker patent and copyright protections. From the 1980s on, as developing world markets became more important, several US corporations including Pfizer, IBM, and DuPont played important roles in writing new global intellectual property rules that protected their interests.[140]

In the early 1990s, members of the WTO negotiated an agreement on Trade-Related Aspects of Intellectual Property Rights, known as TRIPS. This agreement brought intellectual property law into the multilateral trading system, enhancing the power of corporations to set the rules, and reducing the influence of governments. The biggest beneficiaries of TRIPS were the US transnational corporations that had helped to write them.[141]

The TRIPS Agreement sets minimum standards in the international rules governing patents, including those on medicines. The 150 countries that belong to the WTO agreed to certain common standards in the way they enact and implement their patent laws. These standards require that patents be given for a minimum of twenty years, that they may be given both for products and processes, and that pharmaceutical test data can be protected against "unfair commercial use."[142] In 2001, low- and middle-income countries insisted on clarifications of TRIPS that resulted in the Doha Declaration. This add-on asserted that TRIPS should be used, for example, "to promote access to medicines for all," thus reasserting the primacy of health over commercial interests.

In response, at the urging of their national pharmaceutical companies and trade associations, high-income countries began to introduce new restrictions on intellectual property, a process known as TRIPS Plus. Such provisions included extending the term of a patent longer than the twenty-year minimum, limiting the use of compulsory licenses, restricting generic competition, and imposing "data exclusivity," a rule that allowed drug companies to keep data on a drug's safety and efficacy confidential for five or ten years.[143] A 2012 report by the World Health Organization and other international organizations found that TRIPS Plus provisions increased the costs of medicines by tens of millions of dollars, putting essential drugs out of reach of many low-income patients around the world.[144] TRIPS Plus thus rewarded pharmaceutical companies while decreasing the ability of governments to protect public access to affordable medicines.[145]

The pharmaceutical industry is not the only business sector where intellectual property rights sometimes conflict with established human rights. The 169 nations that have ratified the International Covenant on Economic, Social and Cultural Rights, a UN treaty approved in 1966 and enacted in 1976, "recognize the right of everyone" both "to enjoy the benefits of scientific progress and its applications" and "to benefit from the protection of the moral and material interests resulting from any scientific, literary or artistic production of which he is the author."[146] The United States signed but did not ratify this agreement.

By the twenty-first century, the main beneficiaries of intellectual property rights were not the intellectuals who created the property but the corporations that have the political and economic power to bring the ideas to market. The current corporate-driven intellectual property regime has allowed corporations to benefit while also reducing access to essential medicine, making small farmers more dependent on global agribusinesses, and enabling transnational sharing economy companies like Uber and Airbnb to use technology to eliminate jobs and reduce pay, benefits, and control over scheduling for their contingent workforce.

The shared governmental and corporate agenda on intellectual property rights, especially in the United States but also in Europe, shows how governments enable rather than regulate corporations. Instead of abandoning a regulatory role in intellectual property rights or in other domains, governments have changed what they regulate, often seeking to protect corporations from global competitors and to ensure their capacity to use science for their own benefit.

Corporations also look to limit the damage that independent science can inflict on their activities. For corporations, science can be a double-edged sword, both revealing new opportunities for growth while also calling attention to the harms that businesses impose. Scientists' role in uncovering the exorbitant burden of the tobacco industry on global premature deaths and preventable illnesses illustrates the danger science can pose to corporate profits—and also the playbook that the tobacco industry created to counteract damaging evidence.[147]

Indeed, over the last several decades, corporations have developed common strategies to decrease the likelihood that scientific evidence or scientists will jeopardize their business or political goals. First, they have learned that by partnering with academic researchers or establishing their own research teams, they gain greater control of how the findings are framed and used. While the US government paid the substantial costs of creating a science research-and-development infrastructure in the years after World War II, more recently corporations themselves have paid directly for research. By 2010, according to one study of corporate-sponsored science, the for-profit sector conducted or paid for approximately 70 percent of all US research and development. In addition, about 20 percent of US "basic research" is conducted and funded by private industry.[148]

A second strategy seeks to manufacture doubt about the validity of scientific findings. In 1969, a tobacco executive wrote a memo asserting that "doubt is our product since it is the best means of competing with the 'body of fact' that exists in the minds of the general public. It is also the means of establishing a controversy."[149] Energy companies mastered the strategy by supporting scientists to refute the scientific consensus that human energy use was the primary cause of global warming and helped to create a movement denying climate change or the role of energy companies science.[150]

This intensification of the rhetoric of doubt of any scientific evidence that challenges corporate interests reinforces and was magnified by the practice of labeling any critical coverage of President Trump and his allies as fake news. Together these trends and their amplification by social media and right-wing and corporate mainstream media led the critic Michiko Kakutani to proclaim the "death of truth." "Without commonly agreed upon facts," she writes, "there can be no rational debate over policies, no substantive means of evaluating candidates for political office, and no way to hold elected officials accountable to the people. . . . Without truth, democracy is hobbled."[151]

Using these strategies, corporations have appropriated the fruits of scientific and technological discoveries to achieve their business goals, even when such diversion of science harms health, pollutes the planet, undermines democracy, and exacerbates inequalities.

NEW STRATEGIES TO GENERATE IDEOLOGICAL SUPPORT

Capitalism has always needed to produce and sell ideas as well as goods and services. In the twentieth century, authoritarian governments, corporate marketers, and the mass media, with the assistance of academic partners, created new ways to enlist public support for their political, social, and economic agendas. Recognizing that, as the political theorist Steven Lukes has observed, "power is most effective when least observable,"[152] leading institutions found ways to persuade rather than coerce people to want what ruling elites want them to want. By manufacturing consent and engineering credibility, they make their world view seem inevitable.[153]

In 1947, Edward Bernays, a founder of public relations and political propaganda observed:

> The tremendous expansion of communications in the United States has given this Nation the world's most penetrating and effective apparatus for the transmission of ideas. Every resident is constantly exposed to the impact of our vast network of communications which reach every corner of the country, no matter how remote or isolated. Words hammer continually at the eyes and ears of America. The United States has become a small room in which a single whisper is magnified thousands of times.[154]

By the start of the twenty-first century, the din of Bernays's words hammering at the eyes and ears of Americans had become a cacophonous orchestra with Facebook, Twitter, Google, Netflix, and Amazon competing with traditional and digital media, political candidates, think tanks, and independent billionaires to get into not only the eyes and ears but also the minds and consciousness of every American from birth to death.

Corporations themselves played an important role in advancing their ideas and firmly embedding them in American beliefs. In 1971, Lewis Powell, a corporate lawyer who would later become a Supreme Court Justice, wrote a memo to the director of the US Chamber of Commerce urging business leaders to respond more aggressively to what he viewed as an "assault on the enterprise system" by liberals and the social movements of the 1960s.[155] Powell called for more lobbying and campaign contributions, stronger business organizations, and more forceful criticism of people like Ralph Nader, the consumer advocate, who in Powell's view was "the single most effective antagonist of American business."

Powell's call to arms, backed by other business leaders, led to rapid changes. The US Chamber of Commerce soon "doubled its membership, tripled its budget and stepped up its lobbying efforts" in Washington, where it became the dominant corporate voice.[156] In 1971, the National Association of Manufacturers, the voice of corporate producers, moved from Cincinnati to Washington, DC, where it, too, played a growing role in public policy. In 1971, 175 companies had registered lobbyists in the capital; by 1982, the number had increased to almost 2,500. Between 1976 and the mid-1980s, the number of corporate political action committees (PACs) increased from three hundred to more than twelve hundred.

For the eighteen-month cycle of the 2018 Congressional elections, 8,086 federal PACs had registered with the Federal Election Commission, reporting total receipts of $2.6 billion and disbursements of $2.2 billion.[157] Many other actors contributed unreported "dark money" to influence public opinion, legislation, and elections.[158] No other group of learners has a higher per capita expenditure on "education" than the elected and appointed federal officials that lobbyists seek to influence and no other organization spends more on per capita education than corporations and their allies dedicate to persuading public officials to do their bidding.

In the last few decades, corporations and business leaders have devised new ways to influence public opinion and the personal beliefs of ordinary Americans about what changes were and were not possible. Growing consolidation of corporate ownership of most forms of media gave corporate leaders near monopoly control over the messages most Americans saw and heard. In 1983, 90 percent of US mass media was controlled by 50 companies; by 2012, this same share was controlled by just 6: Comcast, NewsCorp, Disney, Viacom, Time Warner, and CBS.[159] In the following years, mergers and acquisitions have further concentrated ownership and tech giants like Amazon, Facebook, and Google have played an increasingly important role in determining what news and ideas make their way into the brains of the American people.

A related disturbing trend was the decline in local news coverage, forced by the bankruptcies of smaller media outlets, some as a result of losing their advertising revenue to Facebook or Amazon or their acquisition by the corporate media giants.[160] According to the Pew Research Center, US newspaper circulation is now at its lowest level since 1940, even as the national population has grown from 132 million to nearly 330 million. Since 2004, one in four newspapers in the United States has closed. These closures harm the public by creating "news deserts" in places farther from media concentrations; taking eyes off corporations and government, making it easier for them to get away with unethical or illegal behavior; and increasing the public's dependence on the stories prepared by the corporate news giants.

The Press Sentinel, a small independent newspaper in southeastern Georgia, illustrates the potential power of this endangered American voice. The paper discovered that Republic Services, an Arizona-based corporation backed by wealthy investors including Bill Gates, had applied to dump ten thousand pounds of coal ash a day in the area. *The Sentinel* published more than seventy articles and editorials about this plan, leading to public hearing and a delay in the plan.[161]

Still another way to influence public beliefs was the establishment of business-friendly think tanks and research institutes. Over the course of the last century, billionaires such as the Koch brothers, Sheldon Adelson, Robert and Rebekah Mercer, Richard Mellon Scaife, and John M. Olin created the Heritage Foundation, the Cato Institute, the American Enterprise Institute, and the Heartland Institute, organizations dedicated to supporting conservative, business-friendly political values and policies.[162] These groups played a powerful, often-hidden role in shaping local, state, and national policies and creating public support for the private interest of their founders.[163] Liberal billionaires such as George Soros, Michael Bloomberg, Pierre Omidyar, and Warren Buffett also created foundations to influence public opinion and, in this century, tech billionaires Mark Zuckerberg, Bill Gates, and Jeff Bezos have also used their wealth to influence social policy and the role of technology in society.[164] While these philanthrocapitalists disagree about how best to reform society, they share the belief that the ultrawealthy have an inalienable right to use their wealth to guide democracy and shape public policy.[165]

In recent decades, corporations have found ways to ride the trends I have described to increase their power and influence. At the same time, other sectors of society that had in the past provided a counterweight to corporate ideological dominance have lost influence. From the 1960s on, families, churches, labor unions, governments, communities, and community organizations lost capacity to shape daily lives and challenge or offer alternatives to corporate messages, creating an empty space into which corporations were eager to enter.

By the beginning of the twenty-first century, these trends had changed how Americans experienced their daily lives. These changes were accompanied by growing signs of discontent that also emerged in the transition from the twentieth to the twenty-first century.

Today two worldviews, each visible at the 2020 World Economic Forum in Davos, compete for the attention of the people of the United States. The first, the dominant one, claims that the nation's and the world's economy and politics are shaped by the inevitable logic of markets and that the best future will result from aligning our individual and collective goals and aspirations with that logic. To these true believers, every crisis, from climate change to the COVID-19 pandemic to systemic racism, proves the inexorableness and resilience of capitalism. Some supporters of this view acknowledge that there are costs to the choices markets impose, but they claim that the burdens are modest in comparison to the benefits. Moreover, they say, the experience of the last fifty years proves that there is no feasible alternative.

But a growing alliance of social movements, disenchanted citizens, young people, and academics argues an alternative view. They assert that pursuing this business-as-usual approach endangers the well-being, even the survival, of humanity and the planet. They point out that today's global predicaments are the result of decisions made by corporations, governments, communities, and individuals. They insist that numerous alternative arrangements—worker and consumer cooperatives; expanded public sector food, healthcare, and housing initiatives; community-centered economic development; mobilizations to dismantle structures that perpetuate racism; and bottom-up global partnerships—are even now being tested around the world. Therefore, claim these voices opposing the status quo, no political and economic configuration is inevitable. Now as in the future, individuals and organizations will make the economic, political, and social decisions that will determine future opportunities for well-being, happiness, and planetary survival.

REFERENCES

Note to readers: Following contemporary referencing practices, in this and subsequent reference notes, I include hyperlinks only for references not readily accessible on common search engines.

PART II

The Pillars of Health

CHAPTER 2

Food

Ultra-processed Products Become the Global Diet

First we eat, then we do everything else.
—*M. F. K. Fisher*

THE RISE OF ULTRA-PROCESSED FOOD

While the twenty-first-century global food system produces more food than ever and has reduced severe malnutrition, it has left the world with four major problems. First, almost one billion people around the world wake up not knowing if they can feed themselves and their children that day. Second, every day about two billion people—the 30 percent of the world's population who are obese or overweight and the hundreds of millions who have diet-related diseases—risk consuming food or beverages that will further elevate their chances of premature death or preventable illnesses. Third, the global food system now contributes about one-third of the human-induced greenhouse gases, the largest single contribution to global warming of any sector.[1] Finally, by paying low wages and offering minimal benefits and no job security, global food companies have lowered the price of processed food but worsened the lives of millions of people who grow, process, sell, and serve food for a living, further exacerbating inequality and poverty. How did the food system that is supposed to feed and nurture people become such a threat to human well-being and survival?

In the decades that marked the transition to the twenty-first century, two trends that began after World War II transformed what people eat and how scientists understand the impact of diet on health. First, an increasing proportion of the diet of Americans and other people around the world came from calories in highly processed food and meat and fewer from fresh produce and unprocessed grains. Second, nutritional and public health researchers began to discover that these changes in diet were associated with a growing burden of premature deaths and preventable illnesses from diet-related diseases such as diabetes, heart disease, high blood pressure, certain forms of cancer, and, more recently, infectious diseases like COVID-19. Unhealthy diets now contribute more to the global burden of disease than unsafe sex and alcohol, tobacco, and drug use combined.[2]

To be sure there has been some progress. According to the United Nations Children's Fund (UNICEF), the prevalence of childhood stunting, a serious form of malnutrition, has been declining since 2000. However, these rates have gone up again since 2015 and nearly 149 million children, one in four children under age five, were stunted in 2018. More than 49 million suffered from wasting, the most dire form of undernutrition that predicts early death.[3]

From 2006 to 2016, according to the American Heart Association, the annual death rate attributable to coronary heart disease in the United States declined 32 percent and the actual number of deaths declined almost 15 percent, a noteworthy achievement. But the overall burden of dietary diseases remains high, still the leading cause of death across age groups and nations.[4]

How did it come to be that as scientists were discovering and documenting the harmful consequences of the modern diet, the world's largest food and agricultural companies were making that diet the default choice for much of the world's population? And how did changes in modern capitalism encourage the global food and agricultural industries to choose this path?

A starting point for answering these questions comes from a study by researchers at the National Cancer Institute that examined changes in the United States food supply from 1970 to 2007. They used a common measure of dietary quality—the Healthy Eating Index—to assess the healthfulness of the US food supply as reported by the United States Department of Agriculture (USDA).[5] They found that on many key indicators, the food supply failed to meet dietary guidelines or had worsened over time:

- Calories from solid fat, alcohol beverages, and added sugars, a triad of unhealthy products, remained high and relatively flat across the years, despite the scientific consensus that these calories contribute significantly to the rise in diet-related diseases and wide publicity about the value of reducing intake. The researchers estimated that calories from these sources would need to decrease by 61 percent to achieve a food supply that could meet expert dietary recommendations.
- Per capita energy (as measured in calories) available in the US food supply increased by about 500 calories per day.[6] Other researchers estimated that increases of 350 calories per day for children and 500 for adults were a primary cause for the doubling of obesity rates in those decades.[7]

- Salt in the food supply, an important contributor to hypertension and cardiovascular disease, would need to decrease by more than half in order to achieve recommended standards.
- The quantity of available fruits and vegetables was lower than needed over the entire period, with fruit supplies needing to double and vegetable supplies to increase by 70 percent to meet dietary guidelines.

While nutritionists continue to debate the precise roles of various nutrients in health and disease, the basic messages for healthy diets have remained essentially the same for more than four decades: eat more fruits, vegetables, and whole grain foods and consume fewer highly processed foods; foods high in sugar, saturated fat, and salt; and less meat. Over this time period, the diet of the American people has barely improved and many of the socioeconomic and racial/ethnic nutritional gaps have widened.

Why is the food system developed here in the United States rapidly becoming the model for producing, distributing, and consuming food around the world, a model that promises to increase the burden of chronic diseases, the main cause of illnesses and death?

One answer comes from investigating how and why ultra-processed foods (UPF) became the dominant product of the global food industry and how the dynamics of modern capitalism favored the growth of ultra-processed food at the expense of other types of food. In her fascinating book *The Way We Eat Now*, Bee Wilson, the British food writer and historian, explains how UPF came to dominate the global diet.[8]

One of the first researchers to call attention to the risks of UPF was the Brazilian nutritionist Carlos Monteiro. He and his colleagues developed a food classification schema they call NOVA. NOVA proposes four food categories: unprocessed and minimally processed, processed culinary ingredients such as salt or vegetable oil, processed, and ultra-processed. Based on the nutritional evidence, these researchers came up with three remarkably simple messages for the world's eaters: eat more unprocessed and minimally processed foods, eat less processed foods, and avoid ultra-processed products.

The procedures that convert food and other products into ultra-processed food include "the fractioning of whole foods into substances, chemical modifications of these substances, assembly of unmodified and modified food substances, frequent use of cosmetic additives and sophisticated packaging."[9]

Monteiro and his colleagues offer some guidance to help eaters to identify UPF. "Check to see if its list of ingredients contains at least one food substance never or rarely used in kitchens, or classes of additives whose function is to make the final product palatable or more appealing," the researchers write. "Common examples," they explain, "are invert sugar, maltodextrin, dextrose, lactose, soluble or insoluble fibre, hydrogenated or interstratified oil." Frequently used additives include "flavor enhancers, colours, emulsifiers, emulsifying salts, sweeteners, thickeners and antifoaming, bulking, carbonated foaming, gelling and glazing agents."[10]

Around the world, UPF are rapidly replacing unprocessed and minimally processed foods as the foundation of the global diet.[11] They are designed to be highly profitable by making them convenient and ready to consume. UPF producers use low-cost ingredients, design products with long shelf lives, use emphatic and catchy branding, often make misleading health claims, and design products to be hyper-palatable, so tasty that eaters find it hard to say no to more.[12]

As it turns out, UPF play to the strengths of today's global food system. The basic crops on which they depend—corn, soy, wheat, rice, and sugar—can be grown on huge tracts of land, require a limited workforce, and serve as foundations for thousands of products, all characteristics that favor the comparative strengths of the world's largest food corporations. They are easy to transport around the world; market across nations and populations; display on shelves in giant supermarkets without spoiling; use profitable agricultural commodities such as palm oil, soy, sugar, and corn; attract loyal, lifetime customers who find the high doses of saturated fat, sugar, and salt irresistible; and bring quick and steady profits to their makers and investors.

Studies show that by 2010, ultra-processed products constituted almost 60 percent of the energy intake in the US diet.[13] This marked the culmination of a century-long transition from a diet in which the majority of food consumed was unprocessed or minimally processed products to one in which UPF dominated. In 2016, the United States had the highest per capita intake of calories from UPF and drink of the eighty countries whose caloric intake was documented by Euromonitor, a business-tracking company. Although overall per capita consumption of ultra-processed food and drink declined in the United States between 2002 and 2016, the US level in 2016 was 33 percent higher than the next highest country, Canada.[14] In addition, consumption of UPF was higher for younger ages, those with lower incomes, whites or Blacks than for Hispanics and other racial/ethnic groups, and those with less education, showing that those with less wealth and power were more exposed to UPF.[15]

Two-thirds of the calories that Americans consumed from packaged foods came from convenient ready-to-eat products.[16] Other studies show that UPF have more calories, sugar, unhealthy fats, and salt than unprocessed or minimally processed foods and less of the dietary fiber, proteins, vitamins, and minerals essential for health.[17]

HEALTH AND ENVIRONMENTAL CONSEQUENCES OF THE ULTRAPROCESSED DIET

Of greatest concern, UPF have been demonstrated to contribute to pathogenic biological processes that lead to diet-related diseases. Studies show that these products have low "satiety potential," meaning they do not make eaters feel full, so they eat more. UPF elicit a high glycemic response, that is, they tell the body to put sugar into the bloodstream, thus elevating the risk for diabetes and other metabolic diseases.[18] They also create a gut environment that, in the words of one research team, is an "evolutionarily unique selection ground for microbes that can promote diverse forms of inflammatory disease."[19]

On the one hand, researchers were discovering how the gut microbiome—the totality of microorganisms, bacteria, viruses, protozoa, and fungi—and their collective genetic material found in the gastrointestinal tract, influences health and disease. On the other hand, the food industry was creating products that compromised the protective effects of the microbiome and magnified its harmful effects.[20]

These biological processes, amplified by product formulation designed to maximize palatability, aggressive marketing, ubiquitous availability, and attractive pricing have exposed billions of individuals to growing amounts of these products. As a result, rates of obesity, hypertension, cardiovascular diseases, metabolic syndrome, gastrointestinal disorders, total and breast cancers, and depression have increased in many places.[21]

Beginning in the 1990s, the Global Burden of Disease consortium, a network of thirty-six hundred researchers in more than 145 countries, has been collecting data on premature death and disability from more than 350 diseases and injuries in 195 countries, by age and sex, from 1990 to the present. This approach allows researchers and public officials to make comparisons over time across age groups and populations about changing causes of death.

In 2019, *The Lancet* published a Global Burden of Disease report on the health effects of dietary risks in 195 countries from 1990 to 2017. The consortium concluded that "suboptimal" diets had become the leading global cause of premature deaths and disability.[22] In 2017, these diets accounted for eleven million deaths and seventy million disability-adjusted life years (DALYs), a measure of the number of years of life lost due to ill health, disability, or early death. The leading causes of these deaths were cardiovascular diseases, followed by cancers and Type II diabetes. Researchers identified fifteen risk factors for diet-related diseases and determined that intake of nearly all types of healthy foods was suboptimal in 2017.

Moreover, they concluded, three ingredients—too much sodium (i.e., salt) and too little unprocessed whole grains and too few fruits and vegetables—accounted for more than half the diet-related deaths and two-thirds of the DALYs. Between 1990, when the study began, and 2017, diet-related deaths increased 37 percent, from 8 million a year to 11 million a year.

The essential ingredients of UPF are highly processed soy and grains such as wheat, corn, and rice and high levels of nutrients such as salt, sugar, and saturated fats and trans-fatty acids, other leading contributors to the dietary burden of disease. UPF contains few fruits and vegetables. When they do, they are also highly processed as with the berries in Strawberry Pop-Tarts.

Sugar is another growing component of the modern diet and a key ingredient of UPF. Excessive sugar consumption from foods and beverages high in added sugars, the sweeteners that food manufacturers add to whatever natural sugars are in a product, contributes to increased risk of type 2 diabetes, cardiovascular diseases, some cancers, as well as nonalcoholic fatty liver disease, dental caries, and obesity. Added sugars also may increase the risk of mental deterioration such as Alzheimer disease.[23]

Between 1950 and 2000, annual sugar consumption in the United States increased almost 40 percent, from about 80 pounds per person per year to about 110 pounds per year.[24] After 2000, annual consumption decreased for a decade then stabilized at about 100 pounds a year. In the United States today, the average person consumes about 2 pounds of sugar a week, the equivalent of a bit more than three twelve-ounce cans of Coca-Cola a day and twice the level recommended by the World Health Organization.[25] About half the sugar Americans consume comes from sugary beverages such as soda and sweetened juices. A study by researchers at the University of North Carolina found that 60 percent of the packaged food sold in supermarkets contained added sugar.[26]

Salt, also a key ingredient in UPF, is a leading risk factor for high blood pressure and cardiovascular diseases, the leading cause of global deaths.[27] More than two-thirds of the packaged products on supermarket shelves contain added salt and about 70 percent of the salt Americans consume comes from these packaged products, not from the table salt shaker, giving supermarkets and their suppliers a dominant role in deciding how much sugar and salt Americans take in.[28] More than half the products on supermarket shelves exceeded the sodium-per-serving conditions for a "healthy food," a US Centers for Disease Control research team found.[29]

Processed meat, another component of the food industry's new diet, includes hot dogs, ham, bacon, sausage, and some deli meats. It refers to meat that has been treated to preserve or flavor it, using processes that include salting, curing, and smoking. The International Agency for Research on Cancer (IARC), the cancer arm of the World Health Organization, has classified processed meat as a carcinogen, something that causes cancer, and red meat as a probable carcinogen, something that probably causes cancer.[30] The meat industry has attacked those designations and hired researchers to cast doubt on the relationship, leaving consumers and policy makers confused.[31]

Despite growing public health concerns about processed meat consumption, US adults have not reduced their consumption of processed meat since 2000, although they have reduced beef consumption and increased the amount of chicken they eat.[32] While people in the US have the world's highest meat consumption, intake of red meat and processed meat is growing most rapidly in low- and middle-income countries, contributing to the rise of diet-related diseases in those nations.[33] Processed meat also increases risk of death from cardiovascular disease. A study in *JAMA* found that processed meat consumption was tied to 57,766 deaths from cardiometabolic diseases in the United States in 2012.[34]

A recent clinical study raised further alarms about the role of UPF in American diets. Kevin Hall and his colleagues at the National Institute of Diabetes and Digestive and Kidney Diseases recruited twenty men and women to live in his clinic for four weeks. For two weeks, they were fed diets high in UPF, the other two they ate mostly unprocessed food. The meals were equivalent in calories and participants were told to eat as much as they wanted. After careful measurements of intakes after each interval, Hall and his team concluded that those on the ultra-processed diet ate five hundred more calories a day, more than enough to gain weight over time. Blood levels of hormones that increase hunger remained high on the ultra-processed diet compared to the unprocessed one, a confirmation that high intakes of UPF can lead to weight gain.[35]

UPF also exacerbate income and racial/ethnic inequities in the burdens of diet-related diseases, in part because the food industry has made them cheaper and more readily available than healthier food. In the United States and other wealthy countries, -low-income, Black and Latinx, and other less well-resourced populations consume higher proportions of processed food than their better-off counterparts, making the low cost and ready availability of UPF an important cause of higher rates of diabetes, cardiovascular diseases, and hypertension among people of color and low-income people.[36] These changes have led some researchers to propose the concept of food apartheid, a system that makes less expensive and unhealthy food accessible to lower socioeconomic groups, especially Blacks, Latinxs, and rural communities, and healthier, more expensive food available to the better-off populations concentrated in urban and suburban areas.[37]

Between 1973 and 2014, the proportion of food spending devoted to fresh fruits and vegetables declined for the four lowest income groups in the United States but increased for the wealthiest fifth. In contrast, spending on bakery products for the lowest fifth of the population increased during this interval. Of interest, total spending in all food categories, healthy and unhealthy, increased for the wealthiest fifth over the forty years, suggesting that they ate more healthier food but also more ultra-processed products.[38]

Gerard Otero, the sociologist who conducted these analyses using data from the USDA, concluded that in this period, low- and middle-income Americans faced greater exposure to unhealthy food while upper-income residents ate more of everything.[39] This suggests that the food apartheid metaphor,[40] in which low-income groups are offered mostly sickening food while the better off can choose healthy diets, is only partially true. Various types of processed foods have become the norm for all sectors of the population, while the wealthiest individuals continue to have better access to the fresh fruits, vegetables, and other minimally processed foods that can counteract some of the harmful effects of the highly processed products.

In reality, all sectors of the population experience diet-related illness as the leading cause of death and illness, even though rates increase significantly for low-income populations and communities of color. In sum, increased income and status protect against, but do not eliminate, the health and social risks of the modern diet. All sectors of society would gain health benefits from a healthier diet.

For populations at highest risk of diet-related diseases, the promotion of unhealthy diets makes daily food choices more difficult. An older man with diabetes living in Appalachia described his view of his food choices to researchers:

> I'm kind of offended by all this advertising that's continually attacking you, saying, "It's good; it's convenient; it's so neat to have it; just have a snack, and it'll make you feel good." I've had to change my approach because I'm diabetic. I can't be seduced by that. I have to be willing to temper my own attraction to food knowing that there are certain consequences that come from that. So how does a diabetic fight all this and try to manage their diabetes? We sit on a teeter-totter. When you look around, you can see that a lot of people are seduced by it. . . . There's stuff that seduces me, and I fall off the wagon. And I eat things I shouldn't, probably because it tastes so good.[41]

His observation also shows how much eaters internalize the responsibility for the choices the food industry offers. Every day the food industry tempts people to fall off the healthy food wagon, yet for the most part food corporations insist their goal is simply to give individuals choices.

The increasing evidence that UPF are contributing to a growing share of the world's caloric intake and its diet-related health problems has encouraged the food industry to generate messages to refute this evidence. Industry arguments include that observed correlations between UPF consumption and health problems are not causal, that processing can make foods healthier, that the definition of UPF is bogus, not based on food science and technology, nor on the reality of the market, and that radical movements are trying to influence society to reject processed foods, labeled arbitrarily as unhealthy, using unscientific criteria. A review of food industry influence on public and scientific discussion of UPF found that thirty-three of the authors of the thirty-eight documents, reports, or other materials criticizing the NOVA classification for UPF had affiliations with ultra-processed food companies.[42]

The production of UPF also has environmental consequences. The food and agriculture sectors—including food transportation, fertilizer, and other industries—contribute almost 30 percent of human carbon emissions.[43]

Several characteristics of the agricultural system worsen the climate effects of this food regime. First, UPF depend on several crops that have led the global transformation from small farms growing many products into industrial monoculture that grows only a few crops: corn, soy, sugar, wheat, rice, palm oil, and a few other grains. This system of agriculture depends on heavy use of fertilizers, pesticides, and fossil-fuel burning tractors and other equipment, each with its own carbon burden. It also encourages de-forestation and soil depletion.

Second, one of the attractions of UPF for food manufacturers is that it can be produced at one location, shipped around the world to sell in other places, and stored on warehouse or supermarket shelves for extended periods. These characteristics require extensive transport by air, sea, rail, and especially trucks, each contributing additional emissions. While not every product can be grown locally or regionally, global food production that depends on global supply chains for the production of packaged foods ensures that additional food miles are a feature of the system, not a glitch.

Third, the diet promoted by the global food industry includes meat, comprising beef, chicken, and pork. Beef requires about twenty-seven kilograms of carbon dioxide for each kilogram of meat eaten, chicken less than seven kilograms of carbon, and lentils less than one kilogram.[44] A 2018 study in *Science* reported that total global consumption of meat had increased from about fifty million metric tons per year in 1960 to three hundred million metric tons in 2010, a sixfold increase. While many factors contributed to this increase, as the authors of the *Science* study drily note, the meat industry "has considerable political influence and allocates large amounts of money to advertising and marketing. Lobbying from the meat industry was intensive during the formulation of U.S. Dietary Guidelines, and civil society organizations claimed that this influenced eventual recommendations."[45] Reducing meat consumption is one of the most effective strategies for slowing climate change and one of the goals most ardently opposed by the many sectors of the food and agricultural industries that profit from food.

HOW TRANSNATIONAL CORPORATIONS CREATED THE WORLD'S NEW DIET

Over the last century, a diet of food grown mostly nationally and regionally, sold relatively unprocessed in a variety of small grocery stores and markets, and prepared and eaten mostly at home changed first in the United States and then around the world. To unpack the multiple causes of this transformation, I examine four sectors of the food economy: supermarkets and food retail, food services sold at fast-food outlets and restaurants, food manufacturing, and agricultural production. For each sector, a story illustrates the rise of the ultraprocessed diet: Walmart's domination of supermarket sales, fast food companies' new strategies for growing market share, the creation of toddler formula, and the rise of palm oil as a global staple.

Supermarkets and Food Retail

The local supermarket is a good place to begin an exploration of how modern capitalism has facilitated the growth of the ultra-processed diet. The nation's more than thirty-eight thousand supermarkets constitute a cauldron where transnational agribusiness and food corporations, store owners and operators, government regulators, and consumers interact to make choices that determine Americans' diet and nutritional health.

Almost two-thirds of the calories people in the United States consume come from supermarkets.[46] Between 1975 and 2008, the number of products for sale in the average US supermarket increased more than fivefold.[47] By 2017, there were forty thousand to fifty thousand products available in supermarkets.[48]

Today, supermarkets are designed more like gambling casinos than the food stores of the early twentieth century. Every feature encourages consumers to stay a little longer, load the shopping cart a little higher, and ring up a bigger tab at the checkout counter. From the perspective of the food industry, supermarkets exist to sell as much food as possible and to yield the highest rate of return. To achieve this goal, supermarkets locate dairy products in back of the store so customers have to pass all the other products on their way, picking up impulse buys as they go; offer supersize shopping carts after they learned that shoppers who used bigger carts spent 40 percent more in the store;[49] place the most profitable and appealing products at eye level and the less profitable ones high or low where they are harder to see; place healthy and unhealthy products next to each other, like fresh apples and caramel sauce, to encourage buyers to reward their healthy choice with a sinful one; and waft smells of cooking rotisserie chicken, brewing coffee, or fresh-baked bread so that customers' salivary glands will be stimulated, to encourage impulse purchases.[50]

New technologies like checkout scanning that give supermarket chain headquarters real-time data on sales to allow instant restocking and surveillance methods that enable stores to use customer cell phones to track their progress down the aisles and send ads for the products they are passing contribute to further increases in sales.

In the twenty-first century, food retailers have replaced food producers as the most powerful component of the global food market. To better understand how and why this change came about—and its implications for the rise of UPF— I take a deeper look at Walmart.

Walmart is the global discount retailer with the highest annual revenues of any of the Forbes Global 2000 corporations. Like many large global food corporations, Walmart sells more than food. It also offers financial services and money orders, prepaid cards, wire transfers, check cashing, and bill payment and specialty services such as auto buying, pharmacy, and tire and battery centers, all designed to draw more customers into their stores. In 2018, food accounted for 56 percent of Walmart's annual revenues.[51]

Walmart's power to influence food choices comes in part from its reach into so many communities. With forty-seven hundred Walmart stores in the United States and almost six hundred Sam's Clubs, the Walmart subsidiary that sells at wholesale prices to members, the company has a store within ten miles of 90 percent of the US population.[52] Overall, Walmart's 23 percent grocery market share has increased over the last decade, despite growing competition.[53] Globally, Walmart operates more than 11,700 retail outlets in twenty-eight countries.

By offering low prices and volume discounts, Walmart brings in customers looking for bargains and offers them deep discounts on enough products to keep them coming back. As a result, other local stores that cannot compete will eventually go out of business, further increasing Walmart sales but also reducing the pressure to keep lowering prices.

Since its founding in Rogers, Arkansas, in 1962, Walmart developed a business strategy that allowed it to dominate markets where competition was limited. Its first stores were in rural communities that had few shopping alternatives. In 2016, Walmart announced it had opened 392 stores in so-called food deserts since 2012.[54] Throughout its history, Walmart has grown by finding underserved markets, then using its size and market power to cut costs and force competitors out of business, a predatory practice that defines modern capitalism.

Walmart has also led the sector in using technology and Big Data to ensure that its distribution and delivery logistics could maximize sales opportunities. By the 1990s, Walmart was already using satellites to exchange data, voice, and video messages between its corporate headquarters and retail outlets. Later, it developed the capacity to use these data to target customers more precisely. For example, in 2004, when Walmart learned that Hurricane Ivan was heading to Florida, its algorithms predicted that customers would want extra packaged breakfast food to weather power outages. Walmart immediately shipped extra crates of Frosted Strawberry Pop-Tarts to the Florida panhandle and sales surged.[55]

Walmart grocery stores in the United States stock a total of 46.1 million products, although each store decides which products to place on the shelf or make available online. Walmart stocks 2.5 million snack and candy products, 2.3 million beverages, 1 million bread and bakery products, 600,000 fruits and vegetables, and 300,000 products to meet special dietary needs.[56] Although

Walmart has made recent efforts to expand the number of healthy and local products it stocks, the vast majority of the products it sells and the revenues it generates come from its packaged highly processed products.

In recent years, Walmart has competed fiercely with Amazon searching for ways to keep its price advantage while also building its online presence and its capacity to satisfy customers with its services.[57] As competition from Amazon increased, Walmart expanded its "click-and-collect" system in which customers could order online and then pick up the order at a nearby store. One business analyst estimated that Walmart's grocery sales in this category will increase by 154 percent each year from 2017 to 2021.[58]

By 2019, Walmart offered curbside pickup at eighteen hundred stores that reached 40 percent of the US population.[59] Curbside pickup allows customers to get their online preordered food brought to their cars in the store parking lot, a service that allowed sales to grow even during the COVID-19 pandemic. To collect these orders speedily, Walmart is testing automated carts that zoom around the stores picking up items, a process that saves time and labor costs.

Walmart wants every customer visit to be a satisfying experience, but a review of Walmart's customer service website shows, not unexpectedly, a mix of reactions:[60]

I'm so pleased with the whole ordering process and delivery. Walmart provides such easy ordering, problem resolutions and quick delivery system. I order for three different addresses and I'll choose Walmart every time! I am so thrilled I don't have to be forced to go with other, less efficient, and dishonest, companies. —A of San Diego

Self-Checkout issues at Wal-Mart are almost always a problem. . . . Today's visit took me at least 20–25 minutes to check out with 3 items. A manager had to be called to override something on the order and 18 minutes later he did not show up. . . . No apologies or acknowledgment from manager until I confronted him, and he responded with an excuse rather than a true apology. —Linda of Barrington, IL

Walmart does not train their employees well. They are not friendly and not at all willing to help me find a product. That is if you can find an employee. They hide somewhere. The prices are not that good. I can find same or better at other stores near my house. All in all, I don't go there anymore. —Pat of Edgewater, FL

Walmart pledges its customers will "save money" and "live better." The reviews suggest that some customers believe that Walmart's logistics, corporate culture, and low prices deliver on this claim while others find the company fails to meet this promise. Customers expect both lower prices and saved time, requiring Walmart to balance its effort to provide these desired commodities against its profits. Clearly, many Americans visit Walmart.

According to one business analyst, 59 percent of US grocery shoppers purchase groceries from Walmart in any three-month period, giving the store a place in millions of households.[61] Globally, 275 million people visit a Walmart store each week, more people than live in all but four of the largest nations of the world.[62]

Walmart has also created alliances with big and small business around the world, allowing it to compete with Amazon and others. It has teamed with Google for online shopping, with Microsoft to purchase Flipkart, an Indian e-commerce service, and with Uber to make home deliveries of groceries.[63] Like other giant corporations responding to the pressures of modern capitalism, Walmart creates these partnerships to amplify its power to create an environment in which it can better pursue its business goals.

Walmart's low prices are part of what makes the store attractive to low-income consumers. More than 52 percent of Walmart customers have household incomes of less than $50,000.[64] Two factors contribute to Walmart's ability to offer low prices. First, its huge size allows it to bargain with food growers and manufacturers around the world. In fact, Walmart has acquired such a dominant voice in the nation's food system that it can force other big companies to acquiesce to its demands. For example, Walmart's insistence that Kraft Foods lower its prices led Kraft, according to one analyst, to "shut down thirty-nine plants, let go 13,500 workers, and eliminate a quarter of its products"[65] because it was no longer able to compete with other Walmart suppliers. For farmers and food workers, Walmart's bargaining power means lower prices for their produce and lower wages.

How do Walmart's decisions influence its role as a purveyor of UPF? One study found that increased Walmart store density was associated with fewer adults meeting the recommended fruit and vegetable intake;[66] another that a 1 percent increase in market share for Walmart supercenters was associated with a small but statistically significant decrease in healthy food purchases in the area.[67] Other evidence suggests that low-income and African American customers are more likely to shop at Walmart[68] and those who shop for bulk items prefer the low pricing that Walmart offers rather than healthier but more expensive food.[69] Whether Walmart's choices convert healthier shoppers into less healthy ones or simply attracts those already committed to less expensive, less healthy products, it does put low-cost, mostly unhealthy food within reach of millions of shoppers.

In 2012, to gain a larger share of healthy food purchases and respond to public and consumer pressure to make healthy food more available, Walmart announced a partnership with Humana Vitality, a rewards program affiliated with the health insurer Humana. The goal of the partnership was to enable the more than one million Humana Vitality members who shop at Walmart to be eligible for a 5 percent discount on fresh fruits, vegetables, and low-fat dairy products.[70]

But Walmart promotes products to appeal to every age and population group. Riding the wave of the intensive promotion and marketing by the makers of toddler formulas and other prepared baby foods, Walmart added thirty thousand new baby products to its online ordering system.[71] Parents visiting Walmart's online ordering system can choose among seventy-two toddler formula and "baby beverage" products, available in powder or ready-to-use, with varieties for those wanting lactose-free, milk-based, soy-based, or kosher products.[72]

The Partnership for Healthier America, an alliance of private foundations and major food companies, was created in 2010 to partner with the private sector to "ensure the health of our nation's youth by solving the childhood obesity crisis."[73] The partnership worked closely with Michelle Obama's Let's Move Initiative. In 2012, Walmart made a commitment to the partnership to take action to improve the nutritional quality of the food it sold.[74] Three years later, Walmart reported to the partnership that it had reformulated packaged food items to include 18 percent less sodium, 10 percent less added sugar, and 6 percent of products with no industrially produced trans fats. The company also reported it had cut prices on "better-for-you" food items and saved customers more than $1 billion per year on fresh fruits and vegetables, making, the company claimed, healthier foods more available and more affordable. Walmart also reported it had invested nearly $15 million in nutrition programs that educate consumers about how to make healthier choices.[75]

An independent evaluation of Walmart's Healthy Food Initiatives by a team led by Barry Popkin, a researcher at the University of North Carolina-Chapel Hill, found some support for Walmart's claims but also provided a context that calls the significance of its accomplishments into question. The researchers assessed whether the nutritional quality of packaged foods purchased at Walmart had changed between 2000 and 2013. Over this interval, investigators found declines in overall energy and energy from sugar and reductions in the sodium in the food purchased, changes with the potential to improve nutrition. They also found a decrease in the volume of purchases of sweets and snacks and small increases in fruit and vegetable consumption.

Based on this study, they concluded that the nutritional profile of Walmart purchases had improved over time, becoming more similar to packaged foods sold at other retail chains.[76] However, they also determined that these improvements were similar to or smaller than what would have been observed had trends observed prior to Walmart's Healthy Food Initiative continued.[77] In other words, Walmart seemed to be riding a wave of national food trends in which people chose healthier food, rather than initiating changes in what its customers bought.

The authors concluded that "food retailer-based Healthy Food Initiatives may not be sufficient to improve the nutritional profile of food purchases." While Walmart has expanded its offering of fresh produce, it has also stocked new processed products including exclusive rights to sell snacks such as Oreo O's cereal and Jelly Donut Oreos.[78] Moreover, by claiming to be a purveyor of healthier food, Walmart deflected attention from its main nutritional role— he country's largest supplier of the lower cost highly processed products that returned high profits to food makers but imposed additional disease burdens on their customers.

Other independent analyses of the Walmart and Partnership for a Healthier America's Healthy Food Initiative had additional criticisms. The very concept of a food desert suggests that only supermarkets can solve the problem of food access in low- income communities.[79] LaDonna Redmond, a longtime food justice advocate, argued that "Walmart is using the term 'food desert' as a Trojan horse to get into our communities and bring about more corporate control of our food system."[80]

FOOD SERVICE

After supermarkets, fast-food chains supply the next largest source of calories in the American diet, accounting for about 15 percent of US caloric intake, more than twice the proportion of calories consumed at full-service restaurants.[81] Thanks to these chains, most Americans now have 24/7 access to ultra-processed products away from home. Across the United States, almost 250,000 establishments sell fast food, half of them quick-service franchises like McDonald's, Subway, or Kentucky Fried Chicken.[82] Between 2004 and 2018, the number of outlets increased by 23 percent, making them one of the fastest-growing sectors of the American economy. According to the United States Centers for Disease Control, between 2013 and 2016, 37 percent of US adults ate fast food on any given day.[83]

And like supermarkets, fast-food outlets offer enough choices to ensure that every customer can "have it your way," as Burger King promises. Between 2007 and 2013, McDonald's menu increased from 85 choices to 145.[84] In an effort to attract or retain health-conscious millennial customers and young moms who wanted to nibble while their children gulped down Big Macs, fast-food chains added salads and apple slices to their menus. However, the best-selling and most profitable items continued to be calorie, salt, and fat-laden French fries, Big Macs, and Happy Meals.[85]

The recent rapid growth of fast food establishments was precipitated in part by an influx of capital from investors looking for more reliable profits after first the collapse of early dot-com startups and later the 2008 recession. By the early years of the new millennium, banks, private equity firms, and other financial institutions had invested billions of dollars in fast food. But as the number of outlets increased, so did competition. "Everybody thinks their brand has what it takes to succeed in the marketplace, Victor Fernandez, a fast-food industry analyst, told a *New York Times* reporter. "You look at a location that looks good, but everybody is looking at the same place and they all come in, and the result is oversaturation."[86]

As competition increases, the bigger, more successful chains buy up smaller chains or drive them out of business. In 2018, for example, Inspire Brands, which also owns Arby's and Buffalo Wild Wings, acquired the drive-in fast food chain Sonic, with thirty-six hundred locations.[87] By 2012, the top-four fast-food chains controlled about 43 percent of the market.[88] Growing concentration and growing competition enabled the biggest companies to spend more on advertising and product design, allowing them to lower prices to drive remaining competitors out of business and to target new markets. A few years ago, for example, McDonald's and Taco Bell identified a new market, "nocturnivores," young often inebriated males who wanted to eat after a night of drinking. Midnight to 5 A.M. became the fastest-growing time segment for US McDonald's locations, and a new opportunity for growth.[89]

Between 1986 and 2016, fast-food companies increased the number of products they served, the size of portions for entrées and desserts, and the number of calories and amount of salt and sugar in most products.[90] As Americans became more concerned about the costs of diet-related diseases for individuals and society, fast-food companies chose to double down on their core business strategy. They offered more products that contributed to the nation's rising rates of obesity, diabetes, and high blood pressures and the growing gap in rates of these conditions between low-income, Black and Latinx, and better off populations.

After the Great Recession of 2008, consumer spending fell and fast-food sales declined, leading to increased competition and industry consolidation. In more recent years, spending on fast food has returned, but the chains are fighting for a stagnant market. And in most cases this fight has been won by the largest companies. In 2018, the ten largest fast-food chains—McDonald's, Starbucks, Subway, Taco Bell, Chick-fil-A, Burger King, Wendy's, Dunkin', Domino's, and Pizza Hut—together accounted for 90 percent of the sector's growth.[91] The COVID-19 pandemic has had a devastating effect on fast-food businesses, leading many outlets to close down for months. As the economy recovers, the major chains will need to market heavily to reverse the sharp declines in revenue following the 2020 economic collapse.

Two practices of the fast-food industry illustrate how corporations respond to reduced demand for unhealthy but profitable products. Predatory marketing refers to marketing unhealthy products to vulnerable populations using techniques that are aggressive and ubiquitous, appeal to emotions, and are misleading.[92] A study by researchers at the Rudd Center for Food Policy and Obesity found that fast-food companies disproportionately targeted Black and Latinx children and young people with their television advertising and that the majority of these ads promoted nutritionally poor products.[93] In this way, these companies contribute to higher rates of obesity and diabetes in communities of color. Overall, food, beverage, and restaurant companies spend almost $14 billion per year on advertising in the United States and more than 80 percent of this advertising promotes fast food, sugary drinks, candy, and unhealthy snacks.

A second strategy for addressing falling fast-food sales in the United States market is to expand globally. According to the industry publication *Restaurant Dive*, the fast-food industry is reaching saturation levels in the US, so in order to grow, many chains are expanding their international footprints.[94] Taco Bell plans to open six hundred restaurants in India during the next ten years. Restaurant Brands International also plans to grow Burger King, Tim Hortons, and Popeyes abroad. In the United States, average annual growth rates are about 2 percent while the expected global growth rate from 2017 to 2021 is expected to be more than double the US rate.

Food Manufacturing

A third sector of the food industry—the companies that manufacture food such as Unilever, Kellogg, and Nestlé—also influence what we eat. A closer examination of one product, toddler formula, a product that introduces babies and young children to highly processed food, shows how changes in globalization, financial pressures for higher profits, and weakened government regulatory capacity contribute to the growth of unhealthy diets.

Toddler formula is designed for one- to three-year-olds after they stop breastfeeding. No nutritional science nor knowledge of child development justifies the need for such products. Yet toddler formulas do serve the purpose of helping Nestlé, Abbott, Mead Johnson (bought in 2017 by the global conglomerate Reckitt Benckiser), and Danone, the four multinational corporations that account for 50 percent of global sales in this sector, to regain sales lost by the increase in breastfeeding. Conveniently, this decision to create new products also prepares young children for a lifetime diet of highly processed foods.

Curiously, the creation of toddler formula resulted from a public health success story—the promotion of breastfeeding. In the last half century, the proportion of new mothers choosing to breastfeed their infants increased significantly. In the late 1940s, only 25 percent of women in the United States breastfed their babies. By 2010, 77 percent of new mothers were breastfeeding. Globally, between 1995 and 2011, according to UNICEF, the proportion of babies who were exclusively breastfed for their first six months increased from 34 percent to 43 percent.[95] The potential impact of optimal breastfeeding practices is especially important in low- and middle-income countries with a high burden of disease and limited access to clean water and sanitation.[96]

Over the last fifty years, a boycott of Nestlé for its role in promoting infant formula and growing public understanding of the health and economic benefits of breastfeeding contributed to these increases in breastfeeding. The boycott targeted Nestlé, the world's largest infant formula company, for its aggressive and deceptive promotion of formula in developing nations. Nestlé misrepresented the benefits of formula, promoted its use in communities where clean water was not available, and falsely led customers to believe its sales agents were health professionals.[97] In 1981, the World Health Assembly approved a new global treaty, the International Code of Marketing of Breast-Milk Substitutes, that restricted marketing of infant formula.[98] Since then, eighty-four countries have enacted legislation implementing the code and its subsequent amendments.[99]

For infant formula companies, however, this health success presented a business problem. With more mothers breastfeeding, fewer purchase infant formula. For the Big Four formula companies, sales fell. To solve this problem, these companies developed "toddler" formulas, packaged breast milk substitutes and a variety of other processed baby foods that blend grains, fruits, vegetables, and other ingredients in products designed to appeal to young children and their parents. With high levels of processing, multiple ingredients, and aggressive, often misleading advertising, these new products meet the definition of UPF.

To market these new toddler foods, the producers make two claims. First, they assert these products promote health. The added prebiotics, the companies allege, aid digestion and probiotics enhance brain and cognitive functions. Other additives such as the fatty acids omega-3 and omega-6 are said to promote healthy infant development and play a role in preventing chronic diseases. Enfamil, for example, boasted that its new NeuroPro line of formula provided "brain-building nutrition inspired by breast milk."[100] Advertisements for another toddler milk, S-26, proclaim it the "perfect mix of science and love."[101] Between 2011 and 2015, overall US ad spending on toddler formula increased by 73 percent.[102]

Second, these companies tout the convenience of their new products, a characteristic that Walmart and fast-food chains also claim. For busy working mothers, single-size portions and disposable pouches made it quicker and easier to feed their toddlers and packaged processed baby foods made meal preparation simpler.

Some companies targeted upscale parents. Nestlé created BabyNes, an adaptation of its Nespresso system for coffee, so that parents could purchase a machine that would prepare disposable single portions of various formula mixes (See Figure 2.1). A review of BabyNes by City Dads Group, a support group for fathers, wrote, "BabyNes infant formula capsules comes in age stages that ;evolve' like breast milk does with changes in calorie, fat and key ingredient levels to meet specific needs of your child's stage of development. This

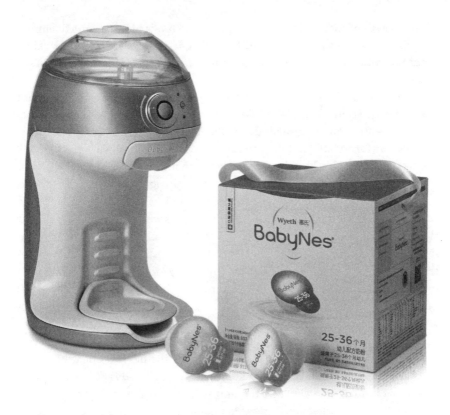

Fig. 2.1 The BabyNes machine based on the Nestlé's Nespresso coffee pod machine, is designed to deliver custom-tailored formula to meet a baby's specific needs. Mom or Dad presses a button, and the custom-designed formula comes out thirty seconds later.
Photo: "BabyNes," by Nestlé, licensed under CC BY-NC-ND 2.0

is done by producing seven different types of formulas, the most of any brand on the market. . . . Each capsule is BPA-free, hermetically sealed and contains a built-in filter to trap water impurities. . . .The BabyNes machine features built-in WiFi that pairs with an app on your computer or mobile device."[103]

Aggressive marketing of these new products brought new revenues to baby and toddler food makers. Between 2011 and 2015, toddler milk was the fastest-growing sector in infant foods. In the key Asia Pacific market, toddler milk accounted for more than 50 percent of revenues from formula.[104] Between 2015 and 2020, industry analysts predict that the global value growth in toddler milk in developed markets such as the United States and Europe is expected to increase by 20 percent, five times faster than standard baby formula.[105]

So what is the problem? Isn't this simply a classic story of free markets leading companies to shift from one product for which demand is falling to another for which demand can be increased? Several unintended consequences of the growth of toddler formula and processed foods illustrate the dilemmas that companies, governments, and the public face when corporations gain a dominant voice in deciding what goes to market and educating consumers about these products.

First, most health claims that toddler formula companies make are not supported by scientific evidence. Several studies have failed to show benefits to infant health from the prebiotics, probiotics, and other additions to infant and toddler formula.[106] In 2015, the *British Medical Journal* withdrew a 1989 article funded by Nestlé making false claims about infant formula.[107]

Second, these companies' advertising campaigns confuse the public, leading to less informed and perhaps riskier choices. By using similar brand names and logos on infant and toddler formula, some mothers believed that the less expensive toddler formula was the same as the more expensive infant formula, and then fed their babies an inappropriate product.[108] Like other industries, these companies established front groups to disseminate their message.[109] Some companies paid "Mommy Bloggers," mothers running social platforms for hundreds or thousands of new mothers, to tout their products without disclosing these payments.

Third, feeding these products to toddlers contradicts the nutritional evidence that eating healthy table food constitutes the best and healthiest way to make the transition from breastfeeding to solid foods. Choosing table foods that are safe and easy to chew and swallow lets parents introduce their children to fruits, vegetables, and other components of a healthy diet and to maintain control of what their toddlers eat. It sets the precedent of families eating together and counteracts food marketers' desire to establish a new market niche for toddlers.

Toddler products are also laced with enough sugar or salt to keep children coming back for more. Like Walt Disney's version of Mary Poppins, who used a spoonful of sugar to help the medicine go down, toddler formula makers learned that sweeteners keep their customers loyal and parents discovered that children already conditioned to sweet food would fuss less if they acquiesced to that taste. A recent report from the US Centers for Disease Control found that packaged toddler foods exceeded recommended standards for sodium, sugar, and fat.[110]

Early childhood, as pediatricians and toddler formula makers know, is a key developmental stage for acquiring food preferences. Children develop their tastes for sugar, salt, and fat in early childhood, setting them up to be lifetime consumers of high levels of these ingredients. Highly processed baby and toddler foods are easy to chew and swallow. Many are sold in pouches, liquids, or gels, normalizing ingesting without chewing, which discourages some children from choosing healthier, less processed foods as they get older.

In addition, growing evidence suggests that diet-related chronic diseases begin much earlier than previously recognized. Obesity-induced metabolic inflammation begins in early childhood and elevates life-time risks for type 2 diabetes and other metabolic diseases.[111] Nonalcoholic fatty liver disease is a chronic liver disease resulting from excessive fat accumulation in the liver that used to be seen mainly in adults but now has become the most common liver disease in children in the United States. Within the last decade, it has become one of the leading indications for liver transplantation in adults.[112] By starting infants and toddlers on a diet that sets the stage for earlier onset of chronic diseases, toddler and baby food makers exacerbate the world's leading health problem. To make matters worse, the COVID-19 pandemic showed that infectious diseases as well can put those who are obese at higher risk of illness and death.

From a public health perspective, the question is *not* what ingredients companies should add or remove from a processed product. The more meaningful ask is "What kind of diet and food supply will best protect the well-being of children?" This is a question the global food industry wants to avoid.

Another contribution of infant and toddler food makers to the growth of UPF is their success in defining convenience and making it a main determinant of food choice. In a country where two adults have to work full-time to support most families, where public child care and paid parental leave available in many European countries is scarce, where rigid gender roles preclude most fathers from taking equal responsibility for feeding their young children, where high-quality child care for young children is often not available or affordable, what mother of young children would not want more convenient ways to feed her babies or toddlers? When leisure time is precious, consumption and brands define identity and self-worth, and old foodways and food cultures have been displaced, the convenience of a diet becomes a paramount value.

Recognizing that convenience was a key factor in feeding infants and toddlers enabled infant and toddler formula makers to commodify convenience in ways that bring profit (e.g., Baby Nepressos). In this way, infant and toddler formula makers join Walmart, McDonald's, and other food corporations in making UPF the easiest way to eat. For parents with busy, stress-filled lives, choosing to spend more time and money to give their child a healthier diet requires a courage and determination that can be difficult to muster day after day.

For US policy makers, implementation of child care, wage, parental leave, tax, and other policies that give families the resources and time to purchase and prepare healthy food seems like an overwhelming task, especially when they recognize that the corporate world will oppose these measures. So it is easier to call for families to be more responsible in choosing their diets and perhaps mandate some additional information on food package labels, leaving the UPF industries still in charge of the American diet.

Food retail, food services, and food manufacturing each depend on a fourth sector: food producers—the bedrock of the world's food system. While hundreds of millions of farmers around the world grow food, a handful of corporations now control the transformation of soil, water, seeds, animals, fertilizers, and pesticides into much of the food that people eat.

A few global corporations in this sector illustrate the ties with other nonfood business sectors and the rapid changes in ownership and control. Bayer, a German multinational life sciences company, is one of the largest pharmaceutical companies in the world. Its goal, it says, is to create "products for the health of humans, animals and plants."[113] In 2018, Bayer acquired Monsanto, the American agrochemical and agricultural biotechnology corporation. Monsanto developed Roundup, a glyphosate-based herbicide, in the 1970s and became a major producer of genetically engineered seeds. Shortly after the acquisition, juries began awarding large sums to plaintiffs who charged that Monsanto's Roundup had caused their cancers. Those early verdicts contributed to Bayer's shares losing 40 percent of their value, even as more than eleven thousand other cases worked their ways through the courts.[114] These losses led the *Wall Street Journal* to call Bayer's purchase one of the worst corporate deals in recent times.[115]

BASF, also based in Germany, is a European chemical company that is the largest chemical producer in the world. In agriculture, the company says, its goal is to create "innovative solutions for growers, supporting them with the task of nurturing a hungry planet."[116] BASF operates in more than eighty countries and runs almost four hundred production sites in Europe, Asia, Australia, the Americas, and Africa.

Like the other sectors of the food system, the companies that produce food have played a key role in the rise of the global ultra-processed diet. The increased use of palm oil in the global food system in the last few decades illustrates how companies that produce an agricultural commodity can benefit from and contribute to the rise of UPF.

Palm oil is used in thousands of foods—from cookies and pizza dough to chocolate, bread, and ice cream. It is also used in household products like toothpaste and detergents and in biofuels. Palm oil can be found in about half the products consumers use daily and the food industry is responsible for 72 percent of its use.[117] An estimated 3 billion people in 150 countries use products made with palm oil.

Palm oil is the kind of commodity that global corporations love. The plant is perennial and evergreen, enabling year-round production. It is a remarkably efficient photosynthesizer, grows in soil unsuited to other crops, and gives higher yields than other oilseed crops.[118] It is cheaper and more versatile than other vegetable oils, making it a desirable ingredient for the global processed food industry, which adds it to thousands of products. It is grown mostly in Malaysia and Indonesia, as well as other nations where land and labor are cheap, and governments easily persuaded to promote policies that favor investment and resource exploitation. Should circumstances force palm oil producers to move to or expand in another continent, it can be done.

The product itself can handle frying without spoiling and blends easily with other oils. It raises the melting temperature of ice cream; preserves highly processed foods, extending their shelf life; and provides the foaming agent used in most shampoos, liquid soaps, and detergents. Between 1995 and 2015, yearly production of palm oil quadrupled and by 2050, it is predicted to quadruple again. By 2022, the global palm oil market is expected to reach $88 billion.[119]

Some of the pressure to expand palm oil production originally came from recommendations by public health and environmental advocates to replace trans fat in food and fossil fuels for cars. In 2006, the United States Food and Drug Administration (FDA) required the food industry to openly note the amount of trans fat or partially hydrogenated oils in food on the nutrition facts label. In 2013, the FDA made a "preliminary determination" that trans fats are not recognized as safe. In 2018, the FDA officially banned the use of partially hydrogenated vegetable oils, which were a major source of trans fats in food sold in American restaurants and grocery stores.[120]

Twelve years earlier, the New York City Department of Health had limited the use of artificial trans fat in food served in restaurants because they contributed to heart attacks and strokes. This was followed by a cascade of similar local and state trans-fat limits that provided the scientific and political rationale for the FDA to take national action. A study published ten years after the ban went into effect found that New York counties that had banned trans fats showed a 6.2 percent greater decline in hospital admissions for myocardial infarction and stroke than residents of counties without trans-fatty acid restrictions.[121]

But the decline of trans fat helped set the stage for the rise in palm oil. Palm oil has some of the commercially useful properties of trans fats and it is cheaper than other healthier substitutes such as olive and canola oils. Thus, palm oil helps to keep the UPF that use it inexpensive and plentiful.

A 2015 review of studies on the health effects of palm oil concluded that increased consumption of palm oil was associated with increased rates of diabetes and obesity, but not cardiovascular disease or cancer.[122] Another recent review by Malaysian scientists concluded there was "insufficient evidence to suggest the impact of palm oil intake on weight changes or BMI."[123]

From a public health perspective, however, "insufficient evidence" on the health effects of palm oil warrants caution. Before exposing billions of people around the world to growing amounts of palm oil, public health authorities would want to be confident that the long-term consequences of increasing exposure to palm oil were less burdensome than alternatives and less than the previous toll from trans fats. Industrially produced trans fats caused an estimated 540,000 deaths each year worldwide.[124] With tens of thousands of chemicals in use in the processed food industry, limited regulation of substitutions, and frequent reformulations guided by financial and marketing considerations, "malsubstitution"—substituting one risky product with another untested potential risk—is a growing probability.[125]

But for the agribusinesses operating in today's economy, such caution is unacceptable. Palm oil companies would lose market share to other types of oil producers, their investors would take their capital elsewhere, and the global food companies that bought their palm oil would find alternative supply chains. And so as soon as it became clear that trans fats were on their way out, big food companies like Unilever switched to palm oil, ensuring their supply chains would be in place by the time bans went into effect. At the same time, rapidly expanding global and national fast-food companies in China, India, and Indonesia also increased their purchases of palm oil, often replacing soya oil. By 2019, these three nations accounted for 40 percent of global palm oil consumption.[126]

Once a product has been introduced into the global economy, it becomes difficult to replace it. Should the massive global exposure to palm oil turn out to have serious health consequences, as now seems possible, it would be difficult to shrink its already deep footprint. Food industry opposition to removing trans fat delayed the decision for two decades. Investment firms like BlackRock, the Vanguard Group, JPMorgan and Fidelity Investments have already invested almost $13 billion in palm oil holdings, making them reluctant to put these investments at risk.[127] Producers like Wilmar, a Singapore conglomerate that controls almost half the world's palm oil trade, and Conagra, a major American food producer, would need to find substitutes and then create new supply chains, both operationally challenging tasks.

Supermarkets and food makers would need to address consumer concerns, requiring new labeling or expensive public campaigns to reassure customers, as they launched after public concerns rose about genetically modified foods. Even if suppliers of substitute products eventually found ways to profit from a less damaging commodity, the delays in changing production practices triggered by industry opposition would continue to expose hundreds of millions of people. To be clear, the health problem is not simply palm oil but the lack of any stringent international process for vetting a product before introducing it into the world's food supply.

Instead, this constellation of corporations uses their power and influence to minimize apprehensions about palm oil, make misleading claims about its safety, and lobby to defeat any proposed control measures. And even if some of the largest companies decided to take the high road and reduce or eliminate use of palm oil, their palm oil suppliers would look to sell to other companies, perhaps at lower prices, allowing these competitors to sell their fast food, snacks, and baked goods at lower prices, another threat to market share and profitability. Another possibility, seen in other product reformulations, is that companies develop premium "free from palm oil" products to sell to their upscale or socially concerned consumers, while continuing to use palm oil in their less expensive products.

Although increased use of palm oil in food and other household products was the primary cause for expanded production, its use in biofuels added to further pressure for expansion. To reduce global warming, in 1997, the European Commission called for increasing energy consumption from renewable sources.[128] A decade later, the United States also set the goal of substituting biofuels for fossil fuels. In his 2007 State of the Union address, President George W. Bush proposed to increase the nation's "energy independence" by replacing petroleum with biofuels—ethanol and biodiesel—thus replacing within ten years 35 billion gallons of petroleum and confronting the "serious challenge of global climate change." Between 2006 and 2017, biodiesel production in the United States increased from 250 million gallons to 1.5 billion gallons. Imports of biodiesel also soared.

Not coincidentally, the proposal also satisfied the nation's agricultural industry, which had for years been lobbying for more biofuel research.[129] However, since not enough additional unused agricultural land was available in the US, and diverting land from food to biofuels could increase the price of food, a politically unpalatable outcome, much of the land needed to meet the growing demand for biofuels in Europe and the United States came from palm oil, of which 85 percent came from Malaysia and Indonesia. It also helped that palm oil was considerably cheaper to produce than other biofuels such as soybean, rapeseed, and sunflower.[130] As Kalyana Sundram, CEO of the Malaysian Palm Oil Council put it, "The cost of production is far less than any comparable vegetable or animal fat. Industry is simply palming off the benefits to the consumer."[131] Sierra Leone, Ecuador, and Colombia, among other nations, also seek to develop their capacity to export palm oil.

Other allies of expanded palm oil production were the World Bank and the International Monetary Fund, which encouraged Asian countries to increase palm oil production to pay off their debts, and the governments of Indonesia and Malaysia. Palm oil now accounts for 13.7 percent of Malaysia's gross national income and is Indonesia's top export. Indonesia promised to convert 13 million acres of forest to industrialized palm production,[132] displacing small farmers and endangering tigers, orangutans, and other wildlife.

In these ways, expanding palm oil production—and other commodities essential to the ultra-processed diet—won the support of those promoting nationalist economic development agendas, a useful ally for the global companies profiting from this growth. Malaysia's minister of primary industries, Teresa Kok, told the European Palm Oil Conference that "palm oil is synonymous with poverty eradication," making it the kind of seemingly win-win proposition that attracts foreign investors, governments, and underemployed rural residents.[132]

But expanded palm oil production also created losers, entities that had less voice in the global economy. The most spectacular loser was the earth's climate. To expand production in Malaysia and Indonesia required clear-cutting tropical forests. Globally, forests hold as much as 45 percent of the planet's carbon that is stored on land, far more than the oilseed crops that replace burned forests. When these trees are cleared, most of that carbon is released, worsening global warming.[133] In Indonesia, expanding palm oil production requires burning peatland forests that grow in rotting plant life rich in carbon. The massive fires used to clear peatland create their own hazards. Researchers at Harvard and Columbia universities estimated that the haze from fires in Indonesia in 2015 resulted in 100,300 excess deaths across Indonesia, Malaysia, and Singapore,[134] another example of palm oil's collateral damage.

Also displaced were the many indigenous groups living in the regions where palm oil plantations replaced tropical rainforest. In Indonesia, for example, thousands of indigenous communities live in the forest collecting berries, oils, fuelwood, medicinal plants, or animals. For these communities, the forest where they have lived for generations is sacred. When palm oil plantations are developed, these people are displaced.[135]

The push to expand palm oil production has also led to land grabbing, the practice of wealthy investors buying up land to grow crops for the global market or sell for a profit. In parts of Africa, community lands are a main target for the expansion of palm oil plantations. Between 2000 and 2015, more than sixty-five large-scale land deals for palm oil plantations in Africa had been signed, covering more than 4.7 million hectares.[136] Partnerships of multinational companies, local elites, and development banks launched a full-scale attack against communities from Sierra Leone in West Africa to the Democratic Republic of the Congo in Central Africa to take their lands for palm oil plantations.[137]

In a different economic system, corporations, governments, scientists, and voters would have asked some questions before plunging into palm oil. What are the short-term costs and benefits of alternatives to palm oil? What are the long-term consequences of a commodity that enables the global food system to continue to expand production of the cheap highly processed diet that drives epidemics of diet-related diseases and encourages transport systems to continue to rely on fuels with a heavy carbon burden? What policies could encourage producers of palm oil to reduce the health and environmental consequences of palm oil rather than externalize its costs to taxpayers, governments, and consumers? The informal but powerful alliance of agriculture producers, food makers, investors, national governments beholden to these industries, and international lenders such as the World Bank and the International Monetary Fund ensured that these questions were not asked, a failure whose costs have yet to be tallied. Now palm oil is so deeply rooted in the global economy that only transformative changes can reduce or eliminate its use.

HOW CHANGES IN TWENTY-FIRST-CENTURY CAPITALISM CHANGED THE FOOD SECTOR

Today, the raw ingredients of highly processed food are grown and shipped around the world and often consumed outside the home. In this transformation, each sector of the food industry changed in response to changes in capitalism. This cascade of alterations in turn changed the economic and political arrangements that produced food.

Of the ninety-three largest global corporations that play central roles in the global food system, companies that in 2018 each had revenues of more than $10 billion, retailers like Walmart, Amazon, and Kroger accounted for almost 60 percent of food industry revenues. Food and beverage producers (companies like Cargill, Nestlé, Unilever) and distributors (companies like PepsiCo, Anheuser-Busch InBev, and Coca Cola) come in second, with 25 percent and almost 9 percent of annual revenues, respectively. Agricultural and chemical producers (such as Dupont, BASF, and Bayer) account for 6 percent of 2018 revenues, and restaurants and fast-food chains like Compass, Starbucks, and McDonald's account for just over 2 percent.

Several of these companies work in many sectors other than food—for example, Walmart and Amazon sell more than food and DuPont makes chemicals for electronics and transportation companies as well as for agriculture. These intersections between food sector businesses and energy, chemical, retail, pharmaceutical, and other sectors give transnational food corporations even more economic and political power.

Retailers' dominance of the global food economy helps to explain the central role this sector plays in shaping food choices of individuals and the business practices of other food business sectors. In each sector, the top companies by revenue are firmly rooted in the production, distribution, and sales of UPF, both a cause and consequence of the rise of UPF in the last few decades.

Several dimensions of the transformation are rooted in recent changes in capitalism. The rise of the food retail sector, first in developed and then in developing countries, described in detail by the agricultural economist Thomas Reardon[138], follows the growing importance of consumption as the source of capital and growth. In the last fifty years, retail chains like Walmart and now Amazon have shown their skill in selling ever-more products, generating the revenues that keep the food system growing and profits flowing. Given their share of revenues and profits, it is not surprising that food retailers have become the central industry influence in shaping food choices of individuals and the business practices of other food business sectors.

As the food production system globalized, those companies that had the resources and reach to profit in this new environment grew and those that did not failed, were bought up, or developed niche markets. Thirty-one of the ninety-three largest food-related companies have their headquarters in the United States. Only five of the world's wealthiest nations (United States, Japan, Canada, Netherlands, and the United Kingdom) have five or more major global food corporations, showing the critical role that these high-income countries and their governmental food policies play in making decisions about food production, distribution, and sales around the world.

In 1973, Earl Butz, a food industry executive whom President Richard Nixon appointed as secretary of agriculture, advised farmers to "get big or get out"[139] and developed subsidy and export policies that encouraged that trend. The consequent growth of big farms producing commodity crops contributed to the glut of corn, soy, and other basic ingredients of UPF and also to the food industry imperative to find markets for their new products in the United States and globally. For food and beverage producers, cheaper products like high fructose corn syrup, used to sweeten soda and many other products, also encouraged the development of new products and new markets, products that then contributed to the rise in obesity and diet-related diseases.[140]

Another trend that favored the rise of the ultra-processed diet was increasing monopoly concentration across most sectors of the food industry. For example, in 2012, the four largest companies controlled 82 percent of the beef packing industry, 85 percent of soybean processing, 63 percent of pork packing, and 53 percent of broiler chicken processing.[141] In food retail, according to the USDA, the proportion of grocery sales by the twenty largest food retailers increased by 60 percent between 1996 and 2016.[142]

Monopoly concentration enables companies to avoid competition on prices; frees resources for more marketing and product development; drives out smaller, perhaps more innovative, businesses and farmers; and makes it more difficult for government to regulate the remaining giants. In the food sector, bigger companies with more global markets are attracted to shelf-stable products that can be shipped around the world and stored for as long as needed, all characteristics that favor highly processed food over healthier alternatives such as fresh fruits and vegetables and lightly processed whole grains.

A recent study of changes in the food systems in Asia, where food sales are growing rapidly, illustrates this cascade of changes. Based on their study of these changes, public health researchers Phillip Baker and Sharon Friel conclude:

> UPF sales has increased rapidly in most middle-income countries (in Asia). Carbonated soft drinks was the leading product category, in which Coca-Cola and PepsiCo had a regional oligopoly. Supermarkets, hypermarkets, and convenience

stores were becoming increasingly dominant as distribution channels for packaged foods throughout the region. Market concentration was increasing in the grocery retail sector in all countries. Food service sales are increasing in all countries led by McDonalds and Yum! Brands.[143]

Financialization has also contributed to recent changes in the global food system. First, the rise of an agricultural commodities futures market has attracted capital from speculators, replacing human need and environmental factors as drivers of food price volatility. In this century, agricultural commodities have become part of a diversified portfolio of financial investors. According to Barclay Hedge, a firm that provides data to institutional investors, commodity assets under management have increased from $41.3 billion in 2001 to $330 billion in 2013.[144] In their efforts to maximize returns, investors withhold commodities from the market, speculate on crop failures, and flood markets to drive prices down, all factors that increase the volatility of food prices and drive small farmers off their land. These changes in food prices in turn contribute to undernutrition (when many people cannot afford more expensive food), and to over-nutrition (when families substitute readily available cheaper products—often calorie dense ultra-processed ones) for healthier more expensive foods.[145]

Another dimension of financialization is the transformation of agricultural resources, mostly land but also patents on the genetic makeup of seeds or animals, into financial assets that are then sold and resold in financial markets, again shaping food production decisions independently of human need.[146] Land grabs to expand palm oil production in Asia, Africa, and Latin America illustrate this phenomenon.

DISRUPTIVE FORCES

The stories of the growth of Walmart, fast-food outlets, toddler formula, and palm oil show how recent changes in the food industry have made the way people eat more damaging to their health and to the planet. Even as these innovations spread around the world, new disruptive forces are surfacing that will further change what and how people eat in coming decades. These shifts will also shape the clashes between a food industry that wants to maximize revenues and profits and consumers, citizens, and food workers who want healthier, more affordable diets, better pay and working conditions, and food systems more compatible with planetary well-being.

Five changes demand attention. First, the way people acquire food is shifting rapidly. More people are getting more food from supermarkets, both offline and online, and are also consuming more calories at fast-food and other eating places outside the home. Around the world, a few giant supermarket chains are rapidly consolidating their domination of that market. At the same time, supermarket business is being disrupted by online ordering, meal kits, and home delivery.

In many countries, including the United States, places that sell inexpensive mostly unhealthy food are growing rapidly. Dollar stores, which started in the 1950s, are discount variety stores that sell many items, including food, for one dollar or less. After the 2008 economic crisis, these stores grew rapidly in the country's most economically distressed places, the largely rural counties with few retail options. Currently, two main chains, Dollar General and Dollar, operate more than thirty thousand stores nationally and plan to open thousands more, vastly outnumbering Walmart and other retailers.[147] Dollar General, a Fortune 500 company that runs the largest chain, had 2018 revenues of $28.6 billion dollars.

In rural communities, dollar stores are causing full-service grocery stores to close. By saturating communities with multiple outlets, dollar store chains are making it harder for new grocers and other local businesses to grow. In the process, they make the mostly highly processed food they sell more available and cheaper and the healthier food less available.[148] "Essentially what the dollar stores are betting on in a large way is that we are going to have a permanent underclass in America," Garrick Brown, a real estate researcher, told Bloomberg News.[149]

At the same time, in some cities, another sector of the food system is emerging in the public and nonprofit sectors in the United States, the United Kingdom, and several middle-income countries. Farmers markets, regional and community food hubs, community-supported agricultural projects, food co-ops, public and nonprofit institutional food programs, and community-owned "social supermarkets" are challenging the for-profit sector by making healthy low-cost food more available in low income, Black, Latinx, and immigrant communities.[150] Whether these enterprises can eventually compete with the market sector—or provide a viable alternative for some residents—will depend on their ability to engage community residents and local governments in creating sustainable alternatives.

A decade from now how individuals and families around the world buy their food may look quite different. Can those seeking to transform the food system use these changes to make diets healthier and more affordable? Can smart public policy leverage these disruptive market forces to achieve public good? Or will the food industry co-opt healthier and community-driven innovations to maintain their dominant role?

Second, the way food is grown is being transformed. Soil scientists are testing dirt to design the optimal chemical and physical environment for each crop. Farmers are using smart phones to control the precise doses of water, fertilizer, and pesticide that each plant gets every day. Geneticists are designing plants that can resist pests and drought and concentrate micronutrients.

Today, these technologies are primarily controlled by big corporations and used to advance their business interests. Could a different system of control such as more open-source biotechnology (e.g., farmers sharing seeds or breeding healthier hybrid plants or animals without resorting to patents) contribute to transformative changes in the health and environmental consequences of the way food is now grown?

Third, how countries negotiate trade agreements is changing. The neoliberal consensus on trade forged in the late twentieth and early twenty-first centuries is under challenge, illustrated by the Brexit debate and President Trump's efforts to renegotiate trade relationships with China, Mexico, Canada, and many other nations. Around the world, some political parties, governments, and industries are questioning whether the corporate-managed trade regime serves their interests. Long-time labor, health, and environmental critics of corporate-managed trade are again raising objections to the dominant trade regime. To date, no global political force has the power to promote trade policies that make the improvement of diets, health, the working conditions of food workers, and the global environment a priority, but could the new debate create an opening for such a force, leading to the emergence of new bottom-up trade alliances?

Fourth, scientists and health professionals are developing new insights into the complex relationship between diet and health. Some doctors and nutritionists argue that food is medicine and that health professionals should master the power of diet to improve health. Advances in personalized medicine—a practice in which genetic sequencing is used to design drugs for a specific individual—has led some to argue for "personalized nutrition." Clinicians use monitoring devices, data on biomarkers, genetics, and medical history to recommend specific nutrients an individual needs to cure or prevent a specific disease.[151] Who will own and control these new technologies? What will it take to convert these now mostly science fiction concepts into practical strategies for improving health? How will the food industry try to use this potential to consolidate its power and control? And what approaches can ensure that these new technologies will contribute to shrinking rather than widening the big gaps in nutritional health between the better off and the poor?

Finally, more people around the world want healthier and safer food. The growth of organic food, the increasing prevalence of health claims in food marketing, and the media attention to healthy food testify to the growing interest in healthy eating. Can this demand be translated into market power that actually changes what people eat? What is the common ground between individuals who want to eat healthily and companies that want to prosper by selling food? Are the new industries that are developing plant-based meats a solution to the environmental pressures of meat—or simply one more addition of a highly processed product to the world's diet? In practice, the largest food companies have been quite successful in co-opting the vision of organic local food, turning it into a marketing strategy,[152] a strategy that plant-based meat makers may seek to replicate.

The good news is that these disruptions make it likely that in the next few decades the world's food system will look dramatically different from the current one that makes UPF the priority. But whether the billions of farmers, food workers, and eaters who would benefit from such a transformation will be able to effectively and successfully challenge the corporate and financial interests that now control the global food system is the most troubling question of all. To assess the prospects for the outcome of this contest requires a more detailed analysis of the successes and failures of resistance to the corporate effort to universalize the global diet based on UPF.

RESISTANCE AND ALTERNATIVES

Throughout the last fifty years, citizens, consumers, food workers, governments, and social movements have challenged the growing power of giant transnational corporations to shape the global burden of disease and climate change. Sometimes these battles failed but in other cases, the forces opposing the global food industry have won concessions that led to improvements in diet and health, workers' rights, and harmful environmental practices. An examination of a few of these successes and failures complicates a simplistic narrative of uncontested or inevitable growth in corporate power and suggests alternatives to a global diet that relies on ultra-processed products.

Walmart. The world largest seller of groceries has encountered resistance on multiple levels. Communities have resisted Walmart's advances, claiming that its entry forced small businesses to close, lowered wages, and made unhealthy food more available. New York City, for example, banned Walmart from opening big box stores within its borders. In 2014, despite more than three decades of growth, 12 million people in seven of the nation's largest cities had no Walmart stores.[153] The combination of labor, political, and community opposition made it difficult for Walmart to penetrate the nation's densest and most profitable urban markets.

In 2018, Walmart acquired a new home delivery business, Jet, that began to make home deliveries of Walmart food in New York City. But Stuart Appelbaum, president of the Retail, Wholesale and Department Store Union, a group that had previously led successful efforts to bar Walmart from opening stores in New York City, observed, "The fact that Walmart had to acquire another company in order to operate in New York City is a testament to our efforts to keep them out."[154] By 2020, Walmart was forced to close Jet.

To counter this resistance, Walmart has continued to expand its e-commerce business. But an earlier effort to create smaller-footprint Express Stores in dense urban neighborhoods failed, leading it to close all 102 of these small-format stores by 2016[155] and subsequently to scale back its Neighborhood Markets, another small-format grocery store.[156] The challenges that Walmart, the world's largest business, has faced in expanding in cities shows the limits of its power and the potential for alliances of urban residents, public officials, and small-business owners to resist its efforts to penetrate urban markets.

Portland, Oregon, which does not ban Walmart stores, decided in 2014 to remove Walmart stocks from its investment portfolio, a task completed by 2016. In the debates on the disinvestment policy, city councilors noted that Walmart "exerts considerable downward pressure on wages"; it "significantly reduced health insurance benefits for part-time employees" by changing eligibility standards; [and] it "has focused on fast, low-cost production at the expense of basic safety measures for employees." The commissioner who led the push for the do-not-buy list, wrote, "You have to start somewhere—and we might as well start with a company that is openly, notoriously and extravagantly bad to the bone."[157] By refusing to pick up the costs that result from Walmart's low wages, which required many of its workers to enroll in publicly supported Medicaid and SNAP (food stamps) programs, these jurisdictions increased the pressure on Walmart to stop externalizing these costs to taxpayers and workers.

Farm worker and labor groups also demanded changes at Walmart, with varying degrees of success. In 2011, the Coalition of Immokalee Workers, a worker-based human rights organization, launched the Fair Food Campaign, a partnership among farmworkers, Florida tomato growers, and participating retail buyers.[158] The Campaign convinced Walmart—as well as McDonald's, Burger King, and other big food companies—to pay a penny a pound more for tomatoes, an increase Florida tomato growers used to raise the wages for pickers. These companies also agreed to ensure that a code of conduct designed to protect agricultural workers' rights is implemented on the farms from which they but their tomatoes.[159]

Finally, in 2018, Senator Bernie Sanders from Vermont and Representative Ro Khanna from California introduced into Congress the Stop WALMART Act, legislation that would prohibit large employers from purchasing stock buybacks for shareholders unless they meet basic criteria for fair employment practices such as a fifteen dollar per hour starting wage for all employees, the ability for all employees to earn up to seven days of paid sick leave, and limiting CEO pay to no more than 150 times the median pay of all employees.[160]

Although Congress is unlikely to pass the Stop WALMART Act any time soon, the legislation brings the issue onto the national political agenda, enabled the discussion of the issue in the 2020 presidential campaign and subsequent elections, and provides a platform for local and national educational and organizing campaigns.

Toddler Formulas . The development of toddler formula, as I noted, is itself the market-driven response to a successful public health campaign to restrict Nestlé's and other formula companies' aggressive promotion of infant formula in the 1970s and beyond. The organizational alliances, scientific evidence, and message framing that guided the Boycott Nestlé's Campaign has also served as a foundation for resisting the promotion of toddler formula. In 2017, growing public health concern led the World Health Organization to publish a guide for ministries of public health on ending the inappropriate promotion of foods for infants and young children.[161] The guide identified products that were being inappropriately marketed, suggested strategies for reducing conflicts of interest between formula makers and health agencies, and recommended regulations to limit deceptive or untruthful promotion. By preparing this guide, WHO contributed to the effort to control marketing of toddler food.

Researchers and nonprofit groups also contributed to the effort to counteract the marketing of toddler formula. The Changing Markets Foundation, a Dutch nonprofit that works in partnership with NGOs, other foundations, and research organizations, creates and supports campaigns to shift market share away from unsustainable products and companies and toward environmentally and socially beneficial solutions.[162] When it concluded that the four largest formula manufacturers were primarily driven by marketing considerations and not by science and health considerations, the foundation decided to put additional pressure on Nestlé, the largest formula maker.[163]

Its 2018 report called on Nestlé to show leadership, by implementing an independent review of its product range at the global level and ensuring that its marketing aligns with the WHO Marketing Code, including removing any comparisons to breastmilk.[164] The campaign led Nestlé to commit to reformulate its infant formula product range to be in line with some of the group's recommendations, particularly those related to phasing out unhealthy ingredients, such as sucrose and flavorings.[165] Previous campaigns against Nestlé had led organizers to conclude that Nestlé does not always keep its commitments but that company promises can serve as benchmarks that open doors for additional activism. By working with independent scientists and contesting Nestlé's health and marketing claims, the foundation challenged the company's assertion that it was a science-driven organization that brought the benefits of nutritional knowledge to its customers.

While these and other efforts to challenge the aggressive promotion and misleading claims about toddler formula led to growing professional and perhaps some public understanding of the health risks of toddler formula and related products, to date these campaigns have not achieved the public attention or policy successes of the earlier Boycott Nestlé campaigns. This limited success testifies to the immense resources that infant and toddler formula makers can bring to the defense of their products and the difficulty of health professional and civil society groups in maintaining pressure on a particular company or sector over decades.

Palm oil. The most effective pushback against the expansion of palm oil production has come from those worried about its environmental impact. Greenpeace, the international environmental organization, played a leading role in putting pressure on the palm oil industry to change its practices. Demonstrating the versatility that environmental activists have used to confront harmful corporate practices, Greenpeace used both cooperative and confrontational tactics to achieve its goals.

Working with palm oil companies, Greenpeace developed a toolkit for stopping deforestation, a guide intended to help companies integrate palm oil cultivation and conservation. According to Jenifer Lucey, the tropical field ecologist at Oxford University who wrote the toolkit, it helped to conserve half a million hectares of forest in multiple countries.[166] Greenpeace also helped to develop certification standards for sustainable palm oil cultivation, providing palm oil growers, civil society groups, and governments with criteria for monitoring industry practices.

Greenpeace also used more militant tactics. In 2018, six Greenpeace activists were arrested in the Gulf of Cadiz near Spain while trying to board a cargo tanker that was carrying palm oil harvested from plantations grown on bulldozed rainforests. The palm oil on the tanker was distributed by Wilmar International, one of the world's largest food manufacturers. Wilmar is a major supplier of palm oil to Mondelez, a Brazilian company that is one of the world's largest producers of ultra-processed snack foods including Oreo and Chips Ahoy! cookies and Ritz Crackers. The mission of Mondelez is "to empower people to snack right."[167]

Waya Maweru, one of the arrested Greenpeace activists, explained the action. "I'm from Indonesia. I've witnessed the devastating impact of deforestation from palm oil and our cities choking with haze as a result of the forest fires. I'm here to send a message to Mondelez that Wilmar's dirty palm oil is destroying our home and we don't want it in our supermarkets" (See Figure 2.2.).[168]

Retail food chains have also joined the effort to reduce palm oil use. In 2018, Iceland, a United Kingdom food retailer that sells frozen foods, pledged to remove palm oil from all its own-brand foods, a move the store hoped would slow the ongoing destruction of tropical rainforests in Southeast Asia. However, given the pervasiveness of palm oil in the global food supply, Iceland was unable to meet its commitment and instead stripped its store label from

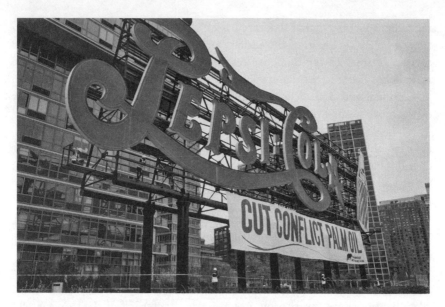

Fig. 2.2 Activists from the International Labor Rights Forum, the Rainforest Action Network, and an Indonesian labor rights advocacy organization call on PepsiCo to stop buying from palm oil producers who use child labor and systemic labor abuses, an illustration of alliances created by fights on commodity supply chains.
Photo: Rainforest Action Network

foods containing palm oil rather than remove palm oil from its branded foods, a less effective strategy for reducing use.[169]

Public health researchers have also contributed evidence to guide policies on palm oil. While palm oil has been linked with higher rates of heart disease and other conditions, it is less harmful than trans fats and cheaper than other trans-fat substitutes, leading some scientists to support its use. But a recent review of the evidence on palm oil in the Bulletin of the World Health Organization urged the public health community to more fully integrate research on health and environmental consequences of palm oil consumption and production and to assess more broadly its role in the expansion of the UPF industry.[170] This broader perspective can contribute to more informed policy decisions in a complex food system.

Opponents of tropical deforestation also acted on the political front. In 2019, eight US Senators, members of the Senate Climate Action Task Force, wrote letters to the nation's largest asset management firms, calling on them to use their financial leverage to stop tropical deforestation. Working with Friends of the Earth, an environmental group, the senators reminded investment firms including BlackRock, Vanguard, TIAA, JPMorgan Chase, Fidelity, and several others, that "addressing risks from deforestation is in line with your fiduciary responsibility," and asked the firms to respond to the senators regarding how they manage these risks.[171] By warning investors that shareholders might hold them accountable for the financial risks of failing to address the climate consequences of destroying tropical forests, the senators hoped to trigger disinvestment in unsustainable palm oil production and to increase pressure on companies like Wilmar and Cargill to improve their practices.

What has been the cumulative impact of these challenges to the palm oil industry? On the positive side, governments, environmentalists, scholars, and investors now know more about the harmful consequences of palm oil production and about some steps that can minimize the damage. A wider alliance of constituencies that are harmed by current palm oil production practices has emerged and has the potential to become a more powerful voice in shaping palm oil policy.

But as in the wider conflict on global warming, the rapid pace of destruction and the overwhelming power of those who benefit from palm oil make optimism difficult. The story of palm oil shows how the dominance of UPF depends on the intersection of complex and powerful systems. Disentangling these systems to open new paths for alternative global diets remains a daunting practical, political, and economic task. Emerging alliances to combat deforestation by the beef and timber industries and to protect the indigenous people whose land and livelihood are being destroyed raises the prospect of a global movement for healthier agricultural practices and respect for human rights.

Agroecology . Ultimately, the foundation for the rise of UPF is the industrial system for food production that emerged in the twentieth century and became fully globalized in recent decades. Creating an alternative to the ultra-processed diet will require transforming this approach to agricultural production. The most developed and tested alternative is an emerging body of practice and science known as agroecology. More recently, some groups have used the term "regenerative agriculture" to describe a system of farming principles and practices that increases biodiversity, enriches soils, improves watersheds, and enhances ecosystem services.[172] Unlike the previous examples, in which civil society groups, governments, and social movements challenged food corporations, the agroecology movement is an example of an effort to demonstrate an alternative to the practices of transnational agricultural corporations.

Agroecology describes the old and new agricultural practices that small farmers in Mexico, Cuba, India, Brazil, and other countries use to grow fruits and vegetables and raise animals, reduce use of pesticides and chemical fertilizers, use water more efficiently, and reduce waste by reusing farm by-products. It also describes the policies that some Brazilian cities follow where schools are mandated to purchase and serve fruits and vegetables grown by local farmers, both to improve the nutritional health of children and to build sustainable markets for local farmers.

Supporters of agroecology include global organizations like La Via Campesina, a network of more than 200 million small and medium sized farmers from 182 organizations in 81 countries who meet to exchange farming practices and develop political strategies to challenge industrial agriculture. Other proponents include a growing body of interdisciplinary scientists from agronomy, soil science, botany, entomology, climate science, systems science, and nutrition. Together, these scholars produce evidence that can help farmers and societies to adopt healthier, more sustainable, and more equitable farming practices.

While there is no single accepted definition of agroecology, one useful characterization calls it the "ecology of food systems."[173] Agroecology is at once a science, a social movement, and a practice.[174] Each of these three descriptions distinguishes agroecology from the industrial agriculture to which it provides an alternative.

As a science, agroecology emphasizes the interactions among different scales and levels of food production; the importance of the biological, environmental, economic, and social causes and consequences of food production; and the agency of farmers and farm communities in choosing how to grow food. The science of agroecology seeks to apply the methods of modern science to understand and inform the practices farmers use in different settings and under different conditions.

As a social movement, agroecology seeks to mobilize the power to replace industrial agriculture as the leading mode of food production. It seeks to identify, promote, and implement public policies and programs that support small farmers and more sustainable food production. It seeks to level the playing field on which Big Food now dominates and to give small farmers, disenfranchised communities, and those suffering from hunger and diet-related diseases a more equitable voice in shaping agricultural and food systems. To date, agroecology has focused on small farmers, food production practices, and the environmental impact of various food-growing regimes, rather than on the food labor force as a whole or the marketing practices of transnational food corporations.

Finally, as a farming practice, agroecology seeks to give small and middle-sized farmers the knowledge, skills, and resources they need to make a living by growing food that supports human and planetary well-being.

To make further progress, the agroecology movement will need to consider several questions. How have the science, movement, and practice of agroecology challenged the global system that produces UPF? How can conventional farmers make the transition to agroecology? What obstacles block further progress? In what ways will Big Food seek to co-opt agroecology and how can its advocates resist such efforts? And what is a realistic plan and time frame for developing a food system based on the principles of agroecology?

Agroecology presents intellectual, organizational, and political challenges to Big Agriculture. Agroecologists contests the conventional wisdom that asserts that the Green Revolution, an approach to farming developed by scientists and agribusinesses that depends heavily on monoculture and intensive use of pesticides and fertilizers, can solve the world's food problems. The evidence and practice that agroecological practitioners have accumulated dispute the accomplishments of the Green Revolution; highlight its environmental, economic, and other limitations; and demonstrate that alternatives in fact exist.

At a 2018 International Symposium on Agroecology held in Rome, the director general of the United Nations Food and Agriculture Organization, Jose Graziano da Silva, called for "transformative change towards sustainable agriculture and food systems based on agroecology,"[175] a sign that agroecology was inching its way into the mainstream.

In Mexico, President Manual Lopez Obrador has pledged to make agroecology the guiding force for Mexico's agricultural future. Prior to his election, more than a hundred Mexican farmer organizations developed the Plan de Ayala 21, which proposed land reform, new methods of agricultural production, and improvements in public and environmental health, grounded in the rights of farmers, farmworkers, women, indigenous people, and youth. In endorsing this plan, Obrador embraced the goal of food sovereignty, the concept that agriculture should serve local communities first, based on local decision making. "In short," the Plan de Ayala groups proclaimed, "we need food and nutrition sovereignty to be public policy, based mainly on small and medium-scale agricultural production, with strategic planning and developed with full participation of both producers and consumers, and guided by agroecological criteria."[176]

In the United States and other high-income countries, agroecology continues to face skepticism. Those in agribusiness believe that new technologies, not agricultural practices tested over centuries, hold the promise for increased food production and they believe that technical rather than social and political solutions can reduce the adverse climate consequences of industrial agriculture.

Recently, proponents of the Green New Deal, the national proposal to integrate climate change, community development, and workforce strategies at the community and national levels, have begun alliances between climate change, food justice, agroecology, and other movements, a promising development that could unite the energies and power of several now-separate movements.[177]

Some observers advocate blending the best of Big Agriculture with agroecology to get the benefits of both approaches. But agroecologists in general reject that approach. A recent report by Friends of the Earth concluded that "agroecology and industrial agriculture are not interchangeable concepts nor practices and cannot coexist. They represent two fundamentally different visions of development and well-being."[178]

To date, agroecology has acknowledged but not emphasized the health and nutritional benefits it can contribute. By highlighting and linking the health and environmental costs of the corporate food system that makes UPF the priority, a food justice movement can create a new foundation for promoting nutritional health, reducing hunger and food insecurity, and protecting our planet.

For some food activists, the COVID-19 pandemic offers an opportunity to create alternatives to vulnerable globalized food supply chains, a diet that increases the risk of coronavirus infection, and the destruction of food sovereignty based on local and regional farming, goals consistent with agroecology.

The pandemic also highlighted the failure of the global food system to end hunger and food insecurity. In mid-2020, the World Food Program predicted that the number of acutely food insecure people in low income nations could increases from 149 million pre-COVID-19 to 270 million by the end of 2020.

Over time, food producers, workers, and eaters working at multiple levels have begun to create alternatives to the current capitalist food system. To bring these alternatives to scale and make them a viable force in people's daily lives will require more unified and grounded food, environmental, and labor movements than exist today.

CHAPTER 3

Education

Private Capital Goes to School

Education is the most powerful weapon which you can use to change the world.
—*Nelson Mandela*

Nothing better promotes lifetime health than education. At every stage of life, more education leads to better health. The reverse is also true: throughout the lifespan, healthier people achieve more academic success and learn more easily. If pharmaceutical companies could bottle and sell education, they could get rich while truthfully making the most extravagant claims. The amazing elixir of education extends life, prevents hospitalizations, improves quality of life, increases income, promotes healthier behavior, and makes people happier.

For more than a century, people of all classes and racial/ethnic groups in the United States have pursued education. Freed slaves, recent immigrants, families living in poverty, residents of rural areas, those aspiring to move into the middle class and above—all saw education as an individual ticket to success or an aspiration for their children or grandchildren.

But there is another story to tell about education. Education is also a tool those with power and wealth use to maintain their privileges, to exclude others from pursuing better lives, and to track people into the slots that maintain an inequitable and unhealthy status quo. Violent attacks on Black and integrated schools after Reconstruction; the creation of vocational schools that diverted females, Blacks, and immigrants from academic programs into those that prepared students for work in factories; boarding schools for Native American children seized from their families; the school-to-prison pipeline for children of color; and the inequitable funding of Black and White schools are examples of education that maintains and widens rather than shrinks inequitable life chances and perpetuates the systemic racism that has characterized the United States.[1]

Over the course of the nineteenth and twentieth centuries, most Americans came to agree that education was mainly a responsibility of the government and the public sector. A strong educational system supported both private and public good and therefore it was fair and smart to use taxpayer dollars to support the public education system. Yes, there were private and religious elementary and high schools and many colleges were private not-for-profit institutions, but business had a limited role and little political and public support for claiming a voice in shaping our educational system.

In the last few decades, however, the wall between public and private has become porous and especially recently the private sector and big corporations have claimed a bigger voice in shaping education policy, spending, and practices. This chapter explores this trend, assessing how changes in modern capitalism have modified the role of markets in education, how these changes have influenced the role of education in promoting well-being, and to what extent parents, students, and communities have resisted these changes. The bottom-line question: has the recent growing presence of private capital in early education, K-12 schools, and higher education in the United States reduced the positive impact of schooling on well-being, equity, and democracy?

In 2017, the US market for educational products and services—across K-12, higher education, and corporate learning—was more than $1.75 trillion and growing.[2] For-profit child care providers, textbook publishers, chains of charter schools, online educational providers, tech companies, testing companies, financial companies that make or service college loans, and for-profit universities—all encourage schools, parents, and students to make decisions that increase the quarterly returns of their companies, often with little regard for the educational and social impact of these choices.

In 2011, News Corp's CEO Rupert Murdoch showed the private sector's interest in this new opportunity, observing that "when it comes to K through 12 education, we see a $500 billion sector in the US alone that is waiting desperately to be transformed by big breakthroughs."[3] By 2019, the market capitalization of the world's listed educational companies was about $190 billion, with the most companies in China and the United States.[4]

HOW CHANGES IN MODERN CAPITALISM INFLUENCE EDUCATION

Capitalists have always cared about education. They look to schools for workers with the skills they need, consumers with the desire to buy their products, and citizens who respect the belief that capitalism is the best system possible.

They also need schools to train the managers who operate their businesses and educate their own children.

Several trends in modern capitalism explain why corporations, financial institutions, and other businesses have found appealing opportunities within the educational system. First, slowed growth in manufacturing and the production of goods has led investors to seek new, more profitable places to put their dollars to work. The service sector offers a large, expanding, and promising arena for investment. In the long economic expansion that followed World War II, manufacturing industries reached saturation of their markets, limiting opportunities for maintaining the pace of growth. In addition, efficiencies due to new technologies and cheaper labor in low-income countries reduced their need for new capital. So investors turned to the service sector to find higher rates of return. A 2017 analysis by Sageworks, a financial information company, found that compared to private companies making things, companies that provided services, from healthcare to education to home care, had higher returns on investment.[5]

Education was an attractive site for new investment because taxpayers had already paid for the infrastructure and were committed to funding the day-to-day expenses of running this system, at least in the K-12 years. By taking over some parts of this public system, investors could find new ways to extract profits from this public revenue stream.

Privatizers also introduce another rationale for shifting services into the market economy. In this view, public services that have been undermined by austerity and disinvestment—public schools and public hospitals, for example—can be offered more efficiently by the private sector. Online charter schools and walk-in private clinics can offer lower-cost alternatives than the public sector.

Another measure of the growing importance of the service sector comes from changing employment patterns. Between 1939 and 2015, private non-farm employment in good-producing industries increased by 8 percent while employment in service-providing private industries rose by 76 percent and in the government sector by 20 percent.[6] Over the last forty years, the number of US workers employed in manufacturing has declined from 19.6 million to 12.5 million.[7] As companies in Europe and Asia challenged US manufacturers of autos, food, electronics, and other products, these American companies automated jobs and moved plants overseas—and posted lower returns. For many investors, it was a no-brainer to put their capital in the rapidly expanding service sector rather than sticking with stagnant manufacturing companies.

Moreover, as more people moved into the middle class in the United States and other high- and middle-income countries, these better off people wanted more education, healthcare, financial services, and food and hotel services, creating new opportunities for economic growth and profit in services. The education sector provides a prime example. In 1980, total US government spending on education was $152 billion; by 2018 it reached $1.1 trillion, a more than 700 percent increase.[8] Like flies to honey, this new public investment in education attracted private investors. Often these patrons borrowed the accountability and racial justice arguments of activists to justify their investments in education, despite the lack of evidence that school privatization contributed to either of these goals.

The growth of the knowledge economy puts new demands on employers. In this economy, the production of goods and services is based on knowledge-intensive activities that contribute to an accelerated pace of technical and scientific advances as well as rapid obsolescence.[9] Business leaders see students, the products of the educational system, as an essential input that will influence their profitability. To ensure that schools turn out the products they need in this new era, they seek a larger and more direct voice in educational policy.

Following the global economic downturn of the late 1970s and beyond, privatization attracted the attention of conservatives, some economists, and some elected officials, who promoted selling healthcare, transportation, housing, telecommunications, and other services to private investors. Prime Minister Margaret Thatcher in the United Kingdom and President Ronald Reagan in the United States claimed that privatization was more efficient, less expensive, and less intrusive to freedom than maintaining these services in the public sector.[10]

In both countries, numerous local, state, and national government agencies invited private companies and nonprofit organizations to assume responsibility for educational services that in the past had been wholly public.[11] Privatizers argued that creating high-tech charter schools, for example, would enable more children to attend charters, improve the quality of education, and, by the way, create new profit opportunities for the companies that sold these technologies.

Austerity, another policy response to economic contraction, provided further incentives for privatization. In 1978 in California, for example, nearly two-thirds of California voters approved Proposition 13, a ballot referendum that reduced property tax rates on homes, businesses, and farms by about 57 percent and capped future increases to no more than two percent. Soon counties and states around the country were also slashing taxes and public revenues, adding a new impetus for private investment.

Former California governor Ronald Reagan described Proposition 13 as a rebellion against "costly, overpowering government" and urged Republicans to use Proposition 13 as their core message for the 1980 presidential contest.[12] In 1977, California spent about $7,400 per pupil, about $1,000 above the national average. By 1983, California's inflation-adjusted per pupil spending had dropped to $6,700, dipping below the national average, where it has generally stayed.[13] These austerity measures led parents, school districts, and public officials to turn to the private sector for relief, leading to the growth of private schools, private universities, and privatized educational support services.

Privatization offered new streams of funding that could mitigate the impact of austerity. But replacing public with private funds risked widening gaps in educational quality available to low-income communities compared to the better off. As Michael Fabricant and Stephen Brier ask in *Austerity Blues*, their book on the privatization of public higher education, "Can that privatized system offer the same promise of quality to the poor or working class student that it does to the wealthy who have priority access to . . . enriched forms of service?"[14] Privatization influenced each level of education, from early education to K-12 to higher education, but the rationale and impact differed by level.

Together, privatization and austerity have contributed to further racial segregation of all levels of education, widened inequitable funding of Black and white schools, and diminished the concept that schooling is a public function that should be used to achieve national values. The combination of the adverse effects of austerity and privatization on education with the rise of a white nationalism that justifies overt racism and is endorsed by mainstream political actors has set back the nation's progress toward a more equitable educational system achieved through the civil rights movement of the mid-twentieth century. Once again, corporate pursuit of self-interest uses racial divides to find new streams of revenue using the discourses of privatization and accountability via student testing.

The growing financialization of the US and global economies is a third trend that extends to many services that used to be wholly in the public sector. As economic transactions are financialized, profit making occurs increasingly through financial channels rather than through production of goods and services.[15] In the education sector, among the funding streams that can be used to bring financial returns to investors are tuition and fees from child care, K-12, and university education; rents from leased spaces; and interest on bank or private equity loans to college students, corporate chains of charter schools, or universities.

In the United States and around the world, schools at all levels have increasingly used these mechanisms to gain new resources for operations or expansion, often to replace funds reduced by privatization or austerity. Schools invest their revenue in financial markets to grow their current support but in doing so they incur debt and give their investors a voice in shaping their policies and practices. What used to be a modest flow of private wealth into the education system has now become a flood of capital that seeks to influence the shape of schooling at every level and create new profit centers that enable investors to extract public dollars into private pockets.

In early child care, for example, social impact bonds have been used to finance expansion of programs in at least twenty US cities, counties, and states. These bonds provide private financing for public programs, with the expectation that child care revenue streams—and public savings from these programs—will be used to pay back investors.[16] While social impact bonds increase funding for child care expansion, one analyst has noted that "the monetization of policy goals . . . transforms substantive social outcomes from the status of ends in themselves to a means for reducing government spending and producing a financial return for investors."[17]

A study of social impact bonds for early child care expansion in Salt Lake City, Utah; Chicago, Illinois; and Greenville, South Carolina, concluded that in Chicago and Salt Lake City, the mechanism led to overpayment of investors and the extraction of funds from the very education programs the bonds were designed to support while in South Carolina and Utah the bonds also contributed to political support for broader public funding. The authors suggest that cities seeking new sources of funding for early child care should be wary of the bonds' marketizing framework, as they can undermine social objectives through their financializing metrics.[18]

In K-12 education, investments from private foundations have helped to launch bonds to raise public money to expand charter schools. In 2009, the Gates Foundation provided collateral to help secure $300 million in tax-exempt bonds to expand such schools in Houston, Texas, giving private investors a way to profit by lending money for this expansion.[19] According to a 2016 report, about 40 percent of children in Detroit and Washington, DC, are in charter schools, and 100 percent of children in New Orleans attend charters, some for-profit and other not, schools with limited or no oversight and public accountability.[20] In each of these systems, Black children constitute the overwhelming majority of students, and are thus the subjects in this experiment in privatizing and financializing education.

Financialization has been best studied at the college level. A review estimated that between 2003 and 2012, college endowment investments grew from $16 billion to $20 billion and the financing costs of college tuition expanded from $21 billion to $48 billion. The former benefited mostly wealthy colleges while the latter left students at less well-off colleges with much higher levels of debt.[21] Proprietary colleges, another site for financialization of education, grew rapidly between 1997 and 2012, then shrunk as a result of bankruptcies and criminal charges, but more recently have grown again as US Secretary of Education Betsy DeVos rescinded many of the Obama-era regulations on for-profit colleges.

At their peak in 2011, those for-profit colleges in which Goldman Sachs was the dominant owner enrolled more than 150,000 students, captured $486 million in federal Pell grants, and netted an operating profit of more than $501 million.[22] As with charter schools, state cuts in funding for higher education in Wisconsin, California, Alaska, and elsewhere set the stage for the intrusion of private capital. Conservative elected officials justified these cuts with austerity arguments, often skipping over the fact that it was the federal and state tax cuts to the wealthy that led to budgetary shortfalls. Also left out of the public narrative was the new opportunity for profit in privatized higher education, an opening that did get renewed media attention as Secretary of Education DeVos sought to dismantle the federal system for regulating and monitoring for-profit colleges.[23]

The COVID-19 pandemic may breathe new life into for-profit higher education. As students struggle with rising tuition, poorly organized online classes, and budget cuts at public universities, for-profit colleges have the marketing expertise and the capital to target this new market. "Predatory for-profit colleges thrive on economic vulnerability and unemployment, which so many people are facing because of the COVID-19 pandemic," said Toby Merrill, director of the Project on Predatory Student Lending. "These schools prey on people looking to improve their career opportunities, using aggressive false advertising, misleading information, and empty promises."[24] Expanding DeVos's quest to subsidize for-profit colleges with public funds, the 2020 federal COVID-19 relief program provided more than $32 million in direct cash assistance to ten of the largest for-profit universities.[25]

Fourth, the globalization of the economy created opportunities to export US educational models, goods, and services, and financing to other countries. Pearson, a United Kingdom–based global testing and textbook company with 2018 revenue of $5.2 billion and more than twenty-four thousand employees in nearly sixty countries, meets the global demand for testing and books created in the United States and United Kingdom.[26] Chris Whittle, founder of Channel One, a company that created a television network to target advertising to children in schools and a founder of Edison Schools, a company that hoped to capture the charter school market, is now creating a new company to open private schools in wealthy cities around the world, starting in the United States and China. By attracting parents from around the world who can afford the $40,000 a year tuition, Whittle hopes to leverage the early investments from private equity firms in China into a global operation. "This is a long-term investment, said Whittle. "Eventually we'll take the company public."[27]

Globalization also provides universities with new markets for students and consulting firms like Bain and Company and McKinsey & Company with new markets for school systems. In the last five years, McKinsey has deployed 175 consultants to work on 600 education projects in 50 countries.[28] These opportunities help to spread US practices on involving the private sector in education, establishing university-corporate partnerships, and ensuring that schools meet the workforce needs of global corporations.

Capturing new developments in science and technology to support business goals constitutes one of the great successes of modern corporate capitalism. In education, this trend has contributed to both innovation and disruption of established practices. New discoveries in neuroscience and cognitive sciences, for example, have led educational researchers to study the origins of atypical development, the biological processes that play a role in learning school-relevant skills, and predictions of educational outcomes that can be tested in educational research.[29]

The findings of this research have contributed to the creation of personalized learning systems, which, like precision medicine and personalized nutrition, promise help for some individuals but also create opportunities for profit. Moreover, in many cases, the corporate implementation of personalized learning undermines schools as communities and educators as knowledge producers. These systems can further segregate low-income, Black, and Latinx children, particularly those with learning problems into more segregated, underfunded settings while the children of wealthier parents get personalized learning environments and private tutoring.[30] The greater challenges low-income families at all levels of education experienced as a result of expansion of online education during the COVID-19 pandemic further illustrated the potential adverse equity impact of these technologies.

Leaders of the personalized learning business at McGraw Hill, a global corporation that distributes digital and other educational products in more than one hundred countries, explain the appeal of personalized learning:

Teachers have always known that teaching to the middle meets the needs of few students. The problem has been that it is difficult to personalize at scale. But now, with the support of technology and more widespread accessibility, addressing students' needs is more possible than ever.[31]

Discoveries in computational computing and artificial intelligence have contributed to the development of hardware, software, and networked platforms that have the potential to make all levels of learning more efficient and tailored to individual need—and to generate profits for tech companies like IBM, Google, Microsoft, and others.[32] As Kirill Pyshkin from Credit Suisse, the global financial services company, observed, "So far only 2 to 3% of the 5 trillion USD spent globally on education is digital. This, combined with EdTech's sudden vital role during COVID-19 and the significant differences seen up to now in its geographical investments, intensify the previously unseized global growth opportunities."[33]

For high schools and universities, online learning systems allow schools to enroll more students, fit schooling into the busy lives of learners, and, in some cases, reduce labor costs. Although the record of educational institutions making money from distance education and online learning is mixed, Forbes estimated that the global e-learning market will reach $325 billion by 2025, up from $107 billion in 2015.[34]

How does the deployment of these technologies influence education? Ben Williamson, an educational researcher in the United Kingdom who studies the role of tech companies in educational reform, observes that the "Silicon Valley discourse of innovation, entrepreneurship, startup culture, makerspaces, crowdsourced solutions, platforms and philanthrocapital is becoming a new language of schooling. These schools are the prototypical products of venture philanthropy and are consistent with the increasing centrality of business terms to describe educational reforms and policies."[35] Williamson goes on to note that corporate involvement encourages a "technocratic mentality that value-free technical expertise is preferable to political conflict—in the institutions of schooling."

Finally, demographic, and socioeconomic changes are changing global education markets. Declining birth rates, especially in high-income countries, mean universities must compete for students with more choices, and also find ways to attract and meet the needs of emerging markets, including returning, older, and non-English-speaking learners. Many companies have defined new market niches by helping public and private universities to build and furnish upscale dormitories, dining halls, and sports centers, the must-haves for universities to attract more full-pay students. This profitable "amenities arms race" raises costs, which are passed on to students, further widening the affordability gap and reducing the number of lower-income students who can afford college.[36]

As the number of manufacturing jobs shrink, more workers need retraining. For corporations, ensuring that their own workforce development programs and those they support through philanthropy and taxes will provide them with the human capital they need to compete effectively in the global economy is a key concern. Winners in the workforce development contest get the educated just-in-time workforce they need and losers end up with overpaid, inadequately educated employees that burden their bottom lines. It is not surprising that business owners want a bigger say in designing the workforce development system that will determine their fate in this lottery.

Changes in the economy also influence educational decisions from child care to university. As more women go back to work after giving birth in order to support their households, early child care becomes important for working families and their employers. Of course, most Black, Latinx, and immigrant women have always had to work after giving birth and the lack of publicly funded early child care imposes added burdens and widens gaps in income and well-being. If economic downturns lead cities and states to cut school budgets, more parents who can afford private schools will use them, further diminishing public support for underfunded public schools. Improvements in the economy make it more attractive for some people to work rather than go to school, and economic downturns send unemployed people back to college. Parents and students respond to these changing economic conditions based on their personal circumstances but always their choices are constrained by the stratifications by race/ethnicity, class, gender, and immigrant status that characterize modern capitalism. In this way, the choices educational corporations offer end up widening gaps in educational access and quality.

Finally, capitalist ideology further influences changes in education. In the longer run, the knowledge economy, a term first popularized in the 1970s, portrays education as the foundation for individual and national economic success. Countries compete to create educational systems that lead to prosperity, and testing companies sell them products that will allow them to assess their success. Every corporation selling educational products, from toys for infants to college certificates and degrees for young and no-so-young adults, can count on their customers already believing that more knowledge will lead to a better life. Despite intense academic debate about the complex interactions between education and economic success,[37] this prevalent belief simplifies the marketing task for sellers, requiring them to convince parents, students, and other buyers that only their product, not their competitors' product, will ensure greater success in the knowledge economy.

Several key tenets of modern capitalism contribute to these changing views on education. The ideas that competition is good, that markets are better at solving social problems than governments, and that individuals are best equipped to make the decisions that shape their destinies have profoundly influenced the practice of schooling at all levels. Another influential capitalist tenet is that unions are bad and that many of the problems of today's educational system are caused by bureaucratic and self-serving unions, especially teachers unions. Former governor Scott Walker's campaign to cut funding for and privatize public education in Wisconsin depended on the rhetoric of greedy, incompetent unions.[38] Demonizing unions has played a critical role in enlisting wider public support for the corporate privatization agenda.

In education, as in other sectors, the trends described here are not distinct separable developments. Rather, together they define the face of twenty-first-century capitalism. Privatization supports financialization, globalization enables worldwide dissemination of new technologies, and capitalist ideology makes all these developments seem natural and inevitable. Together, these changes have transformed how parents, children, and young people make decisions about their education.

These changes in our economic and political system have also changed the role of corporations, investors, real estate developers, and publishing companies in setting educational policy. Tech companies, private equity firms, financial institutions, venture philanthropy, textbook and testing companies, and others have all claimed seats at the tables where educational policies are decided. As the former Google CEO Eric Schmidt observed in a book he coauthored, *The New Digital Age: Reshaping the Future of People, Nations and Business*:

> Modern technology platforms, such as Google, Facebook, Amazon, and Apple, are even more powerful than most people realize, and our future world will

be profoundly altered by their adoption and . . . the speed at which they scale. Almost nothing short of a biological virus can spread as quickly, efficiently, or aggressively as these technology platforms, and this makes the people who build, control and use them powerful too.[39]

In the past few decades, private equity and venture capital investors; financial institutions; wealthy individual and corporate philanthropists; business organizations; for-profit school operators; and educational management, textbook, and testing companies have coalesced to constitute a new corporate educational sector. As education activist Howard Ryan has noted, this sector weaves together several strands of influence, each with distinct priorities.[40]

The first strand is "edubusiness,"[41] the companies that seek to profit by privatizing previously public or nonprofit educational institutions or services. The second strand, venture philanthropy, illustrates that reducing corporate influence to seeking more revenue oversimplifies a more complex story. This strand, which education scholar Diane Ravitch calls "The Billionaire Boys Club," includes Bill Gates, Jeff Bezos and his ex-wife, MacKenzie Bezos, the Walton Foundation, and the Eli and Edythe Broad Foundation (See Figures 3.1a and 3.1b). Their goals are to remake the American educational system to be more efficient, more competitive, and more market driven.[42] They favor more testing, accountability, competition, and measurable standards. They often see teachers, and especially teachers unions, as an obstacle to improving education. The businesses that made their fortunes may also benefit financially from the educational policies they propose, but their aims are framed in loftier terms.

Corporations and their trade association (e.g., Business Roundtable and the US Chamber of Commerce, both strong proponents of No Child Left Behind) constitute the third strand, the corporate educational sector.[43] Their goals include ensuring that corporate America gets the workforce it needs both for new tech jobs and the growing number of low wage less skilled jobs. This strand also seeks to finance education in ways that do not put an unreasonable burden on corporate taxpayers.

Finally, a fourth heterogenous strand, conservative Christians, wealthy right-wing activists, and white supremacist organizations seek to preserve or restore an educational system that maintains class stratification, racial segregation, and conservative values on sexuality, gender, and markets. Groups like the Foundation for Traditional Values, which seeks to break down the separation between church and state, the Home School Legal Defense Association, which defends home schooling, the American Federation for Children, a school choice advocacy organization, and others work with conservative Republicans and Christians to link education reform with other right-wing and nationalist movements.[44]

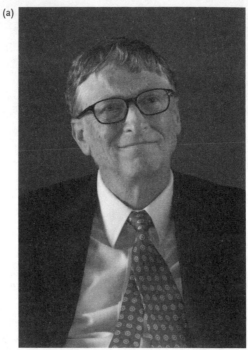

(a)

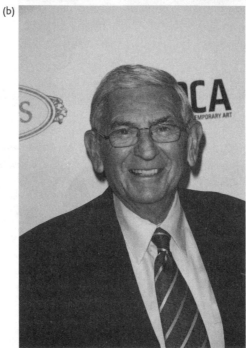

(b)

Figs. 3.1a and 3.1b Eli Broad and Bill Gates are two of the billionaire philanthropists who support charter schools.

While these different strands of market-friendly educational reform do not agree on everything, together they have brought a powerful new voice into the ongoing American debate about the proper role for government and markets in education. These reformers are Democratic and Republican, urban and rural, and Black and white. They are not homogenous and some strands (e.g., some proponents of charter schools) frame their goals in the language of racial justice and equity.

Many voices participate in the national discourse on education reform, but no parties have more resources, deeper connections in corridors of power, or more shared affinities in worldview than the leaders of education corporations and the billionaires who dominate educational philanthropy. To understand recent changes in education requires understanding the goals and methods of these groups. It also requires understanding the infrastructures these reformers have created to advance their goals. For example, the State Policy Network, an alliance of sixty-six right-wing "ideas factories" that span every state in the nation used its $80 million war chest—funded by the Koch brothers and the Walton Family Foundation—to create a "messaging guide" that can facilitate coordination of conservative strategy across the country.[45] Other education alliances, for example those supported by the Bill & Melinda Gates Foundation, align more with Democratic causes and groups but share the commitment to educational reforms that protect market values.[46]

In her recent book on resistance to privatization, education scholar Diane Ravitch summarizes the ideology of what she calls "the disruption movement," her term for the spectrum of advocates of privatization. The movement, she writes, relies on two dogmas, "first, the benefits of standardization, and second, the power of markets, at scale, to drive innovation and results. Their blind adherence to these principles has been disastrous in education. These principles don't work in schools for the same reasons that they don't work for families, churches and other institutions that function primarily on the basis of human interactions, not profits and losses."[47]

I now turn to exploring how these disrupters exert their influence, how they profit, and their impact on how learners and their families experience the changed landscape at three different levels of the educational system.

Early Child care

If education is the wonder drug that prevents or reduces the impact of multiple health problems across the life span, then early childhood education is that drug on steroids. A growing body of evidence shows that children who receive high-quality child care in their early years, compared to those who do not or those who have only lower quality care, gain the following benefits:

- improved mental health throughout childhood;[48]
- fewer deaths by age twenty-one; better self-reported health; lower rates of binge drinking alcohol, smoking, and using illegal drugs; and better mental health;[49]
- in their thirties, a lower risk of heart disease and its associated risk factors, including obesity, high blood pressure, high blood sugar, and high cholesterol; and[50]
- quality preschool also improved short-term and longer-term educational attainment, itself a lifetime health benefit, and lowered crime rates in participants compared to nonparticipants.[51]

Services for young children include two related but distinct categories: child care and early childhood education. The former, a broader concept, emphasizes the goals of enabling parents to work while keeping children safe and happy, the latter also includes education and experiences that prepare children for school and life success.

Quality child care and early childhood education bring benefits to families and communities, allowing parents to work more, thus increasing family income, reducing parental stress, and preparing children for school success, every parent's aspiration. More than schooling in later life, early care is both a social service that benefits families and allows parents to work, while at the same time providing education, promoting healthy development, and teaching new skills to children.

While the costs of comprehensive early childhood education are high, the rate of return suggests that it is a good investment. The cost of ABC/Care, a well-studied model of comprehensive early child care, was $18,514 in 2014 US dollars, about midway in the US average price of basic child care, which ranges from $9,589 to $23,354, with little evidence that more expensive care is necessarily better care. For disadvantaged children, this comprehensive model produces a 13 percent annual return on investment.[52] Some studies estimate that for every dollar spent on high-quality pre-kindergarten education as much as $10 is saved in costs for other government services over the child's life span.[53] Custodial child care, often delivered in homes, is less expensive but delivers fewer long-term social benefits.

Moreover, failing to provide affordable child care generates its own costs. American businesses lose an estimated $12.7 billion annually because of their employees' child care challenges and nationally, the cost of lost earnings, productivity, and revenue due to inadequate child care totals an estimated $57 billion each year.[54]

In addition, inequitable access to quality child care contributes to persistent class, racial/ethnic, and other gaps in health and education and to higher levels of criminal justice involvement, making new investments in care a promising strategy for shrinking the class-based, racial/ethnic, and other gaps in health, education, and life prospects that characterize the United States today.[55] Already in twenty-eight states, a year of daycare on average costs more than getting a year of public college education.[56] Fortunately, evidence suggests that disadvantaged groups benefit most from comprehensive early childhood education, further bolstering the case for additional support.[57] Such support could help to close the large and growing educational achievement gap that divides children from low-income households and communities of color and their better-off peers.[58]

Despite these powerful benefits, parents face formidable obstacles in finding affordable high-quality childcare. In 2017, two-thirds of children under six lived in households where all available parents (mother and father or single parent) were in the labor force.[59] One in three families spend 20 percent or more of their income on child care, almost three times the recommended maximum of 7 percent of income. For an individual earning minimum wage, the average annual cost of full-time child care would require 64 percent of their income.[60]

Half of families who looked for child care in 2016 reported difficulty finding it, and nearly one million families never found the program they wanted. Major reported obstacles were high costs, low quality, or no open slots.[61] In 2016 alone, an estimated two million parents, mostly women, were estimated to have made career sacrifices due to problems with childcare.[62]

Even families who consider themselves middle class find paying for child care a struggle. Patricia Bauer, who lives in San Diego with her husband and two young sons, told an NPR reporter, "We are struggling."[63] Bauer's entire take-home pay of $2,400 a month goes to paying for child care for her two children. "We feel like we're working so hard," Bauer explained, "but any minute we could lose everything—you know if we had some emergency, we don't have savings." Bauer considered quitting her job to stay at home to care for her kids but after finding out what she would have to pay to replace her employer-provided insurance, she decided "that's another huge bill we couldn't afford." "We joke that as soon as our boys are in public school, we'll be rich!" says Bauer, highlighting the value of publicly funded education.

Another problem facing early child care is the low pay for staff and teachers. Teachers in early childhood education earn on average about $29,000, less than half of what kindergarten teachers in public schools earn. In every state, median annual earnings for a child care worker qualify that worker for benefits such as SNAP or Medicaid, an indication of how our current child care system depends on the public safety net system created for the unemployed and low-wage workforce.[64] Low pay for child care workers leads to high turnover, a reality that disrupts the education and care of the children, distresses parents, and damages the lives and well-being of the workers.

The gap between the benefits that early child care could offer families and communities and the availability of such care has recently persuaded some elected officials, philanthropists, and employers to advocate for the expansion and improvement of child care programs. Cities like New York have created new programs for preschool children. Overall, between 2016 and 2019 public funding for early child care increased by 17 percent, an impressive gain in an era when many public programs were being cut.

But given the past modest public funding for early childhood education and the continued resistance of many local, state, and national elected officials to approve more spending on public services, especially those that benefit low-income people, it seems unlikely that the gap between child care supply and demand will be filled any time soon. Even less likely is the prospect that public funding will become available to close the quality gap—the difference in costs between comprehensive child care and custodial care. Such improvements would require substantial investments in lifting teacher salaries and training, expanding and improving facilities, and adding the nutritional, health, and other services that constitute essential components of quality care.

If modern capitalism in the United States cannot solve problems in the public sector, it turns to private business, the solution I examine here. These profiles of a few companies, entrepreneurs, investors, and philanthropists who are forging an expanded private-sector role in early childhood education highlight the potential and limitations of this strategy.

KinderCare. KinderCare Education is the largest for-profit provider of early childhood education in the United States. It operates more than 1,380 early learning centers and more than 560 afterschool programs at elementary schools. It also manages child care programs and benefits for more than four hundred corporations. It educates 185,000 children each day, employs thirty-two thousand people of whom about thirty thousand are teachers. Its 2019, its annual revenues were $968 million.[65]

KinderCare was founded as a public company in 1969. It expanded rapidly by taking on debt to acquire new centers but after the 2007 financial crisis, when higher-than-usual unemployment led to a decline in children needing care outside the home, growth and revenues faltered. After the company had not seen a profitable quarter in three years, it turned to private equity (PE), funds and investors that invest directly in private companies, for additional financing. It closed underperforming and underutilized centers and developed an aggressive strategy of acquiring new centers in promising markets.[66] One of its early investors was Betsy DeVos, the wealthy Republican activist and fundraiser who later became Donald Trump's Secretary of Education. In her ethics review before confirmation, DeVos reported her KinderCare investment of $500,000 to $1 million as one of the 102 potential conflicts of interest that she was required to divest.[67]

In 2015, KinderCare was acquired by PE firm Partners Group, a Swiss-based private markets investment manager with $83 billion in assets under management and serving more than 850 institutional investors.[68] To make this purchase, Private Partners obtained financing from Credit Suisse, Barclays, and Bank of Montreal. Between 2014 and 2017, according to Bloomberg News, Partners Group outperformed industry leaders like the Blackstone Group, the Carlyle Group, and KKR & Company. Overall, its return increased tenfold since 2005.[69] Partners Group, according to Steffen Meister, its executive chairman, invested in companies suited to long-term growth, category leaders with significant market share in their niche and continued growth potential ahead.[70] By making KinderCare a private company, Partners Group contributed to the national trend of fewer publicly listed and more private corporations.

Tom Wyatt, who continued as KinderCare's CEO after the takeover, observed that Partners Group "recognized how its experience and knowledge of brick-and-mortar and multi-business-unit companies could translate to the growing private equity sector of education."[71] In addition, he noted, Partners Group "informed our approach to re-financing debt to access dollars to invest and negotiate an attractive investment rate."

The new capital from Partners Group also enabled KinderCare to look for new investment opportunities. In 2018, KinderCare acquired Rainbow Child Care Center, a company that owned 140 centers in sixteen states.[72] To buy Rainbow, KinderCare borrowed $205 million, a loan the rating agency Moody's called credit negative, based on its adverse impact on the company's leverage, but noted the added debt did not change the company's credit rating or outlook.[73]

By 2019, KinderCare had reported twenty-two consecutive quarters of growth. Its return to profitability depended on the Partners Group private equity financing and KinderCare's leaders using tested strategies from the retail sector. Before joining the company, CEO Wyatt had served as president of Gap Inc.'s Old Navy division.[74] In 2012, KinderCare hired Wei-Li Chong, who had worked for a decade with fashion retailer Ann Taylor, making him president in 2017. Using data analytics and a staff survey, Chong created profiles of KinderCare's best teachers and redesigned the hiring interview to find the right staff.

"In retail," Chong said, "they're obsessed with emotional connection to the brain. There's never been a focus on that with early learning. . . . But if you do that, great things happen with their children." KinderCare's new data-driven hiring algorithms sought out teachers who could connect to parents and children, rather than those with more training or experience in early childhood education, a lesson borrowed from managers with expertise in operating multi-site retail businesses. Chong attributed higher staff retention to the redesigned hiring process, and also in part credited staff with emotional connection skills to KinderCare's return to profitability. At the completion of the hiring process redesign, he observed, "We're experiencing unprecedented growth right now."[75]

How does KinderCare's deep roots in the private sector influence the experience of children, parents, and staff? In such a large and complex organization with so many levels of management (i.e., learning center, region, and corporation as a whole) no simple or homogeneous answer is available.

But several websites provide opportunities for parents to describe and rate their experiences at KinderCare. A few comments illustrate the range of opinions and also the challenges parents face in finding the right child care placement:

> The daycare my sons (4 years and 8 weeks) goes to was bought by KinderCare and I absolutely love it. Yes, it's expensive but they do so much with the kids. They really work on education with the kids and are always making sure they have fun while learning. Casey

> I send my baby to a KinderCare center that's offered through my work as a work benefit. I can only speak for the infant room, but I will say . . . that her two main teachers are absolutely top notch. They are very loving and sweet and truly try their best. However, they are extremely over worked and there is obviously tons of pressure on them to do more with less. . . . I walk in the infant room and everyone is crying and there are two teachers tending to 8 kids with no additional support. At least one day a week when I pick up my baby, she's crying . . . or literally zoned out staring at the ceiling like she's been left alone forever while the teachers are taking care of other kids. . . . I am looking for a center that wants to go above and beyond. As I mentioned, this place I send my baby to is a company benefit. I don't feel that it benefits me or my baby in any way to send her there. . . . I'm currently trying to reconcile my feelings to see if I should continue to bring my baby here. Julia[76]

National studies show that only about 10 percent of child care centers provide "high quality care" and most offer fair or poor care.[77] Marcy Whitebook, the director of the Center for the Study of Child Care Employment at the University of California, Berkeley, told a reporter, "We've got decades of research, and it suggests that child care and early childhood education in this country is mediocre at best."[78] A 2015 report from the US Department of Education found that children from low-income families are less likely to be enrolled in preschool than their more affluent peers and those low-income children who are participating are less likely to be enrolled in high-quality programs.[79]

KinderCare claims "educational excellence in each and every brand" and cites the accreditation status of its learning centers—almost all are accredited by the National Association of the Education of Young Children, a national group that accredits about ten thousand early child care programs.[80] Its proprietary curriculum is used in all sites and KinderCare claims that its approach makes the children it enrolls, on average, four months ahead of their peers in kindergarten readiness. On its website, the company reports that "the longer children are enrolled, the better they'll do." But the data they cite do not provide meaningful evidence to support that claim and no independent or peer-reviewed reports documenting KinderCare's record are publicly available. At KinderCare and other child care centers, parents seeking to assess quality lack readily available credible guidance.

But they can find assistance online. Like retailers that pay Mommy Bloggers to promote their products, KinderCare sponsors satisfied customers to post testimonials. A few excerpts from one such blog post, by Rachel P, describes on her own blog why she chose to enroll her son and daughter in KinderCare:

> So for me, I am comforted by knowing that KinderCare is a large and trusted network with an incredible reputation across the country. . . . They are builders . . . creating confidence in children. Instilling an unshakable self-worth. Imparting a conviction that they carry with them as they take their first steps . . . and every step towards taking on the world. They rise, so they can shine. They are KinderCare. An amazing place to go to learn and play, to laugh and cry, to grow and mature. Creating confidence for life.[81]

A child care business that answers to investors and whose survival depends on meeting their expectations has to ensure that its primary revenue stream— tuition and fees from parents—is steady. At KinderCare, while cost varies by site and age, a full year of care for an infant or toddler is just under $20,000 a year and for a pre-kindergarten age child about $17,000 a year.

What happens when parents can no longer afford these fees? Two stories from Houston—one sad, the other tragic—illustrate the possibilities. Shauna enrolled her daughter Hadley in KinderCare the day she returned to work from maternity care:

> We had our daughter there from 3 months to about 1 year. Unfortunately, I was laid off and we no longer can bring her there. However, I wish almost every day I could! Not because I don't want to spend time with my daughter, but because it was a wonderful experience for her. She benefited from great education, wonderful teachers, and socialization. She learned independence from me, and to be comfortable around others outside of the home. I loved the structure, the fun, and the creativity, and I know she did, too. I very much recommend bringing your child here![82]

Child development experts agree that for young children, stability provides a key foundation for healthy development. The combination of precarious work arrangements for parents, forcing them to change child care arrangements as their work and finances change, and child care center instability, due to cuts in funding or disinvestment, can undermine that foundation. In contrast to children enrolled in stably public funded programs, children in the for-profit sector suffer when KinderCare or other child care business executives adjust their expansion and contraction plans to realize new opportunities.

The New Republic journalist Jonathan Cohn told the child care story of Kenya Mire, a low-wage worker and her daughter Kendyll.[83] After enrolling her infant daughter in a few different home child care centers and then having to drop out because she lost work, Mire scraped together enough money to enroll her daughter in a local Houston KinderCare. But her part-time $10 an hour job as a hostess at a steakhouse was not sufficient to keep up with payments so KinderCare asked Mire to withdraw her daughter. Later, when her work situation improved with a new oil company job, she tried KinderCare again, but the center would not take Kendyll until Mire paid her debt. By the time she did, no openings were available.

Shortly after, however, Mire found a spot in a local home-based child care run by a woman who seemed experienced, warm with children, and charged a price Mire could afford. All was going well until one day the proprietor left the napping children unattended to go shopping. A fire started and Kendyll and three other children died. The owner ended up with a long jail sentence, but the story highlights the perils of both the low end of home-based child care and the high end of for-profit chains like KinderCare. While deaths in child care centers are rare, a study found that the death rate for infants in home child care settings was seven times higher than in centers.[84] Had publicly funded child care been available or had KinderCare set its tuition policies to benefit families as well as investors, these deaths might have been averted.

Acelero. Another approach to corporate involvement in early child care is privatization of formerly public services. Acelero Learning is a private company with about $85 million in annual revenues that operates previously publicly managed Head Start centers serving five thousand children in four states and sells management services to Head Start providers serving an additional thirty thousand children across the country. As Kim Syman, a managing partner at New Profit, an investor in Acelero, observed, the company has "the potential to disrupt a stagnant $10 billion Head Start system and set higher standards across the field."[85]

Acelero seeks to have "systemic impact by harnessing technology and developing a proprietary database to help other providers achieve better results." It cites third-party evaluation studies that show that the children it serves achieve roughly twice the gains of the average Head Start center—higher than any other provider in the field. A report by an independent educational consulting firm identifies the best data practices of Acelero Learning and other

Head Start programs,[86] but as with KinderCare, the evidence on which Acelero makes its claims of effectiveness or publicly available reports on these claims are not readily available.

KinderCare, Acelero, and many other large and small companies working in child care have helped to create new ways to expand the number of child care placements, bring data science to making the operation and management of multiple child care programs more efficient, and apply lessons from other sectors such as retail and sharing economy services to the urgent task of scaling up child care expansion. They have also attracted—and been attracted by—powerful new partners to the early child care sector: private equity, venture capital, and social impact investors; technology companies; major philanthropists; educational consulting firms; and politicians with national aspirations.

Early child care has the potential to bring enormous benefits to young children, their families, communities, and society as a whole. The current supply of early child care is woefully inadequate, quality is usually low, and those families who could benefit most from good early child care face formidable affordability barriers.

It would be appealing to affirm twenty-first-century capitalists' response to every social problem: bring in the private sector. Use their know-how, capital, and ability to drive policy to expand and improve early child care, especially at a time when political opposition to more public funding seems nearly insurmountable.

Before going down this road, however, the evidence on private sector engagement in early child care suggests several caveats. First, what makes early child care attractive to investors—rapid expansion, high return on investment, and cost savings—undermines three essential elements of effective child care: high quality and comprehensive programs, high staff-child ratios, and affordability even to low-income families. Small and middle-size private child care companies have only two strategies to make ends meet: enroll more children or charge higher fees, both strategies that compromise quality or access. Big corporations like KinderCare can better meet these challenges by achieving economies of scale, sacrificing current profits to increase market share and drive smaller competitors out of business, or buying up competitors.

Second, private investment is always vulnerable to changing economic circumstances. An economic downturn, a pandemic, or another investment opportunity with higher returns could lead private investors to flee the child care field, jeopardizing the infrastructure they had created and further disrupting the lives of the children and families served by the programs in which they invested.

Finally, a fully integrated educational system, one that is designed to enable children to move from early childcare programs to elementary, middle, and high schools, and then college or technical schools, offers the best hope for helping all children develop their lifetime health, social, and educational potential. Building an early care system that answers to private investors rather than the public sector responsible for most K-12 education seems to undermine that vision.

The bottom-line question that the American people must answer is whether the benefits of high-quality public early care and education for all young children outweigh the costs of imposing higher taxes on wealthy businesses and individuals to pay for these services and restricting the rights of companies to profit from early child care. The United States is alone among wealthy countries in choosing not to create a public system for early child care.

K-12 EDUCATION

In early child care, prospects for profit lie in expanding a small, underdeveloped sector to meet growing parental demand for more child care placements. In K-12, however, opportunity requires capturing a bigger share of the more than $670 billion that US taxpayers contribute to public education annually.[87] To better understand this potential, I describe a few of the companies that have found ways to tap into this lucrative revenue stream.

K12 Inc . K12 Inc. is a technology-based education company that, with its subsidiaries (including K12, an education management organization), provides online curricula, software programs for schools, and educational systems to promote personalized learning for students in grades K-12 in the United States and internationally. It sells its services to public, charter, and private schools; early childhood programs; and others and employs forty-six hundred people. Its 2020 revenue was just over $1 billion.[88]

K12 Inc.'s CEO and chairman is Nathaniel Alonzo Davis, who previously served as CEO and president of XM Satellite Radio Holdings, Inc. His cash compensation from K12 in 2019 was $2.2 million with an additional $4.2 million in compensation from restricted stock awards. Board members include John M. Engler, president of the Business Roundtable and former governor of Michigan; Steven B. Fink, CEO of Lawrence Investments, LLC, and the founder of KinderCare; Eliza McFadden, president and CEO of The Barbara Bush Foundation for Family Literacy; and Elanna Yalow, chief academic officer at KinderCare.

In 2016, California's then--Attorney General Kamala Harris announced that the California Department of Justice had reached a settlement with K12 Inc. over alleged violations of California's false claims, false advertising, and unfair competition laws. Harris charged that "K12 and its schools misled parents and the State of California by claiming taxpayer dollars for questionable student attendance, misstating student success and parent satisfaction, and loading nonprofit charities with debt. . . This settlement ensures K12 and its schools are held accountable and make much-needed improvements."[89]

K12 Inc. paid a $2.5 million settlement and reimbursed the Attorney General's Office another $6 million to pay for the investigation. However, when Harris disclosed that K12 had also agreed to expunge the $160 million debt it had imposed on its California charter school customers, K12 fired back that Harris's claim of debt relief was "shameless and categorically incorrect."[90] The dispute highlights the complex and financialized relationships between for-profit companies like K12 Inc. and nonprofit charter schools. Since California forbids for-profit companies from operating charters, K12, the educational management company, works as a "service provider" for nonprofit schools, who pass on substantial portions of their revenue to K12. The company charges charters a single flat fee for its services (e.g., leasing space, purchasing supplies, human resources), then adjusts the bill according to what the state actually pays the school, an unusual "pay-what-you-can" approach. The $160 million was the difference between K12's bills and what the charters actually paid. While these charges did not show up on the balance sheets of either the schools or K12, their contracts require them to be repaid if the school has a surplus or if it terminates its contact with K12, leading Harris to claim savings from the settlement.

In 2019, K-12 Inc. had a conflict with the state of Georgia that illustrates some of the ways that its goals of seeking profits and educating children can compete. For years, K12 ran the Georgia Cyber Academy, a fully online public institution that was the state's largest school, with ten thousand students enrolled in 2018. However, under K12 management, the school had poor academic performance and its board severed the relationship with the company.[91] So K12 Inc. proposed a new school in Georgia, Destination Career Academy, and sought approval to enroll eight thousand students and receive as much as $160 million in taxpayer support for a five-year charter. However, the State Charter School Commission rejected this application. Its chairman, Tom Lewis, said, "I have never seen an application as bad and ill-prepared as this one." And in disengaging from Cyber Academy, K-12 temporarily cut off student use of their computers and the school lost access to emails and student records.

Pearson Education. With a 2019 market value of $8.6 billion, annual sales of about $5.5 billion, and almost seventeen thousand employees, Pearson PLC, based in London, is the world's largest educational services company.[92] Its product lines include an online charter school chain, Connections Academy, that enrolls more than seventy thousand students in twenty-eight US states; book publishers; educational media brands including Addison-Wesley, Peachpit, Prentice Hall, and eCollege; and technological services for digital learning at universities.

Pearson's best-known product is its tests. The average American child in a public school now takes 113 standardized tests by high school graduation—sometimes as many as 20 a year[93]—and many of those tests and the books and online programs that help teachers and students prepare for them are sold by Pearson. In 2015, Fortune reported, Pearson controlled 60 percent of the US testing market.[94]

How did Pearson capture this lucrative stream of public funding? And how have the imperatives of modern capitalism contributed to the spectacular growth of what critics call "high-stakes testing," tests where a single student score can determine a child's advancement or failure, public funding for the school system, or the salaries of teachers?

On his third day in office in 2001, President George W. Bush announced No Child Left Behind, a new federal education program based on the premise that to overcome the supposed failures of American schools that put the "nation at risk,"[95] the country needed to set high standards and establish measurable goals to improve individual outcomes. The law mandated states to develop assessments in basic skills and made federal school funding conditional on the implementation and reporting of tests. In a briefing for Wall Street investment analysts a month after Bush signed the law, Pearson's CEO at the time observed that No Child Left Behind's requirement for annual testing and school report cards "reads like our business plan."[96]

Although educators, parents, and some elected officials criticized the implementation of No Child Left Behind, eight years later, President Barack Obama created Race to the Top, a revised educational approach that required performance-based evaluations for teachers and principals based on multiple measures of educator effectiveness, common educational standards, policies that did not prohibit the expansion of high-quality charter schools, and the creation and use of data systems to complete these assessments. Under the American Recovery and Reinvestment Act of 2009, Race to the Top received $4.35 billion which the US Department of Education then competitively awarded to state and local school systems to achieve its goals.

This bipartisan consensus that federal dollars should support expanded testing created the business opportunity that Pearson grabbed, an opportunity facilitated perhaps by the $8 million the company spent on lobbying from 2009 to 2014.[97] The case for clear outcomes and objective assessment of results is compelling. As he was leaving office in 2009, President Bush explained No Child Left behind:

> Local schools remain under local control. In exchange for federal dollars, however, we expect results. We're spending money on schools, and shouldn't we determine whether or not the money we're spending is yielding the results society expects? So states set standards. . . . And we hold schools accountable for meeting the standards. . . . The key to measuring is to test. . . . Testing is important to

solve problems. You can't solve them unless you diagnose the problem in the first place. Testing is important to make sure children don't slip too far behind. . . . Measuring results allows us to focus resources on children who need extra help. And measuring gives parents something to compare other schools with. . . . Nothing will get a parent's attention more than if he or she sees that the school her child goes to isn't performing as well as the school around the corner.[98]

Obama's Race to the Top changed some of the rules—it turned responsibility for testing to state governments and added testing of classrooms and teachers to testing of individual students. But it did not renounce the importance of standardized testing as the path to educational improvement. Between 2001 and 2014, public spending on testing and testing contracts tripled from $882 million to $2.5 billion.[99] As Pearson's executive vice president Steve Dowling told investors in 2006, "One of the great advantages of having these contracts is you get in and, as contracts change, and they pretty consistently do, you have an opportunity to build scope in those contracts and also increase your margins."[100]

In the real world, the reasonable goal of assessing educational progress confronted some hard truths. First, neither federal nor state governments had the will or expertise to develop national tests, so the task fell to that default solver of any social problem: the private sector. Some education experts proposed that local schools should come up with their own ways to document their record in meeting federal standards, using performance standards and the assessments of teachers. But supporters of a strong private sector role objected. Why "throw money at government" for something like testing when that is exactly what industry does best?

What elected officials would want to take responsibility for investing the billions of dollars in taxpayer funds needed to develop, field test, and score national assessments and also train teachers to prepare their students for these tests? A safer route would be to farm out more modest allocations each year to states and school systems to enable them to make these decisions. And, in part as a result of this decentralized decision making, who but a global corporation could amass the capital to develop tests, lobby legislators and public officials to use their test, and sponsor researchers to vouch for the validity of the tests? Thus, some of the genuine concerns about equity and accountability were diverted into a scheme that ended up benefiting big corporations. This example illustrates a wider problem—when the public sector is unable to respond to public concerns about a social problem such as public school accountability, some commercial organization (in this case testing companies) will step in promising to be responsive to the unmet need but in fact is searching for new revenue streams.

And Pearson did profit from the new interest in school accountability. The company's renewed focus on testing was part of a broader restructuring of

Pearson that John Fallon, who became CEO in 2013, instituted to restore diminished profitability. He closed the unprofitable adult education unit in the UK, a company that provided apprenticeships to put adults back to work;[101] cut four thousand jobs, saving $215 million in costs; and acquired Brazil's Grupo Multi chain of English-language centers for $721 million. Fallon likened Pearson's push into data-driven education to IBM's successful move from hardware into services, a move Fortune called "a smart strategy."[102] In 2019, Pearson sold its US school course materials business to the private equity group Nexus Capital Management, consolidating its move from books to what Fallon calls its "digital first strategy that will drive our future growth."[103] Due to Fallon's success in this strategy, Pearson gave its CEO a 70 percent pay rise in 2018, increasing his total pay from £1.7 million to £3.1 million, his first bonus after five years of profit warnings during the restructuring process.[104]

To win the testing market, Pearson had to battle other companies, including McGraw Hill, Educational Testing Service, and Questar. But the biggest vendors generally do better in getting contracts for standardized tests.[105] In 2014, a nonprofit competitor sued Pearson over its tactics to win a contract worth as much as $1 billion for developing testing programs for a consortium of states. A judge dismissed the complaint, ruling that the nonprofit lacked standing to sue over the contract.[106] In 2015, McGraw Hill, a main competitor, decided to leave the testing business, helping Pearson consolidate its dominance.[107] As in other sectors, as the testing business concentrates, schools systems and public officials have less power to negotiate with multinational corporations. Rather than tailor their services to individual school system customers, these firms prefer to standardize practices to save costs. In the decade after No Child Left Behind was passed, Pearson Education's profits increased by 175 percent and between 2000 and 2006 test sales jumped fivefold. By that year, 60 percent of schoolchildren in the United States lived in states giving Pearson tests.[108]

But Pearson's practices provoked a litany of complaints. In Texas, a coalition of opponents of the state's testing system disclosed that Pearson was advertising on Craigslist for graders of its state exam, looking for college graduates, "any field welcome," who would be paid $12 an hour for doing the job. "Prior to seeing this ad," the critics wrote, "we have heard concerns from across the state about the state's standardized testing system, the rigidity of the state's accountability system, and the quality of the people grading the written portion of the state's test and the consistency of the results. Now we have a better idea why."[109]

Nor was testing limited to students. Private companies were also hired to assess teacher value and the eligibility and credentialing of new teachers. In Chicago, a combination of low enrollment and "poor test results" led to shutting down fifty schools in low-income Black neighborhoods and the firing of a substantial percent of Black teachers and principals.

Pearson also sought to engage academia in building support for its testing business. It hired Sir Michael Barber, a former professor of education at the University of London as its chief education adviser. Barber had also served as chief education adviser to UK Prime Minister Tony Blair and has worked for the global consulting firms McKinsey & Company and the Boston Consulting Group. Fortune has called him "the single most influential educator on the face of the earth."[110]

Like other private education companies, Pearson hires researchers to demonstrate the superiority of its products. After academic researchers at Stanford University published a report documenting high failure levels at on-line charter schools,[111] Pearson commissioned several studies of Connection Academy, its online charter school that is the second-largest provider of on-line charter schools after K12 Inc. These reports were reviewed not by academic researchers but by SRI International and PwC, consulting firms that work for global corporations. In these and other cases, the research that drives policy is purchased by the company and the data and findings are not scrutinized by independent peer review.

Pearson claimed its studies showed that Connections Academy matched the performance of brick-and-mortar schools and did significantly better than other online schools in teaching reading. But outside experts said the company's method of comparing schools rather than individual students undercut its argument. "You can't make these claims of effectiveness with school-level data. Period," said Ruth Curran Neild, director of the Philadelphia Education Research Consortium, a partnership between Philadelphia public and charter schools and universities.[112] To illustrate, the outcomes of high-performing charter schools are impressive if researchers look only at the percent of seniors going on to college, rather than the proportion of incoming ninth graders who go on to graduate and enroll in college. By developing policies that encourage academically struggling ninth graders to drop out, a school can graduate a persistent college-bound group.

Finally, Pearson used aggressive lobbying to win contracts and persuade state governments and the US Department of Education to set policies that favored its business interests. Between 2002 and 2019, Pearson reported spending $8.6 million on federal lobbying.[113] In Alabama, after Pearson won a six-year $22 million no-bid contract to supply a digital curriculum to the Huntsville school district, *Politico* reported that the company made Huntsville school superintendent Casey Wardynski a spokesperson and Huntsville its showcase. Wardynski was listed as one of Pearson's team of experts and gave talks to visiting educators from other states.[114] Pearson also hired staff from state agencies to assist in its efforts to win new business. In Texas, for example, eleven staff left the state Education Authority to work for Pearson.[115]

How well did school systems use the technologies that Pearson and other EdTech companies marketed? A fascinating study by Glimpse K12, an education technology company that analyzes school spending, provides some disturbing answers. The company analyzed the use of $2 billion worth of total spending in 275 K-12 schools across the United States. It then tracked actual student and teacher use of the software licenses that these schools had purchased. The study found that on average 67 percent of the licenses had gone unused, suggesting they were purchased and never utilized. Based on this finding, Glimpse K12 estimated that $5.6 billion of the $8.4 billion that US schools spend on educational software may be wasted each year.[116] The study did not assess what role aggressive marketing, technologically unsophisticated administrators, or other factors played in this wasted spending. However, unrealistic expectations for technology clearly benefit tech companies but not necessarily schoolchildren, a point emphasized by the limitations and glitches of the technologies schools purchased from Amazon, Google, Zoom, and other Big Tech companies after COVID-19 closed schools.

UNIVERSITY EDUCATION

One of the great policy successes in the United States in the last few decades has been increased enrollment in college, including groups previously often excluded from higher education. Between 1990 and 2009, US college enrollment increased by 148 percent. By 2010, for the first time in US history, more than half of eighteen- and nineteen-year-olds were enrolled in college. In the last thirty-five years, the number of Blacks, Latinxs, and other racial/ethnic populations attending college has more than doubled and about one-third of the entire adult population now enrolls in college.[117] By 2016, 39 percent of college students were from households with incomes at or below 130 percent of the federal poverty line, an increase from 28 percent in 1996.[118] Since a college degree offers lifetime health, social, and economic benefits,[119] this increase constitutes an important success for improving health and democracy and reducing inequalities in health, education, and income.

But two parallel developments, each associated with the changing face of capitalism, reduced the equity impact of increased college enrollment. First, college became much more expensive, making it difficult for students from lower-income families to stay enrolled and graduate. Between 1989 and 2016, the price for a four-year degree doubled, even after inflation. Between 2005 and 2016, prices for undergraduate education at public institutions rose 34 percent and at private nonprofit institutions by 26 percent, after adjusting for inflation.[120]

Among the factors that contributed to higher costs were a significant increase in the ratio of administrators to faculty; new construction, especially of amenities like sports centers and elegant dormitories, designed to help win ratings wars; increased costs for recruiting and attracting desirable (i.e., paying) students; and increased legal costs to protect against liability for sexual harassment and sex or disability discrimination. Together these changes constitute a corporatization of higher education, with more attention paid to financial than academic goals.[121] State funding for higher education has decreased by 25 percent per student over the last thirty years and states have cut $9 billion from higher education in the last ten years alone.

Second, federal student aid, which had expanded in the 1960s and 1970s, was essentially frozen, the victim of austerity at the state and national levels and tax cuts for the wealthy and corporations that began in the 1980s. In 1972, Pell Grants, the main federal subsidy for low-income undergraduate students, covered more than four-fifths of the cost of attending the average four-year public university. By 2018, it covered less than one-third of the costs. The original Pell Grant covered all costs of the typical community college; today it covers only about 60 percent, making it especially hard for the 6 million students, mostly from low-income households, to maintain enrollment.[122] These declines in student aid contributed to the rise in student debt.

To solve the public and private college affordability problem, public policy makers turned to the private sector to make the investments they were unwilling to take on. And because growing college enrollment, the rising cost of college degrees, and declining student aid also offered big opportunities for financial institutions, other lenders, and for-profit colleges, emerging edubusinesses were happy to lend a hand, sometimes in concert with other sectors of the corporate educational sector.

Through changes in national lending rules in the 1990s and early years of the new millennium, federal policy made lending money to college students a lucrative new profit center. By 2018, 45 million US college students owed more than $1.6 trillion, more than the nation's credit card and auto loan debt combined. Each year one million student borrowers default and by 2023, 40 percent of students are expected to default on their loans.[123] In 2017, about $120 billion (10 percent) of outstanding federally held student loan debt was in default.[124] Some analysts predict that student loan debt may trigger another financial collapse, much as the collapse of the housing loan mortgages balloon did in 2008. Once again, the COVID-19 Recession is likely to spotlight prior vulnerabilities, in this case by accelerating student loan default.

One company that plays a key role in student loans is Navient, created in 2014 as a private spin-off of a public spin-off. Its story illustrates how government and edubusiness have blurred the line between public and private. Navient was born in 1972 as part of a government entity known as Sallie Mae, an agency charged with oversight of federal student loans. Sallie Mae became a private company in 2004 and in 2014, it spun off the Navient Corporation as a publicly traded corporation that serviced and collected on student loans. By 2017, Navient serviced more than $300 billion in federal and private student loans for more than 12 million borrowers.[125]

What impact do student loans have on the well-being of college students, dropouts, and graduates? Studies show that student debt contributes to food insecurity, housing instability, delayed healthcare, depression and anxiety, increased dropout rates, poorer credit, and increased likelihood of returning to the parental home.[126] Low-income, immigrant, and Black and Latinx students experience these debt-related problems at higher rates than white and better-off students.

A few stories that student borrowers told to Student Debt Crisis, a non-profit organization dedicated to reforming student debt and higher education loan policies, illustrate some of these consequences:[127]

> I live in San Diego and have a three-year old daughter. Just to support us, I had to go back to school so that I could put my $70k+ student loan balance ($500+ monthly payment) in deferral . . . until I make more money. So now, I work full time and go to school full time. I hardly see my daughter. . . . Meanwhile, my current student loans will still be accruing interest while in deferral. Not to mention, I am on the "extended graduate repayment program" which means every two years my payments increase by 20 percent and I have 25 years to pay them off. *A student from California*

> I am a stay at home mom who can't work because I can't afford to pay for childcare if both my husband and I work at the same time. My student loans have caused me to sit at a standstill and constantly pray that they don't increase. I live on the income driven repayment plan and I pray that my required amount doesn't go up because I can barely afford to get by when it's at 0. Knowing that I have such a huge debt with nothing I can do about it is the worst feeling of all. *A student from Tacoma, Washington*

> I have $48,000 of student loan debt dating back to 2011 and cannot get hired in the field of my degree. I will never be able to pay it off while making next to nothing in a customer service job. *A student from St. Petersburg, Florida*

Perhaps most poignantly, for millions of young people current student loan practices call into question the most basic tenets of the American dream—that a college degree is a sure-fire path to lifetime success; that with hard work, a college degree is attainable for most high school graduates; and that after college, buying a home or a car or having children are reasonable aspirations. Again, the voice of a borrower tells the story:

> I went back to school for engineering when I was in my mid-20s. I feel lucky to have chosen a career that allows me to pay off my debt. However, I've felt the burden of this debt. I've put off purchasing a home, contributing to retirement, and having children in order to make good on my promise to pay back what I borrowed. —*Scott from California*

Education and Health: Virtuous or Vicious Circle?

A fundamental truth in public health is that more education leads to better health, better health leads to more academic success, and more academic success leads to more life success. The United States and other countries of the world could find no better policy goal and no better site for additional investment than to build this virtuous circle between education, health, and personal and community success.

But at every level of this country's educational system, the growing role of private capital has instead accelerated a vicious circle. Educational opportunities not offered contribute to the rise of preventable health and social problems. Inequitable access to quality preschool, K-12, and university education widens class and racial/ethnic gaps in income, wealth, life success, and health. Twenty-first century capitalism has privatized schools, imposed austerity budgets, funded education by financializing tuition and fees, and blocked teachers from organizing unions that could better get them the pay, working conditions, and health benefits that make teaching a respected and life-satisfying career. Together these acts have undermined the capacity of the nation's educational system to achieve its health, academic, and democratic goals.

Unaffordable child care, private schools, and for-profit universities push children and families into lower-quality alternatives, debt, or psychological distress, all contributors to poor mental and physical well-being. These pressures widen already deep stratifications, making our nation more segregated and inequitable and compromising the capacity of education to bring people together to achieve social goals.

In coming years, the American people will need to decide whether to change course, to make the virtuous circle between education and well-being the driving force in education and social policy. The default is business as usual, giving private capital an ever-growing voice in shaping our early childhood, K-12, and university education systems and thus allowing the vicious circle of missed opportunities and widening inequalities in health and schooling to accelerate. Recent battles on the future of education provide some insights into how this contest may play out.

RESISTANCE AND ALTERNATIVES

At each level of our education system, the corporate education sector has used its wealth and power to find ways to make money from students and their families and from taxpayers and governments. It has won a bigger voice in shaping educational policy and institutions and used that voice to advance its economic, political, and ideological agendas.

In some cases, however, this sector's goals of changing school practices to increase its revenues, capture public funding, modify curricula and texts, and set public policy have come into conflict with the aspirations of students, families, communities, taxpayers, and public officials. A few stories of this resistance and search for alternatives—the push to expand public funding of early childhood education, teacher strikes and organizing, the battles over charter schools and high-stakes testing, and the efforts to regulate college student loans—illustrate the accomplishments and limitations of recent battles on the proper role for markets in education.

Expanding public early childhood education. The health and moral arguments for more public investment in child care and early childhood education are compelling. Better-paid child care workers have lower turnover rates and deliver higher–quality, more consistent services that in turn improve the health and educational and life success of children. Expanding child care also helps women to make progress in their careers by finding a higher-paying job, applying for a promotion, seeking more hours at work, or finding a job in the first place.[128]

And significant proportions of American voters support expanded public funding for early child care, according to a 2018 public opinion poll by the Center for American Progress. Nearly eight in ten voters support increasing funding for quality, affordable child care or early childhood education programs—and about seven in ten voters agree that they would be "more likely" to vote for a candidate who supports increasing funding. A strong majority of voters of all parties—70 percent of Republicans and independents, and 90 percent of Democrats support additional funding for child care.[129]

This support had helped move expanded child care support higher on the national political agenda. In the 2018 election, eighteen successful candidates for governor had talked about child care and early childhood education in their campaigns.[130] In the 2020 presidential primary elections, every Democratic candidate had a policy proposal or statement calling for expansion of federal investment in early childcare.[131] Many of these proposals also for the first time move child care from being solely a siloed women's issue into one that connects to improving education, strengthening the economy, and reducing inequality.

Another voice for improving the quality and availability of child care comes from labor unions and worker groups. In California, Child Care Providers United (CCPU), a joint venture of two national labor unions, Service Employees International Union (SEIU) and American Federation of State, County and Municipal Employees (AFSCME), formed in 1998 to organize child care workers in child care centers as well as in family day care, a setting where wages were lower, hours longer, and benefits fewer. The mission of CCPU is to offer child care providers "a powerful voice to improve our livelihoods and the services we provide, for working families whether white, Black, Asian, or Brown. We are working for childcare for all and unions for all."[132]

In 2019, California governor Gavin Newsom signed a law allowing family day care workers to bargain collectively, marking a major victory for the mostly women of color who had organized the campaign. The bill had been vetoed by his five predecessors. In California, private home child care operators are paid directly by the state as part of the subsidy system for child care for low-income families. The newly organized home-based child care workers bargain directly with the state government, a novel arrangement that gives some level of public protection to self-employed workers.[133] Under the new law, California's twenty-seven thousand licensed family child care workers can bargain for higher pay, better benefits, health insurance, and more education and training. Some of these benefits will also be available to the thirteen thousand additional license-exempt careers such as family members, friends, or neighbors who care for children.

In Los Angeles County, where financial pressures have closed sixteen hundred family child care centers with fifteen thousand slots over five years, advocates hope the new law will slow that loss and perhaps encourage others to open new home-based programs. Eleven other states now allow home-based child care workers to sign collective bargaining agreements.

New York City expanded child care and early childhood education in another way. In his 2013 run for mayor, Bill DeBlasio, elected with the support of labor unions, African Americans, and progressives, promised to make prekindergarten available to all of the city's four-year olds whose families wanted it. This move effectively doubled the number of free, public slots of this age group and removed the financial barriers and bureaucratic mazes that the parents of the city's seventy thousand four-year-olds encountered in finding child care. The mayor wanted to fund the program with a new tax on those making more than half a million dollars a year, but the tax-averse governor refused. Finally, after political pressure, the governor offered instead to pay the added cost out of state tax revenues. Thus, universal publicly funded pre-K was established, and most observers agreed the program was implemented quickly and effectively.

In 2017, the city began to implement universal 3-K—offering free public education to all three-year-olds, implemented over a few years starting in neighborhoods with the highest need. By fall 2018, about five thousand students were enrolled in six community districts that offer 3-K, and the city plans to expand to a dozen districts by fall 2021, a move that may be delayed by budget cuts in response to the COVID-19 Recession.[134] Three-K proved more challenging than pre-K for four-year-olds as space for new classrooms ran out, three-year-olds needed different services than older children, and some of the new programs were initially operated by community providers with child care experience, rather than schools. Eventually, all these programs were transferred to the city's Department of Education and teachers for three- and four-year-olds were paid the same salaries as regular public school teachers and had the same rights to unionize.

Pre- and 3-K also opened doors for additional reforms. In 2019, Jessica Ramos, a state senator elected in the 2018 Democratic sweep of the New York State Senate and a labor activist from an immigrant family, introduced legislation to add a payroll tax on large businesses to expand 3-K and raise wages for teachers of three-year-olds, enabling the tripling of slots in 3-K proposed by a candidate for the 2021 mayoral election.[135] A broad coalition of community and labor organizations faulted the slow pace of state investments in early childhood education.[136]

For the tens of thousands of parents who no longer had to pay $10,000 or more per year for private child care, for the thousands of assistant teachers and teachers who were now earning up to $20,000 more per year and for New York City's three- and four-year-olds who now had safe places to spend the day, qualified teachers to help them learn, and an educational program that would prepare them for the later grades, pre-K and 3-K were extremely popular. In addition, as one journalist noted, "At a moment when the nation's democratic organizations from the courts to the free press were under attack, the egalitarian goal of pre-K for all—of *anything* for all—becomes only more valuable, and only more worthy of cherishing."[137]

The diverse constituencies that support expanded childcare—business groups, philanthropies, teachers' unions, parents groups, and advocates— agree on several goals, including the need for expanded public funding, higher pay and more and better benefits and training for teachers and other staff, and a sharp focus on the quality of care. On the most basic questions, however, there is not much discussion or consensus. Is child care and early child education a charity for the needy like food pantries or free clinics or is it a universal right in any civilized society? And what is the role for government and business? Should the United States rely on the private sector to develop innovative models of child care, accepting their right to earn a profit from their ingenuity, even if such profitable activities exclude the most in need or widen inequities in educational achievement?

For those who accept some public role in early childhood education, two quite different models present themselves. The first is based on the mid-twentieth-century vision of public schools in which these schools are publicly supported, available to all, not an appropriate arena for profit-making, and having a social mission of advancing national goals related to democracy, racial integration, equity, and civic engagement.

The second model looks more like the current healthcare system. After the massive public investment of federal dollars that followed the creation of Medicare and Medicaid in 1965 and the 2010 Affordable Care Act, which provided new guarantees for access, the United States healthcare system is much bigger and provides some level of services to more people. But it is a system totally shaped by private sector insurance, pharmaceutical, medical device, hospital, and other industries. Their continued dominant voice in healthcare ensures that medical care continues to widen rather than shrink inequities in health status, extract significant resources from the system for management and profit, and contain costs by under-paying low-wage workers and denying care to some who need it.

After many decades of business and conservative marketing of the ideas of privatization, deregulation, austerity, tax cuts, and individual rather than social responsibility for success, few powerful players in the current political climate are willing to propose the public investments needed for the public school model for early childhood education. That makes the default scenario the healthcare model, with subsidies, tax breaks, employer incentives, and other market mechanisms as the levers for change. To realize the profits that a public private partnership for expanded child care requires, this approach requires lowering costs by sacrificing quality, keeping wages down, or charging parents more. Unfortunately, these very measures make early childhood education unlikely to fulfill its potential to improve health, education, and equity.

Organizing teachers and teacher strikes. In 2018, teachers opened another front in the battle against corporate education. The state-level strikes began in West Virginia, where many teachers had seen their wages, job security, and benefits fall as education was contracted out. They went on strike for higher pay, better benefits, and new restrictions on charter school expansion.[138] Although West Virginia teachers, like those in many states, have no legal right to bargain collectively or to strike,[139] twenty thousand teachers in all fifty-five West Virginia counties stayed out for more than a week, the first teachers' strike in that state in thirty years. In many towns, these strikes were supported by students and their parents.

Ultimately, the union won a 5 percent pay raise, not only for teachers but for all state workers. A year later, West Virginia teachers authorized another strike if legislators continued to pursue school choice measures.[140] Teachers in other cities and states including Los Angeles, Oakland, Oklahoma, Arizona, and Kentucky also went on strike, winning both pay hikes but also new funding for smaller class sizes, school nurses, legal support for immigrant students, and limits on charter schools and performance pay.

In Los Angeles, the teachers' union allied with parent and community groups (See Figure 3.2). As Alex Caputo-Pearl, the leader of the LA teachers' union, explained, "We are fighting to show that we are willing to be bold, to show that we are willing to work with parents and community and share the steering wheel with them. This foreshadows what the labor movement needs to do to go forward."[141] In other groundbreaking actions, teachers at charter schools in Los Angeles and Chicago organized and threatened strikes, winning

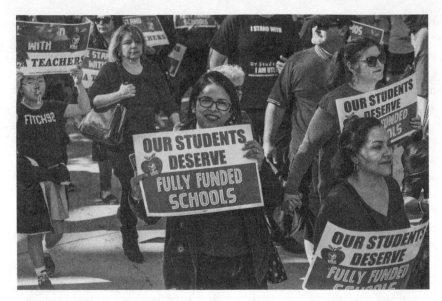

Fig. 3.2 Parents and teachers demonstrate in support of the 2019 strike by thirty-four thousand teachers in Los Angeles.
Photo: © John Doukas / Shutterstock

settlements that included pay increases, added protections for undocumented students, and other concessions.

While increases in pay and improvements in working conditions were key goals of striking teachers, other objectives included reversals of the privatization of public schools, limits on the expansion of charter schools, and reduced reliance on high-stakes testing.[142] Teachers and teacher unions played a critical role in helping Democrats retake the House of Representatives in the 2018 Congressional election, creating new openings to oppose the efforts by Secretary of Education Betsy DeVos and the Trump Administration to privatize education and deregulate edubusiness.[143] In these ways, teachers helped to set the stage for a deeper national discussion on the future of schooling and alternatives to privatization, austerity, and the role of testing. The strikes and organizing also set new models for social justice organizing and new ways of aligning the labor interests of teachers, the desires of parents and communities for better schools, and the struggles of Black communities to diminish the pernicious impact of racism.

Perhaps most important, the new focus of teacher organizing helped to transform disaffected teachers into an enduring social movement. "In 2012, Chicago teachers went on strike and introduced a new phrase to their fight," explained Rebecca Tarlu, a scholar of teacher organizing. "They said, 'We're fighting for the schools that Chicago students deserve.' During that strike, the Chicago teachers' union and the Teachers 4 Social Justice network joined forces to merge education and racial justice. You had communities of color where schools were getting shut down and the union helping to fight against that."[144] From this movement emerged a broad coalition that went on to pressure Rahm Emanuel, the privatizing, pro-charter mayor, to withdraw from running for a third term in 2019 and to elect a new progressive mayor, Chicago's first African American female mayor, Lori Lightfoot. In these ways, teacher organizing has shown the ways that labor organizing can open new paths to wider transformation and move beyond the narrower trade unionism of previous decades.

Limiting charter schools. Another trigger for school activism has been closing public schools and shifting funds into private charters, often operated or managed by private corporations. In Chicago, Mayor Richard Daley's 2004 proposal to close and then privatize public schools sparked a grass-roots opposition movement.[145] Similar movements emerged in Philadelphia and Newark, as well as in New Orleans, after corporate reformers used Hurricane Katrina to privatize New Orleans schools almost wholly. As education scholars Julia Sass Rubin, Ryan Good, and Michelle Fine observed, these struggles to keep public schools open and resist increased privatization often played out at the community, municipal, and state levels; brought together parents groups, civil rights organizations, teachers unions, and progressive elected officials; formed alliances with the NAACP, Black Lives Matter, and other national organizations; and worked to elect new voices to school boards, city councils, and mayors offices.[146] In these ways, community resistance to privatization serves as a model for building successful multilevel social movements that can fight for alternatives to corporate intrusion into people's daily lives.

Ending high-stakes testing. The Partnership for Assessment of Readiness for College and Careers (PARCC) was created in 2010 as a consortium of twenty-four states and the District of Columbia to meet the testing mandates of President Obama's Race to the Top. In 2014, Pearson was hired to create the exams that PARCC school systems would use to test achievement of Common Core standards.[147]

By the end of 2019, only five of the original twenty-four states participating in PARCC still used the Pearson test, a demonstration of the power of a movement to resist corporate intrusion into school affairs. The demise of PARCC also showed the potential for local, statewide, and national organizing of schools, with high-stakes testing serving as a starting point for engaging young people, parents, teachers, and communities in claiming a voice in creating the schools they wanted. It also shows the potential for contesting who gets to collect, use, and interpret the data needed to monitor social progress.[148] State education officials as well as parent and youth testing opt-out groups and schools challenged the rights of Pearson and other testing companies to determine what markers of educational progress are collected, who gets to interpret the results, and who profits from these policies.

Regulating college student loans. In the last days of the Obama Administration in early 2017, the Consumer Financial Protection Board, with the attorneys general of Illinois, Pennsylvania, and Washington State, filed a complaint in a federal court alleging that Navient, the organization that managed college student loans, had violated the Fair Credit Reporting Act and Fair Debt Collection Act. California and Mississippi have also sued Navient. The suits charged that Navient "systematically and illegally [failed] borrowers at every stage of repayment" with "abusive interest charges, hurting disabled military veterans by making inaccurate reports to credit companies about them and making repayments harder than necessary."[149] According to the court filing, "Navient has failed to perform its core duties in the servicing of student loans, violating Federal consumer financial laws . . . and misreported information to consumer reporting agencies about thousands of borrowers who were totally and permanently disabled, including veterans whose total and permanent disability was connected to their military service."[150]

A subsequent 2019 report by the inspector general of the Department of Education found the Department of Education failed to provide proper oversight of Navient and other loan servicers and that these companies failed to properly inform their student borrowers of repayment options.[151] Similarly a report by the Government Accountability Office found that Navient encouraged borrowers to use a loan repayment method called "forbearance," a process where students can defer any repayment for several years but still incur interest charges, a choice that benefits Navient, by increasing its total repayment, and the college, which isn't penalized for students in forbearance as it is for those who default.[152] For students, however, the choice of forbearance over other options means additional lifetime debt.

In the first two years of the Trump Administration, the president and Congress proposed new, more lenient rules for Navient and other lenders; appointed a former official of a for-profit university to the senior position in the US Department of Education, responsible for oversight of student loans; and weakened the Consumer Financial Control Board. Federal enforcement declined dramatically. Secretary of Education Betsy DeVos claimed that federal law preempts states from suing loan servicers like Navient, but a judge dismissed her objection while the Department of Education Inspector General and GAO reports provided independent evidence of the state attorneys general claims.[153]

In 2020, Navient settled another lawsuit brought by teachers who had been rejected for loan forgiveness based on their public service and supported by the American Federation of Teachers. Navient had created a maze of complex rules that disqualified all but 3,200 of the 146,000 applicants who had applied for forgiveness. The settlement required Navient to change its screening practices, retrain its staff, and pay $1.75 million to fund a new, independent organization that will educate and counsel borrowers in public-service jobs.[154]

This several-year history of federal involvement in monitoring the college student loan industry illustrates both the potential and limitation of regulation and litigation to counteract corporate efforts to profit from, in this case, students' needs to finance higher education. Rising student debt, media focus on the disparate racial and class impact of lender abuses of the system, and the growing awareness of public dissatisfaction with the high cost of college education brought the issue to national attention.

In the 2020 presidential primary, Democratic candidates and President Trump released plans calling for various new programs to reduce or relieve student debt.[155] And the idea that college education should be free in the same way K-12 education is entered the national discourse, setting the stage for ongoing activism to achieve this goal.

Students themselves became activists against abusive lending practices. The Debt Collective organizes people facing many kinds of debt. It acknowledges:

> Today most of us are in debt. No matter how much we work or how hard we try to get ahead, we are barely getting by. We are struggling to get out from under student debt, medical debt, payday loans, housing debt, criminal justice debt, credit card debt, and more. For too long, we've experienced these debts in fear and isolation, while others get rich off of our monthly payments. The Debt Collective is here to say, no more![156]

The group conducts direct actions and campaigns of noncooperation with the finance industry, seeking broad debt cancellation while fighting for policies to end mass indebtedness, including free public higher education, universal healthcare, worker-owned business, fair wages for everyone, and decarceration and reparations for racial justice. In 2015, the collective helped students from the for-profit Corinthian College to go on strike by withholding loan payments. With some help from Obama's Department of Education, they won forgiveness for $480 million in debt. This protest popularized new loan-forgiveness plans now under consideration.[157] Other student groups fighting debt include The Strike Debt network, which mobilized borrowers to go into default to mandate student loan reform, while another group, Rolling Jubilee, used seven hundred thousand dollars in donations to buy up and cancel almost $32 million of student loan debt.[158]

Several states have also sued Navient for its misleading marketing and processing of college student loan repayment options. These and other cases won damages from educational corporations and compensated its victims. Equally important, like state attorneys general legal settlements with the tobacco industry, the court cases have revealed the shady practices of edubusinesses and perhaps contributed to de-normalizing the acceptability of making a profit at the cost of pushing low-income and middle-class college students into debt.

WHAT DIRECTION FOR PUBLIC EDUCATION?

In the aftermath of the 2008 fiscal crisis, education has become a key battleground for competing visions of the future. On one side, parents, children, teachers, unions, college students, and communities demand schools that engage, educate, and open new doors to a social order based on human need, improved well-being, decent jobs, and equitable access to paths to success. On the other side, elites seek to hold onto and expand their control of the education sector and find additional opportunities for investment and profit. In many cases, they have enlisted parents, students, and policy makers dissatisfied with the inequitable status quo but skeptical that the more transformative changes that social justice advocates seek are achievable.

More than a decade after the 2008 fiscal crisis officially ended, those seeking an alternative to market dominance of schooling can claim some victories— and acknowledge some losses. Child care activists have moved universal early childhood education and care higher on the national agenda, winning support from labor unions, teachers' groups, women's rights organizations, and some elected officials. Cities such as New York, Washington, DC, and Philadelphia are working to make free early childhood education universally available, and a few candidates in the 2020 presidential primary elections called for universal free child care. Thus, models for early childhood education wholly or mostly in the public sector will continue to evolve.

Teachers unions have won important victories in Nevada, West Virginia, Chicago, Los Angeles, and elsewhere and have moved into the mainstream the idea that paying teachers more and treating them with respect improves schools for children. While charter schools are still growing, more elected officials and communities are questioning this approach, especially the role of corporations and financial institutions.

In 2016, the NAACP, the African American civil rights group that had supported charter schools, called for a moratorium on further expansion until charter schools are subject to the same accountability as traditional public schools and develop a funding system that does not hurt other schools. The NAACP called on charter schools to end harsh discipline practices that push out students and segregate high-performing children "from those whose aspirations may be high but whose talents are not yet as obvious." The resolution urges that instead of giving students access to charter schools through school choice, policy makers increase their support for improving the quality of traditional public schools.[159]

At the college level, free college education has become a popular political goal, and both liberal and conservative politicians are searching for ways to reduce college debt. In addition, state attorneys general, public interest lawyers, and investigative journalists have focused attention on the crass conflicts of interest that President Trump and his family, Betsy DeVos and her family, and the lobbyists and industry insiders they have appointed to high positions in the Department of Education report between their private investments in educational ventures and their public roles.[160] The ethical and legal violations already disclosed have strengthened the resolve of some public officials to monitor and limit such conflicts.

These advances have helped to inform a still sometimes inchoate vision of a different, more public, democratic, and equitable educational system. This vision has served as a rallying point for a still-often siloed and heterogeneous alliance of forces working to transform education.

But there have been losses too. The movement of capital into education continues at a rapid pace, at all levels, funding for education varies widely by state, city, and especially class and race, leaving the educational structures that produce inequality in place. In most places, racial segregation of schools at all levels has yet to be reversed. As Black Lives Matter, its sister organizations, and white supporters expand their focus on systemic racism in policing to public education they have the potential to raise such a challenge.

While the participants in the corporate educational complex have disagreements, they concur on two fundamental beliefs: that market solutions are always better than public solutions and that they have the right to use their wealth and power to shape the American educational system as they see fit. These beliefs contradict American democratic traditions and accelerate the transformation of education from a social good to an individually purchasable commodity.

As movements emerge to resist the corporate education sector's agenda of privatization, financialization, and globalization, they will need to find new ways to coalesce their support across preschool, K-12, and university. Together, these movements will need to bring together the voices and collective power of children, young people, feminists, racial and social justice activists, union members, parents, teachers, education reformers, and public officials who are searching for alternatives to corporate-dominated education.

CHAPTER 4

Healthcare

The Medical Care Industry's War on Cancer

Of all the forms of inequality, injustice in health is the most shocking and the most inhuman because it often results in physical death.
                                        —*Martin Luther King Jr.*

In 2020, cancer was expected to strike more than 1.8 million Americans and kill more than 600,000.[1] Presently, the risk of an American man developing an invasive cancer over his lifetime is almost one in two, and for a woman the risk is about one in three.[2] Overall, cancer is the second-leading cause of death in the United States, but the leading killer for women aged forty to seventy-nine and men aged sixty to seventy-nine.[3] More than 15.5 million living Americans have a history of cancer and 40 percent can expect a cancer diagnosis in their lifetime.[4] Heart disease kills more people but has declined significantly over the last few decades. While new cases of cancer have dropped overall, largely because of successful public health campaigns to reduce cigarette smoking, the decline has been slower than for heart disease. Liver cancer, melanoma, and cancer of the uterus continue to rise in incidence and five-year survival rates for cancers of the lung, esophagus, liver, and pancreas are less than 20 percent.

Cancer is also an important driver of health inequalities. A recent study estimated that one-third of cancer deaths among US residents twenty-five to seventy-four could be averted with the elimination of socioeconomic disparities.[5] Although racial disparities in cancer care are narrowing, the American Cancer Society found that Black men were still twice as likely to die of cancer as Asian/Pacific Islander men and 20 percent more likely to die of cancer than white men.[6]

On the emotional side, despite advances in treatment, cancer continues to cause overwhelming pain and suffering both for those with cancer and for their families and friends. The threat of cancer strikes fear into millions of Americans. Researchers on the fear of cancer have found that people view the disease as "an enemy," not just a disease, but as a sentient persona with traits, such as viciousness, unpredictability, and indestructibility. People described cancer as lurking inside you, spreading stealthily and inescapably. Cancer betrays; one person observed "cancer is a traitor. . . . You can be examined all the time . . . and nothing comes up, and then when you find out you have cancer it's too late.'"[7] In 2020, the COVID-19 pandemic wreaked havoc on the world's health, caused levels of fear and anxiety to shoot up, and overwhelmed the US healthcare system but cancer has caused many more deaths in the past and will do so into the foreseeable future.

Globally, cancer cases increased by 28 percent between 2006 and 2016, with the largest increases in low- and middle-income countries.[8] Limited access to treatment and less developed healthcare systems in lower-income countries also led to higher cancer death rates in these nations than in wealthier ones, further exacerbating the well-being gap among nations. For many poorer nations, cancer imposes a continuing and increasing burden on health, medical costs, and productivity.

Researchers estimate that more than 70 percent of cases of cancer may be preventable,[9] but that only half of those who get cancer can be cured with existing therapies; the other half will die of their disease.[10] While scientists have made remarkable progress in understanding cancer, to date these new insights have been slow to bring about reductions in cancer incidence or longevity.

In fact, despite the pharmaceutical industry's claims of huge advances in cancer treatment, the vast majority of new findings from laboratory studies have no immediate clinical impact. As Azra Raza, an oncologist at Columbia University, writes, "The failure rate for drugs brought into clinical trials using such preclinical drug-testing platforms is 95 percent. The 5 percent of drugs that reach approval might as well have failed, since they prolong survival by no more than a few months at best. Since 2005, 70 percent of approved drugs have shown zero improvement in survival rates while up to 70 percent have been actually harmful to patients."[11]

Despite its contributions to health inequities, cancer seems far removed from our social and economic institutions. It is a calamity that strikes out of the blue. For some usually unknown reason, cells in our body begin malignant proliferation and too often, despite the best efforts of modern science and medicine, that burst of cell division kills its victims.

But every stage of cancer, from the first aberrant division of cells to who gets what kind of care, to how families pay for the last stages of treatment, is profoundly influenced by our social and economic system. In this chapter, I use the example of cancer to examine how changes in modern capitalism have influenced our encounter with basic biological processes. I show how financialization, privatization, corporate capture of science, globalization, and biomedical reductionism have shaped our healthcare system's response to cancer—as well as to other serious threats to health. I consider recent developments in cancer treatment—the rise of precision medicine, private equity's investment in oncology group practices, patent protection for cancer treatments, and the skyrocketing cost of cancer care—to explore how individuals, families, and communities experience cancer in a twenty-first-century capitalist world. I focus on cancer because it teaches deep lessons about the impact of the current social and economic system on who gets what kind of healthcare, but similar insights would emerge from an examination of COVID-19, diabetes, depression, or dementia.

SUCCESSES IN CANCER CONTROL

To be sure, modern science and medicine, fueled in part by private-sector capital, have contributed to important advances in cancer control. Compared to the mid-twentieth century, more types of cancer are treatable, survival time for many cancers has been extended, and new treatment options using genomics (the science that studies the interactions of a person's genes with one another and the environment), targeted irradiation, and immunotherapies have been developed. These provide physicians with alternatives to surgery and radiation, the previous mainstays often characterized by serious side effects, impaired quality of life, and uncertain efficacy. Health insurance, especially after the 2010 Affordable Care Act, has provided new or additional coverage to many people with cancer. In its 2020 report, the American Cancer Society announced that the cancer death rate in the United States fell 2.2 percent from 2016 to 2017—the largest single-year decline in cancer mortality ever reported. Since 1991 the rate has dropped 29 percent, which means approximately 2.9 million fewer cancer deaths than would have occurred if the mortality rate had remained constant.[12]

But the greatest advances in cancer control have come from public health campaigns based on decades of research and a concerted mobilization of citizens, elected officials, and health professionals. These movements led to dramatic reductions in cigarette smoking and subsequent declines in lung cancer and other tobacco-related cancers. Researchers estimate that twentieth-century tobacco control programs and policies were responsible for preventing more than 795,000 lung cancer deaths in the United States from 1975 through 2000.[13] One of the most impressive accomplishments has been the drop in some Black-white disparities in cancer death rates, shrinking from a peak of 33 percent in 1993 to 14 percent in 2016. This accomplishment is largely due to declines in Black teen smoking rates,[14] showing the promise of public health strategies to reduce health inequities compared to the lack of success in shrinking gaps in access to and quality of cancer treatment for Blacks.[15] Advances in public health screening programs and in early diagnosis of breast cancer and prostate cancer have also contributed somewhat to improved survival—but not to reduced incidence. In fact, the failure to make new breast cancer screening programs and treatment accessible to Black Americans may have widened racial inequities for this site of cancer.[16]

As the successes in tobacco control show, the surest path to reducing cancer incidence and mortality is to reduce or eliminate exposure to substances that cause cancer. The principal causes of the rise in cancer around the world, according to the World Health Organization, are increased exposures to tobacco, foods high in fat and calories, alcohol, and physical inactivity. Other research points to the influence of air pollution and other toxic environmental and occupational exposures.

In 1946, Wilhelm Carl Hueper, an early pioneer in the field of occupational medicine and the first director of the Environmental Cancer Section of the National Cancer Institute, wrote that "the continued occurrence of occupational cancers, . . . represents a challenge not only to the intelligence but also to the social conscience of human society, because industrial cancers may be compared with a biologic bomb having a delayed time fuse which may be placed in the body of the victim without his knowledge and realization and which may display its deadly effect many years later when the conditions connected with its introduction are often forgotten."[17] Seventy-five years and millions of occupational and environmental cancer deaths later, the world has yet to meet Hueper's challenge, a marker of the success of asbestos, chemical, tobacco, and other businesses making carcinogenic products in thwarting both intelligence and conscience.

These facts suggest that global success in cancer control will require taking on prevention. Expanding effective implementation of strategies that limit tobacco industry marketing and pricing practices to low- and middle-income countries as well as high-income ones is one obvious proven strategy. Also critical to success will be reducing the predatory marketing practices of global ultra-processed food, alcohol, and chemical industries that contribute to cancer and other chronic diseases. But unlike selling expensive drugs and treatments to treat cancer, preventing cancer by limiting the carcinogenic practices of the tobacco, alcohol, food, and chemical industries is not profitable. And the success of these industries in shaping our political system and blocking initiatives that jeopardize profits has made cancer prevention a less feasible strategy than expanded treatment within contemporary capitalism.

For the millions for whom the cellular changes that lead to cancer have already begun, however, it is the healthcare industry that will shape their encounter with the disease, and these encounters are the focus here. Like our food and education systems, the privatization, globalization, and financialization of modern capitalism have also changed the healthcare system in the United States and around the world. These changes influence who gets what kind of cancer care at what cost and how the costs and benefits of these treatments are allocated. As noted, in high-income countries and increasingly in low- and middle-income countries as well, similar dynamics influence the treatment of other major causes of premature death and preventable illness.[18]

PRECISION MEDICINE

Precision medicine, also sometimes called personalized medicine, applies new scientific understanding of the role of the human genome in the development and progression of diseases to identify and formulate medicines to target the specific form of illness affecting that person. In cancer, precision medicine has contributed to dramatic improvements in survival for melanoma, the most serious type of skin cancer, and in some other forms of cancer but, so far, its overall impact on the burden of cancer has been modest. One study found that only 9 percent of patients with metastatic cancer will be eligible for genome-targeted precision drugs and only 5 percent will actually benefit. And many of those patients who do benefit from therapy relapse after two years.[19]

Yet precision medicine has attracted intense interest from venture capital and big pharmaceutical companies. What has made this particular advance so attractive to capitalism and what are some of the consequences of the growth of precision medicine for the prospects for cancer control? In some ways, precision medicine is a marketers' dream come true. It enables—even requires—the creation of thousands of niche market segments of cancer patients whose tumors have a distinct genetic profile as generated by the analytic power of big databases. Since the development of each niche requires substantial investment, precision medicine creates multiple opportunities for capturing a market of cancer victims willing and able to pay high prices for what they hope will be life-saving treatment.

Precision medicine also generates support for a variety of other technologies that have their own profit potential: multi-gene assays to test for tumor characteristics, manufacture of the many drugs and biologicals identified as having a potential for treatment, and the expansion of electronic health records that can aggregate data on precision medicine treatments and their impact. Given the strong protection of intellectual property rights for the pharmaceutical industry, including for biologic precision medicines, the discoverer of the precise formula to target a particular tumor will enjoy a monopoly for many years, a legal protection that ensures high prices and quick profits.

In previous decades, pharmaceutical companies looked for blockbuster drugs, products that could generate a billion dollars or more in profits because the targeted conditions affected millions of people and required lifetime treatment. Tagamet, a heartburn and stomach acid treatment; Lipitor, which treats high cholesterol; Advair, an asthma treatment; and Nexium, which treats gastroesophageal reflux disease (GERD), are examples of blockbusters.[20]

Another strategy to find blockbusters was to create, then market diseases to generate sales, a process labeled "disease-mongering."[21] Drugs for social anxiety disorders, male pattern baldness, and some female sexuality problems are examples of this approach. When these drugs have side effects, needlessly reinforce anxiety about these common conditions, or divert capital from more serious threats to public health, they add to the costs the pharmaceutical industry imposes on society.

But as many new patent-protected drugs for common conditions were brought to market, the potential for new blockbusters declined. And as patents on the original ones ran out, ending monopoly rights, pharmaceutical companies needed a new way to make money.

Niche busters—drugs that could completely capture a smaller market and promise dramatic improvements in cure rates or longevity—offered a new way to restore profits lost to faded blockbusters. "The economics are much more attractive for rare diseases than they were in the past," explained Usama Malik, Pfizer's head of business innovation.[22] Drug companies can charge higher prices for these products to help recoup development costs for a small market, so niche drugs make a growing contribution to pharma's bottom line.

Serendipitously, precision medicine's contribution to the development of niche busters for rarer diseases also helps the pharmaceutical industry to overcome increasingly negative public perceptions. Bernard Munos, a former advisor on corporate strategy for Eli Lilly, observed that with few new drug entities emerging from the industry's pipeline, and more than six thousand diseases affecting an estimated 25 million Americans still without a therapeutic option, "society is turning away from us and saying, 'this is a raw deal; this is not the covenant that we agreed to.'" "Ultimately," Munos says, "the acid test of success for the industry is our impact on public health."[23]

Precision medicines offer benefits to those suffering from the few types of cancer that respond—help anyone would want if they or a loved one had this type of cancer. But the reason precision medicine attracted financial capital and substantial public investment from the National Cancer Institute had more to do with its potential for increasing returns on investment than for improving public health.

As is often the case with modern capitalism, the ability to capture capital for an innovation that makes money always risks losing opportunities for other investments that would contribute more to human well-being although without offering the same return on investment. As health decision making shifts from doctors, hospital directors, and public health agencies to the executive suites of the health insurance, pharmaceutical, medical device, hospital chain, and private equity businesses, the bottom line is not the patients' or community's health but the financial health of these businesses and their investors.

ONCOLOGY PRACTICES

Increased corporate penetration of the healthcare system changes not only what treatments and medicines are available but also who delivers care, in what setting, and at what cost. In the last decade, the organization of clinicians treating cancer has changed significantly, from physician-owned community oncology practices to hospital-owned and private equity–fund owned or managed practices. For those who grew up getting their care from family practitioners like Dr. Marcus Welby and Dr. Steve Kiley, the stars of the 1970s television show *Marcus Welby, M.D.*, the thought that your doctors were accountable to a private equity firm for how many patients they saw and what cancer treatments they prescribed is understandably alien.

In 2018, the professional organization of community oncology practices reported that over the past decade, 1,653 community oncology practices had been closed, acquired by hospitals, undergone corporate mergers, or reported that they were struggling financially. Overall, since 2008, about fourteen practices per month have suffered these fates.[24] "All across the country, I hear from practicing community oncologists that they can no longer afford to keep their practices open and continue treating patients," said Dr. Mark Thompson, an Ohio oncologist and president of the Community Oncology Alliance.[25]

While market forces jeopardize these practices, research findings indicate that they deliver more affordable, patient-centered, and comprehensive care and better integrated end-of-life palliative care than hospital-based programs.[26] Anyone who has supported a cancer patient through treatment can imagine the wrenching disruption that results from an oncologist having to go out of practice or raise fees because the private equity owner ended financing for the oncology center.

Several factors have precipitated these changes. First, as the costs for equipment, treatment, and the expertise needed for cancer care increased, fewer physician practices could on their own generate the capital needed to keep up. Two willing suppliers of capital stepped in. First, hospitals and hospital chains bought up oncology practices, hoping to capture wider markets, collect the higher reimbursements they could generate compared to non-hospital–based outpatient practices, and use the increased patient load to bargain more effectively with insurers for more reimbursement.

Private equity firms also bought up oncology (as well as dermatology, radiation, and other high-revenue specialty) practices. These companies acquired between 60 and 80 percent ownership in practices, paying between $1 and

$2 million per physician, leaving the remainder of the business with physician owners so they too would have a stake in generating higher revenue. Annual returns for these investors were 20 percent or more.[27]

For private equity investors, oncology practices were attractive, as one business analyst wrote, because the high demand for oncology services due to population aging and the rising number of people with cancer meant that providers could count on "steady cash flows for oncology practices for years to come." Another attraction, according to VMG, the nation's leading healthcare valuation firm, was:

> the low-competition environment. While investors have crowded other subspecialties (dermatology, ophthalmology, and orthopedics, among others), significant consolidation and roll-ups have not yet made waves across oncology. Private equity firms who are the first movers in the space will have the opportunity to acquire the best assets at more attractive valuations with less competition from other buyers.[28]

How did the majority owners (the equity investors) and the physician owner-managers modify their practices in this new arrangement? To increase revenue, firms would buy up other smaller practices; hire new high-income-generating physicians and replace those who generated less revenue with lower cost physician assistants or other practitioners; and encourage use of equipment, procedures, and treatments that increased revenue. In other words, the decisions about who to hire, what treatments to offer, and what equipment to buy were not dictated by what was best for each patient but balanced against what was best for the financial health of the firm.

Private equity firms claimed that they provided needed capital, more autonomy than a hospital would provide, and the opportunity to profit from the future sale of the practice. These new owners generally aim to sell practices within three to seven years after buying them, a process they call a "liquidity event," an opportunity to cash out their gain to make more profitable investments elsewhere.[29] In fact, for some equity investors, their interest in physician group practices replaced prior investments in for-profit hospitals, which turned out to be less lucrative than anticipated.[30] For doctors and patients, "liquidity events" mean finding a new job or a new oncologist.

How did these changes in ownership affect care? One study found that urologists treating prostate cancer who were employed by the larger practices associated with hospital or investor ownership, compared to those working in smaller multidisciplinary group practices, charged higher prices for treatment. In addition, urologists working in practices that owned their own intensity-modulated radiation therapy (IMRT) equipment—a device that delivers high doses of radiation to the cancer site—charged more than those working in practices that used equipment owned by others.[31] Other studies have shown that IMRT, which costs an additional $15,000–$20,000 per treatment course than surgical or other radiation options, does not consistently result in better outcomes than older, better-studied options, and may lead to undertreatment, raising concerns about secondary malignancies.[32] These studies suggests that corporate ownership contributes to higher costs for cancer care but not necessarily to improved outcomes.

Moreover, this churn in ownership of oncology practices, combined with the organizational changes precipitated by hospital mergers and acquisitions and the fluctuating affiliations with insurance companies and pharmacy benefits managers, creates an instability of care for both patients and providers. One of the most reliable predictors of good medical care is consistency of provider-patient relationships, a quality undermined when some parties to care regularly seek to move their capital to more profitable ventures, even if that means interrupting someone's cancer care.

CHANGES IN ACCESS TO HEALTHCARE AND HEALTH INSURANCE

Who gets health insurance, how much they pay for it, and what benefits the insurance plan offers shape the outcome of a person's encounters with cancer as much as the rate at which cells are dividing. In recent decades, policy debates on healthcare have captured the attention of the American people, their government, and key corporate players. For the last twenty years, about 40 percent of American have said they were very or somewhat worried about not being able to pay medical costs for normal healthcare.[33] Since 1992, public policy on healthcare and its cost have been major issues in every presidential and many congressional elections.

Most of the efforts to improve quality and access to healthcare and to lower its costs—often contradictory goals—have emphasized the necessity of improving management. Unfortunately, substantial research evidence shows that these efforts have not yet led to meaningful improvements in quality or reductions in cost.[34] It is worth noting that despite the differences in healthcare reforms proposed by Presidents Clinton, Bush, Obama, and Trump, none of these presidents was willing or able to make changes that threatened the fundamental power or control of the health insurance, pharmaceutical, or hospital industries. With more transformative changes of control seemingly off the table, a new system evolved through a series of more modest reforms. Each of these must pass through the gauntlet of special interests— physicians' organizations, insurers, hospital chains, medical device makers, equity investors—who work to ensure that implementation does not jeopardize their profitability or control.

The battles between oncology group practices, private equity funds, and hospitals for control of clinical care and its revenue illustrate this process. Continuing conflicts about cancer drug coverage between insurers, hospitals, doctors, patients, and pharmacy benefit managers (the go-between companies that negotiate with drug companies about which medicines insurance plans will cover at what price) provide another example.

CANCER COSTS

The high cost of cancer care prevents many who need care from getting it. Direct medical costs for cancer in the United States exceed $80 billion a year and the costs of premature illness and death from cancer exceed $130 billion a year. In 2017, the cost of cancer drugs alone in the United States was $50 billion, a figure expected to double to $100 billion by 2022.[35]

As a result of the high out-of-pocket costs for cancer care, more than half of people with cancer experience repossession of their house, bankruptcy, loss of independence, or the breakup of family relationships.[36] Some of the newer treatments cost more than $60,000 a month and over the last decade the average monthly cost per agent has more than doubled.[37]

One recent study of 9.5 million people with newly diagnosed cancer found that two years after diagnosis, more than 42 percent had depleted their entire life's assets and after four years, 38 percent remained financially insolvent. Another study, completed before the implementation of the Affordable Care Act, found that more than 2 million cancer survivors did not receive necessary medical services because they could not afford this care.[38] A social worker for the support group CancerCare told a reporter that two comments she hears regularly from callers to the group's hotline are "I don't want to bankrupt my family" and "I can't afford to live."[39]

Another consequence of high costs is that cancer patients delay or forego care they need. One study found that one-third of Medicare patients who were expected to use Gleevec—the lifesaving leukemia medication that costs up to $146,000 a year—failed to fill prescriptions within six months of diagnosis, reducing their chances of successful treatment.[40] John Krahne, a sixty-five-year-old man in California who had been fighting brain tumors for a decade, received bad news from his doctor. Although his brain tumors were stable, his lung tumors had grown, he told an NPR reporter. The doctor prescribed Alecensa, a drug that sells for more than $159,000 a year. Medicare charged Krahne $3,200 for his first copay with a second $3,200 due a month later, as a new year of coverage kicked in. For the first time since being diagnosed, Krahne delayed filling his prescription, hoping that his cancer would not grow quickly while he waited for the new year of coverage. "We hope it doesn't hurt my chance of cure," says Krahne. "It was an educated risk that we didn't take lightly." Ultimately, Genentech, Alecensa's manufacturer, agreed to pay some of Krahne's out-of-pocket costs but these costs could top $10,000 a year.[41]

In some cases, these expensive new treatments led to marked increases in survival. In other cases, not so much. Bristol-Myers Squibb set the price of a newly approved melanoma drug Yervoy at $120,000 for a course of therapy. Studies showed that the drug was associated with an increase in life expectancy of four months.[42] Who should decide whether an added four months is worth $120,000? There is no easy answer to that question but now it is drug companies that decide which drugs to develop and which to ignore, decisions based primarily on the expected revenue the new drug will generate.

Why is cancer care so expensive? First, the emphasis on aggressive intervention and late-stage treatments using new technologies such as precision medicine, intensity-modulated radiation therapy, and immunotherapy contributes to high costs. Each of these treatments has powerful players advocating expanded use, many of whom profit from such expansion. With more than seven hundred cancer drugs now in late-stage development—up 60 percent from a decade ago—sharp increases in cancer costs are expected to continue (See Figure 4.1).[43]

Second, intellectual property rights laws add to the cost of cancer drugs. The 1995 Trade-Related Aspects of Intellectual Property Rights (TRIPS) amendment to the World Trade Organization rules enabled American pharmaceutical corporations to globalize patent protections.[44] TRIPS is the most comprehensive multilateral agreement on intellectual property and ensures long monopolies, usually from ten to twenty years, of protection for both

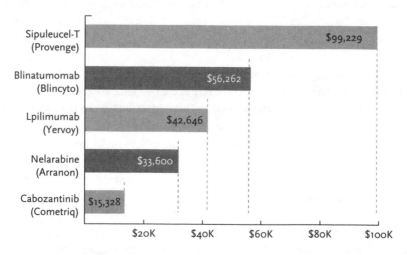

Average U.S. monthly income pre-tax: $3,600

Fig. 4.1 Monthly Costs of Most Expensive Cancer Drugs in the US Market.
Photo: Data retrieved from DrugPricingLab—Memorial Sloan Kettering. (2019). Drug Pricing Abacus.

pharmaceutical and biologic cancer treatments, monopolies that guarantee high prices. In 2001 at its meeting in Doha, the WTO reaffirmed flexibility of TRIPS member states to circumvent patent rights for better access to essential medicines. But today about half the cancer drugs on the WHO's Essential Medicine List still have patent protection, making them unaffordable in many parts of the world.

Recent renegotiation of trade treaties initiated by governments in the United States, United Kingdom, and elsewhere seek to emphasize the rights of national pharmaceutical industries over the universal right to have access to essential medicines. In these negotiations, government officials and industry representatives have pursued what are called TRIPS-plus agreements that reduce government flexibility and extend patent protection. NGOs and public health advocates point to the lack of safeguards in international trade to protect sustainable access to medicines.[45] However, in the trade agreement between Canada, Mexico, and the United States approved in 2020, the provision President Trump had proposed to extend patent exclusivity for drugs was rejected in favor of slightly more restrictive patent protection rules, a move advocated by those concerned about high drug prices.[46]

The story of Gleevec, a treatment for chronic myeloid leukemia (CML), illustrates how such patent protections keep the cost of cancer drugs high in high-, middle-, and low-income countries and how multinational drug corporations use their global power to maintain these prices.[47] In 1993, Novartis, the Swiss drug maker, patented Gleevec and it soon became the company's most profitable product. By 1997, several Indian drug makers began selling generic versions of Gleevec. In 2004, Indian companies were selling Gleevec at a price of about $4,230 per year while Novartis was charging $55,000 per year.

In 2007, Novartis went to the Indian courts with a novel interpretation of patent law, claiming that its modification of Gleevec, patented in Switzerland in 2001, had "evergreened" all previous patents and therefore made the Indian generic versions a violation of Novartis's intellectual property rights. Novartis lost in the Indian courts, but many other national health systems stopped buying the Indian generics, fearful of legal action. In these countries, cancer patients were deprived of access to affordable treatments for CML. This set a precedent for wealthy nations, and reinforced global Big Pharma's control of drug pricing. In a letter published in *Blood*, the journal of the American Society of Hematology, more than one hundred hematologists and oncologists from around the world protested the high cost of Gleevec, charged that Novartis's prices were harming their patients, and called for new rules on generic pricing and limits on intellectual property right protection that prevented profiteering by drug companies.[48]

In late 2017, almost two years after its patent expired, a month's supply of branded Gleevec was priced at around $9,000 a month, while the cost of the generic version was about $8,000 per month. The failure to reduce the price of this remarkably effective drug more significantly, wrote an industry analyst in *Forbes*, illustrates the complexity of the drug market and the ability of big drug companies to game the system. They do this by discouraging competitors, setting up patient benefit programs to divert political pressure for more effective cost containment, and persuading doctors to continue to prescribe the more expensive patented version.[49]

In an analysis of the impact of global trade regimes on the price of cancer drugs, researchers concluded that the real reason for the reluctance of multinational pharma companies to lower prices for cancer drugs in middle-income countries was not profit in those nations, but rather their "broader pharmaceutical global strategy" to protect prices of branded cancer drugs in high-income countries. These prices, wrote Dwaipayan Banerjee and James Sargent, two prominent researchers on the cancer drug industry, "seem to have escaped the limitations of both state regulation as well as market-based forms of cost control."[50]

In 2017, after all the legal wrangling, Novartis still earned $4.7 billion from Gleevec.[51] In sum, to protect markets for expensive and highly profitable cancer drugs in the United States and Europe, these companies aggressively pursue pricing strategies that put their drugs out of reach of health systems and cancer patients in the low- and middle-income countries that are experiencing the fastest growth of cancer burdens.

Myriad Genetics, a multinational company that produces and markets molecular diagnostic tests, provides another example of the impact of patents on prices of cancer care. In 1997, Myriad filed a patent for the BRCA1 and BRCA2 genes, naturally occurring mutations that increase the risk for certain forms of breast and ovarian cancer. Myriad charged $3,000 for the test and breast cancer activists worried that a patent might discourage other companies from developing cheaper and better tests.[52] In this case, however, the American Civil Liberties Union and other groups filed a lawsuit challenging Myriad's right to patent human genes.

Ultimately, in 2013, the US Supreme Court found that naturally occurring DNA segments such as the BRCA genes are "a product of nature and not patent eligible" merely because they have been isolated.[53] However, the court decided that genes or gene fragments created by companies are, as a human invention, patentable. This has led to the patenting of a number of newer biologic cancer treatments, including several priced at more than $100,000 per year.

Pharmaceutical companies argue that extended patent protections and high prices are fair and justifiable incentives for their substantial investments in research and development. However, independent analysts have shown that much of the original research depends on federal funding, not corporate investment, and that a significant portion of what pharmaceutical companies call "research" expenses is in fact marketing and promotion.[54] This includes the costs of designing alternative drugs with minimal differences from the original, so called "me-too drugs" that extend patent and monopoly protection and spending on "education" of physicians to prescribe their products.

One analysis found that the "true" R & D costs for an average drug are about $43 million, rather than the eighteen times larger industry estimate of $802 million.[55] Moreover, much of the evidence supporting the industry narrative of just rewards for taking research risks has been conducted by industry-funded economists whose methodologies cannot sustain unbiased analysis. Another study based on a review of the US Securities and Exchange Commission filings for ten cancer drugs found that these companies overestimated the costs of developing drugs and underestimated the revenue they generated for the company, suggesting that at least some of the industry-sponsored evidence to justify the high costs of cancer drugs is misleading or fabricated.[56]

Such deceptive use of evidence is problematic in itself. Even worse is pharma's claim that their research is advancing cancer treatment and thus justifies what Light and Warburton, two cancer policy scholars, describe as "wasteful and inefficient corporate research structures." These research programs develop mainly "new medicines of little advantage that compete for market share at high prices." These new drugs then become "the medicines the rest of the world wants, because the rich have them and presumably benefit from them."[57]

Pharmaceutical companies also keep prices high by extensive lobbying and campaign contributions to Congress in order to maintain the laws that block Medicare from negotiating on drug prices. The success of pharmaceutical companies in persuading legislators to ban price negotiation through the Medicare Modernization Act of 2003 and the Affordable Care Act of 2010 is like Congress barring McDonald's from bargaining on the price of beef. Recently, both Democratic and Republican politicians proposed new legislation to limit drug prices, setting off the usual frenzy of pharma lobbying.

The Pharmaceutical Industry Labor-Management Association, a coalition that includes major drug makers like Pfizer and Johnson & Johnson as well as large construction-industry unions whose members help build pharmaceutical plants and research labs, spent $660,000 in 2019 to buy Facebook ads and distribute leaflets and flyers at union meetings making the case that the proposed bill to limit drug price increases "threatens thousands of good-paying jobs and restricts access to lifesaving medication."[58] The Facebook ads targeted fifteen recently elected Democrats in Congress.

In contrast, health systems in most other nations do bargain and therefore offer drugs, including cancer drugs, at substantially lower prices. Medicare is the single largest payor of cancer care in the United States. To illustrate the inconsistencies of federal policy, the Medicaid program, which pays for healthcare for low-income people, also cannot bargain but it does get legally set reductions on drug prices and pays much lower prices for drugs than Medicare.

One way that pharmaceutical companies have responded to the criticism of high prices is to expand their philanthropic programs that provide free or subsidized drugs to certain populations in the United States and in low- and middle-income countries. Illustrating the pharmaceutical industry's determined efforts to keep quarterly returns rolling in, even from their patient assistance programs, several drug makers including Johnson & Johnson, Biogen, Celgene, and others settled Justice Department charges that they illegally funneled kickbacks through patient assistance charities.[59] The kickbacks were designed to ensure that the assistance programs funded payment only for the drug they manufactured, not competitor drugs, even if the alternatives were less expensive. Johnson & Johnson's Actelion Pharmaceuticals agreed to settle for $360 million, United Therapeutics for $210 million, and Pfizer for $24 million in similar suits.

The pharmaceutical industry has also used its philanthropic arms to support cancer patient advocacy groups. At first look, this seems like a worthy activity—pharma companies use their ample profits to fund organizations that educate people about cancer and help them find treatment. But a deeper examination suggests that drug companies use these groups to make the case for more public funding for cancer research, drug assistance programs, and other advocacy designed to benefit their bottom line.

As the public reputation of the drug industry has plummeted, companies have found that representatives of patient groups are more credible messengers for bringing industry messages to the media and public officials. Often this financial support is cloaked, leaving the public unaware they are getting industry-sponsored messages. Researchers at Columbia University studied the websites of 161 organizations with grants from the drug maker Eli Lilly. They found that only 25 percent of health advocacy organizations that received Lilly grants acknowledged the company's contributions on their websites and only 10 percent acknowledged Lilly as a grant event sponsor.[60]

Yet another factor contributing to rising costs is the entry of many new corporate players into cancer care, each seeking to win new revenue in this growth market. Amazon is financing GRAIL, a $900 million plan to detect cancer earlier by monitoring circulating tumor DNA in the bloodstream. GRAIL offers Amazon access to genomic data and complex analysis tools that it hopes to use to acquire more customers.[61] Google Ventures, now known as GV, has invested in Flatiron Health, a start-up that organizes oncology data to help cancer patients and doctors, a commitment that Flatiron used to raise $130 million from other investors.[62] With Google's backing, Flatiron will acquire Altos Solutions, an electronic medical records company. This dizzying buying and selling offers more risks of compromising confidential patient data and reduces the likelihood of sustainable improvements in getting data to doctors who need it. But these new ventures do create more opportunities to make money.

Cancer patients and their families increasingly use the internet as a source of information. This can help patients find support, information, and possible sources of care but it can also increase anxiety, confusion, and uncertainty about the reliability of information, spread misinformation, and encourage use of expensive but untested remedies.[63] A 2013 study found seventy-seven cancer care-related smartphone applications on the Apple iTunes platform, of which only 56 percent cited relevant scientific data backing up the app.[64]

The new sources of information that these investments fund may help some cancer patients, but overall they pitch cancer patients to spend more on untested therapies. They also provide an information glut that can overwhelm patients and their families with contradictory and unjustified claims for new treatments and move public and private capital from effective but unprofitable interventions (e.g., encouraging people to quit smoking or consume less highly processed foods), to less effective but more profitable ones.

Every new technology has the potential to aid patients—and to bring profits to the industries selling it. Who controls the deployment of the technology determines who benefits and who pays the costs. The case of electronic health records (EHRs) and precision medicine for cancer illustrate this process. In his 2015 State of the Union address, President Obama declared, "Tonight, I'm launching a new Precision Medicine Initiative to bring us closer to curing diseases like cancer and diabetes—and to give all of us access to the personalized information we need to keep ourselves and our families healthier."[65]

As Frances Collins and Harold Varmus, the leaders of the new initiative, explained, among its goals were to use EHRs of cancer patients to gather data from the medical records on unexplained drug resistance, genomic heterogeneity of tumors, insufficient means for monitoring responses and tumor recurrence, and knowledge about the impact of drug combinations to accumulate data that could more speedily lead to improvements in cancer care.

The use of EHRs increased rapidly because the Affordable Care Act required—and funded—expansion and because this public spending attracted private capital looking for profits. EHRs also help hospitals and insurers to track revenue more closely. By 2018, the federal government had spent $38 billion requiring doctors and hospitals to install electronic health records systems through Medicare and Medicaid.[66] Annual healthcare spending on EHRs was more than $6 billion a year. As tech companies enter this industry and consolidate it by buying up smaller businesses, costs can be expected to increase further, another example of federal subsidies for private corporations.

Although spending on EHRs has increased substantially in the last decade, as yet there is little evidence that in practice, they improve treatment decisions, patient care, or patient satisfaction. One study found that reports of cancer biopsies in EHRs, critical information for treatment decisions, could not be confirmed as fully accurate or inaccurate in 66 percent of the records.[67]

EHRs do, however, burden the work of healthcare providers. A study of almost eighteen hundred physicians in Rhode Island found that 70 percent reported increased technology-related stress and 26 percent reported burnout from this cause.[68] Some physicians report spending more time entering data on EHRs than talking to their patients, a problem exacerbated by revenue-generating hospital rules that mandate many patient encounters per hour.

While new technologies may benefit some patients, investors will support and companies develop only those options that have the potential to yield profits, ignoring the public health opportunity costs of less profitable alternatives, diverting resources to risky ventures, and contributing to the growing inequitable access to cancer treatment for low-income families and people of color.

In the ongoing battle to contain the cost of medical care without unduly compromising quality, public and private insurers deploy various strategies to lower costs. Transferring the financial risks for the cost of care down the line is one favored method of cost-containment. Insurers transfer risk to clinicians mainly by shifting to them liability for high-cost patients and also by paying them for the "value" of the care they deliver and its outcomes, rather than by fees for the services they provide. They transfer risk to patients by imposing high deductibles and co-pays.

Many cancer patients report that these deductibles speed their journey into debt or bankruptcy. V. J., a real estate agent who survived two bouts of breast cancer, the first in her thirties and the second in her fifties, told a reporter that her first treatment cost $40,000 and bankrupted her while the second cost $120,000. Although she had good insurance coverage for the later recurrence, her co-pays and premiums totaled $25,000, putting her in debt at a time her treatment prevented her from working.[69]

The mind-numbing complexity of the rules that determine insurance reimbursement for the various components of cancer care ensure that few patients or clinicians understand them. Thus, they are often unable to disentangle their treatment choices from the financial incentives or penalties that insurers craft. Moreover, these arcane rules give additional power to the pharmaceutical, hospital, and insurance industries that can afford to hire the staff to master them and to lobby and make campaign contributions to shape the policies that set the rules.

For those who survive cancer long enough to go into debt, modern capitalism has devised some ingenious ways for patients to get cash—and in the process for investors to make profits. Coventry First is an insurance company that describes itself as the "leader and creator" of the "life settlement" industry. Investors buy life insurance policies from people with cancer or other illnesses, cover the premiums until the individual's death, and then collect the payout. For desperate cancer patients, the amount paid out often enables them to begin cancer therapy but leaves their families with nothing after they die.

For an insured person with a death benefit of $1 million, a third-party investor may pay $250,000 for the policy, considerably more than the $100,000 cash surrender value of the policy. The investor assumes subsequent premium payments but if his bet on quick death plays out—of course a higher likelihood for someone with cancer—then the investor will collect $1 million at the patient's death, a tidy return on investment. As speculation in housing mortgages collapsed after the 2008 financial crisis and with ten thousand baby boomers turning sixty-five every day, investing in life settlements seemed like a safer haven. Some analysts predicted the market could reach $500 billion.[70] This financial scheme first emerged during the AIDS epidemic and has expanded since.

GoFundMe provides another, perhaps more palatable, option for those with cancer debts. GoFundMe, a private for-profit company, has raised more than $5 billion from 50 million donors around the world. More than a third of its funding drives seek contributions for medical expenses. Making a profit by tapping into people's charitable impulses exemplifies the spirit of twenty-first-century capitalism. Does it actually help cancer patients?

A review of its website finds dozens of pleas for support from people with cancer, usually seeking to raise between $25,000 and $250,000 for their cancer treatment. Stefanie, for example, is a thirty-three-year-old woman with a one-year-old daughter who, after several treatments, now has Stage 3 metastatic cervical cancer. The only hope of significantly extending her life, writes her family, is costly experimental surgery. More than twenty-one hundred people viewed her story and in two months, 719 people contributed $93,180 toward the $100,000 goal, enabling Stephanie to have her surgery at a highly rated cancer center.[71]

While many cancer survivors have gotten life-saving or life extending treatment as a result of GoFundMe, scholars have noted some problems. Two researchers at Simon Fraser University in Canada reviewed 220 cancer campaigns on GoFundMe from cancer patients in the United States, Canada, and a few other countries who reported using their campaign to pay for complementary or alternative cancer therapies. These campaigns requested on average $26,000 and in total received 24 percent of what they requested. At least 28 percent of the patients had died by the time the researchers completed their review. The study found that 38 percent of the individuals using GoFundMe used alternative treatments as well as traditional ones, 29 percent used these alternatives as a substitute for traditional therapy because of the fear of its effects or skepticism about its activity, and 31 percent pursued alternatives for financial or medical reasons.[72]

Previous research shows that about half of cancer patients use complementary or alternative medicines[73] and that patients who use such alternatives have a lower chance of survival than those who do not.[74] Of course, some people use these treatment after they have exhausted other alternatives but the authors of the study were concerned that GoFundMe contributed to the bombardment of cancer patients and their families with unverifiable claims, making them vulnerable to self-interested promoters of ineffective or harmful treatments,[75] a charge that, to be fair, has also been leveled at oncologists and cancer hospitals.

In a healthcare system that has increasingly reverted to the "buyer beware" mentality that allowed snake oil salesmen to flourish before the establishment of the US Food and Drug Administration in 1906, people with cancer and their families have to find their way through a maze of conflicting, self-promoting claims, making the cancer experience even more stressful.

Two other big corporate players also warrant further scrutiny: the hospital industry and medical device makers. Hospital charges are by far the biggest cost in the nation's $3.5 trillion a year healthcare market, accounting for 44 percent of personal expenses of those with private insurance. Between 2007 and 2014, hospital prices increased 42 percent for inpatient care and 25 percent for outpatient care, much higher than the increases in costs for physician care.[76] These increases occurred in both for-profit and ostensibly not-for-profit hospitals. As Elizabeth Rosenthal, the editor-in-chief of Kaiser Health News, has observed, the former use the higher revenue to increase returns to shareholders and both for-profit and not-for-profit systems use their higher cash flow to buy up oncology practices, improve their food services and other amenities to attract high income patients, invest in technologies that increase revenue but not necessarily improve care, and pay their CEOs exorbitant salaries.

Both systems also use their growing revenue to lobby Congress to further increase their government payments. A study by a Yale University health economist and his colleagues showed that hospitals in districts whose congressional representative voted to approve an industry-sponsored measure to allow hospitals to increase charges for government reimbursement collected more money from the government than hospitals in other districts. They also found that these congressional representatives received a 22 percent increase in total campaign contributions and a 65 percent increase in contributions from individuals working in the healthcare industry in the members' home states.[77] Disturbingly, as Rosenthal notes, the increased hospital spending does not lead to improved outcomes. European hospitals spend much less but have better or comparable outcomes.

Finally, the medical device industry contributes to increased costs for cancer care. In 2017, the World Health Organization identified hundreds of priority medical devices that can be used for management of cancer and specifically described medical devices for six types of cancer: breast, cervical, colorectal, leukemia, lung, and prostate.[78] These devices play an important role in screening, treatment, and management of cancer. However, as with cancer drugs, the US government does not regulate the costs of medical devices nor use any of its potentially enormous bargaining power to reduce costs. So, it defaults to pricing whatever the American market will bear.[79] There is no requirement for new drugs or devices to be more effective or less costly than existing approved regimens. Payers, such as Medicare, have adopted these new technologies without considering cost effectiveness or comparative effectiveness.

While medical devices constitute a small share of total medical costs, the Medicare Payment Advisory Commission estimates that spending on devices may be growing at twice the annual rate of drug expenditures.[80] In addition, profit margins for large device companies are in the 20 to 30 percent range, much higher than for other medical sectors.[81] These trends suggest that further expansion of this sector is likely.

In 2019, the US Food and Drug Administration asked Allergan, a global drug and medical device distributor, to recall the textured breast implants it made. These implants were used during reconstructive surgery after mastectomy for breast cancer. The recall was based on data that Allergan implants had caused 481 of the 573 cases and 33 deaths from a rare form of cancer reported from around the world.[82] Other reports of adverse health consequences and defects in breast implants show the high costs that an inadequately regulated medical device industry can impose on people fighting cancer and on public health.[83]

WAR ON CANCER AND THE CANCER MOONSHOT

In 1971, President Richard Nixon declared war on cancer, saying "the time has come in America when the same kind of concentrated effort that split the atom and took man to the moon should be turned toward conquering this dread disease. Let us make a total national commitment to achieve this goal." When he signed the National Cancer Act into law later that year, Nixon said "I hope in the years ahead we will look back on this action today as the most significant action taken during my Administration."[84]

Seventeen years later, Vice President Al Gore announced, "We want to be the first generation that finally wins the war on cancer." He said science was on the verge of a breakthrough and proposed a 65 percent increase in federal funding for cancer research over five years. "For the first time, the enemy is outmatched," Gore asserted.[85]

In 2002, at a White House meeting with cancer researchers and survivors, President George W. Bush reported "the fight against cancer has seen major victories and is on the verge of major breakthroughs. . . Medical science is helping cancer victims survive, and helping survivors lead better lives." Bush announced that his 2003 budget "would increase funding for cancer research by $629 million, for a total investment in cancer research throughout the

National Institutes of Health of more than $5 billion. In order to win the war against cancer, we must fund the war against cancer."[86]

In 2016, forty-five years after Nixon's declaration of war on cancer, President Barack Obama put his vice president Joe Biden in charge of the "Cancer Moonshot," declaring "a new national effort to get it done . . . for the loved ones we've all lost, for the families that we can still save, let's make America the country that cures cancer once and for all."[87]

And in the 2020 presidential campaign, President Trump, Joe Biden, and other candidates vowed to continue the war on cancer, demonstrating that both Republicans and Democrats believe that the war on cancer is good politics, good policy, and good science.

From Nixon's time, however, some scientists and activists have questioned the basic premises of the war on cancer. In this view, the "war on cancer" frame reflects the values of modern capitalism and has actually set back progress on reducing the health and economic burden of cancer.

The notion of wars on scientific problems originates from the successful effort to build an atomic bomb during World War II and to win the space race by landing a man on the moon in 1969. Both of these efforts mobilized government funding and corporate expertise to create focused solutions to technical and logistical obstacles to achieving a single goal.

But applying this approach to cancer ignores the fact that cancer is not one condition but two hundred diseases, each with its own distinct pathways and causes. It overestimates the degree of current scientific understanding of cancer (compared to atomic physics or rocket launching or space travel) and underestimates the complexity of the biological, environmental, and other forces that influence the natural history of cancers. As Sol Spiegelman, a cancer researcher at Columbia University, observed at the start of Nixon's war on cancer, "An all-out effort [to find a cure for cancer] at this time would be like trying to land a man on the moon without knowing Newton's laws of gravity."[88] While more is known today, many researchers continue to emphasize that science is only beginning to understand how various types of cancer start, grow, and kill—essential insights for the development of effective treatments.

The war on cancer assumes that with enough effort, researchers can find a single or a few cures for a single condition. This reflects the reductionist paradigm of Western biomedical science, itself strongly influenced by corporate interests. Reductionism posits that reducing complex biological or medical problems into the sum of their many parts leads to understanding a single cause and finding a cure. In cancer research, this has meant funding a "war" to hunt down the specific genes or subcellular processes that initiate carcinogenesis, then devising a drug or technology to interrupt that process. The last task is assigned to private-sector organizations—mostly drug companies—that can muster the capital to develop, produce, and market these alleged magic bullets, translating the knowledge acquired through public funding into patented products or services that can succeed in the marketplace by generating returns for their producers.

Declaring war on the cells, genes, and subcellular processes that contribute to cancer also makes it easier to ignore the social and political processes that shape cancer and to focus instead on biological and individual-level causes. It is like trying to understand music by analyzing sound waves or literature by counting the frequency of word use.

In 1989, Samuel Broder, then director of the National Cancer Institute, acknowledged that "poverty was a carcinogen"[89] but over the decades, the wars on cancer have never targeted poverty or manufacturers of carcinogenic commodities such as tobacco, ultra-processed food, alcohol, asbestos, or pesticides. (Although to be fair, George W. Bush, in announcing his war on cancer, did jokingly promise to eat more broccoli, despite his well-known distaste for the vegetable.) [90] Focusing on prevention or targeting carcinogenic industries could jeopardize elite support for the war on cancer, a prerequisite for continued public and private funding for research, philanthropic contributions, and the favorable media coverage essential for public support of any war.

Instead, members of Vice President Biden's Cancer Moonshot Blue Ribbon Panel included biomedical cancer researchers but also leaders of Pfizer and Amazon, and Patrick Soon-Shiong, a physician-entrepreneur who invented the blockbuster pancreatic cancer drug Abraxane and founded several biotech and health start-ups. According to Forbes, his net worth is about $7 billion.[91] In 2018, he bought *The Los Angeles Times*.

Like many of those who made fortunes from cancer treatment, Soon-Shiong has faced some legal troubles. In 2019, Sorrento, a small company that manufactured a cancer drug that competed with Abraxane, accused Soon-Shiong of buying up a drug that it hoped to market as a less expensive alternative competitor to one of Soon-Shiong's products. This alternative, claimed Sorrento, might save the US healthcare system more than $1 billion.[92] Soon-Shiong bought the rights to the new drug, then withdrew it from the market. Sorrento is seeking $1 billion in an arbitration complaint and $90.5 million in a civil lawsuit.[93] Drug companies use the process known as "catch and kill" to maintain monopoly rights on patented drugs, a strategy that can be considered a violation of seldom-enforced antitrust laws.[94] The potential for conflicts of interest in cancer drug policy recommendations seems obvious.

On the Moonshot Panel, Soon-Shiong advocated the creation of a massive database of potential genetic factors that could be used to design cancer drugs by conducting genomic sequencing of one hundred thousand patients. Not surprisingly, the Moonshot Panel included only one recommendation for prevention—to focus on individual behavior and access to healthcare—[95] but no recommendations that would jeopardize the industries that produce the carcinogens that permeate the daily lives of people around the world.

The war metaphor has also encouraged the scientists, policy makers, advocates, and businesses who appealed for the public and private funds to support the war to exaggerate its successes and to prematurely claim seeing the proverbial light at the end of the tunnel. The designers and makers of precision medicines, for example, promised their discoveries would dramatically change the course of cancer. Proponents of early cancer screening, such as Susan G. Komen, argued that more screening saved lives. However, as cancer researcher Gilbert Welch has noted, overly broad cancer screening programs that tell everyone with abnormal cells that they have cancer inevitably lead to overdiagnosis and skyrocketing survival rates,[96] but not to improvements in population health.

The rhetoric of the war on cancer, Sol Spiegelman noted, "had raised public expectations of impending breakthroughs . . . by suggesting cancer could be 'conquered' in a matter of years." Instead, he wrote, the war framework "contributed to rising skepticism of modern biomedical science among Americans who had long believed in its inevitable progress."[97]

As corporations, right-wing populists, climate change deniers, middle-class anti-vaxxers, and others attack the capacity of science to provide objective evidence to guide policy and improve human and planetary well-being, the cancer warriors' distortions of cancer science further diminishes the credibility of scientists, healthcare providers, and public health professionals. By squandering this most precious asset of the scientific community, those who misrepresent the evidence on the limited success of the war on cancer jeopardize the capacity of the scientific community to contribute to solving other medical and environmental problems.

False claims about success also reinforce the sometimes accurate perception that scientists and clinicians forge secret alliances with big corporations at the expense of their patients' well-being. In 2018, for example, an investigative team from *Pro Publica* and *The New York Times* found that Dr. José Baselga, the chief medical officer of the internationally recognized Memorial Sloan Kettering Cancer Center, had failed to disclose millions of dollars in payments from healthcare companies in dozens of research articles, violating hospital and medical journal rules (See Figure 4.2).[98] Baselga was forced to resign but the damage to Sloan Kettering's reputation as an objective dispenser of cancer treatment and research will be more difficult to repair.

In response to the rapid spread of the COVID-19 pandemic and its devastating impact on public health and the economy, politicians and corporate leaders called for a war on the coronavirus, returning to the favored metaphor to advocate policies that transferred public resources into private companies that hoped to develop new treatments, vaccines, and antigen and antibody tests. Once again the war metaphor risked distorting science, hiding corruption and profiteering, and masking the underlying causes of the rapid spread of the pandemic such as poverty, racism, lack of affordable housing, lack of

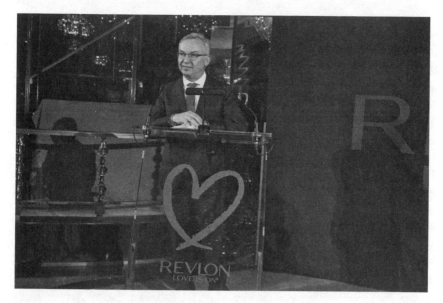

Fig. 4.2 Dr. José Baselga, physician-in-chief and chief medical officer of Memorial Sloan Kettering, a leading cancer hospital in New York City, celebrates the success of a fundraising drive in 2015. In 2018, he was forced to resign after failing to disclose drug industry funding for his research. Soon after, he was appointed head of research and development in oncology at AstraZeneca, the British-Swedish drug maker.
Photo: © Cindy Ord /Getty Images

worker safety protections, a deregulated, austerity-scarred public health system, and understaffed and under-regulated for-profit nursing homes.[99]

PUSHING BACK AGAINST CORPORATE CONTROL OF CANCER CARE

As the pharmaceutical, insurance, and hospital industries consolidated their control of the healthcare system, cancer patients and their families, healthcare providers, and some elected officials have resisted these incursions. Deeper understanding of the successes and failures of these contests yields insights into how corporations respond to challenges from government, health professionals, advocates, and others.

Patient Activism. Beginning in the early 1970s, inspired by the women's and anti–Vietnam War movements, people with cancer began to seek alternatives to the medical/corporate narratives of cancer. Some women with breast cancer rejected the orthodoxy of routine radical mastectomy and the view that physicians should have sole responsibility for making treatment decisions. Rose Kushner, a journalist and activist diagnosed with breast cancer, created the

Breast Cancer Advisory Center, which educated and mobilized women to demand more funding for research on breast cancer and a larger voice for women in treatment decisions. Kushner said, "I think what I did was the highest level of women's liberation. I said 'No' to a group of doctors who told me 'You must sign this paper, you don't have to know what it's all about.'"[100] This earlier activist response to medical domination was later strengthened by the fierce advocacy of people with HIV infection, who challenged drug and insurance companies, government policies, and the research institutions that decided which treatment options to pursue.

The successes of breast cancer and HIV activists in claiming a voice for patients in setting research directions, questioning medical practices, and insisting that patient needs came first helped to change the national conversation about who sets the medical research agenda. The activists created new platforms where they could challenge—or support—the claims and perspective of researchers and industry representatives. These included National Institutes of Health review committees, which now invited patient representatives, and new activist groups such as ACT UP, Breast Cancer Action in the San Francisco Bay area, and the Long Island Breast Cancer Coalition, a group that tackled the environmental causes of breast cancer.[101] Cancer activism also attracted media and policy maker attention, further amplifying its impact.

The role of patients in changing cancer policy continues. As the International Consortium of Investigative Journalists reported in its investigation of implants for breast cancer, more than fifty thousand women around the world have joined a Facebook group, Breast Implant Illness and Healing, whose membership has skyrocketed with new media attention on implants.[102] The reason for the surge, says the group's founder, Nicole Daruda, is that no one else would take their ailments seriously. "Women were having all these problems, and, when they go to their doctors, they get told there's nothing wrong with their implants," Daruda said. In 2019, these activists, together with investigative journalists and health advocates, forced several governments around the world to change their regulation of breast implants and monitor product defects more closely.[103]

Healthcare Reform. For more than fifty years, progressive physicians and grassroots reformers in the labor, civil rights, feminist, and AIDS activist movements have campaigned for a national health system that made affordable, quality healthcare available to all residents of the United States. As historian Beatrice Hoffman observed, these campaigns "contained the seeds of a wider critique of the American health care system, leading some movements to adopt calls for universal coverage" and access to healthcare as a fundamental human right. Making access to healthcare a right rather than regarding it as one more commodity to be allocated by market forces constituted a fundamental challenge to twenty-first-century capitalism.[104] The deep divide between these two views perhaps helps to explain why the fight over healthcare has been so consuming for the American people for more than fifty years.

The passage of the Affordable Care Act in 2010 was an important albeit limited success for this movement. As a result of the ACA, 20 million people gained insurance coverage and discriminatory practices such as refusing to insure people with existing health problems ended, a big win for those with cancer. Despite the claims of opponents, after the ACA, neither waiting time, overall costs, or patient dissatisfaction with care increased significantly. Cancer patients made some specific gains: the uninsured rates for cancer survivors decreased from 12.4 percent to 7.7 percent and uninsurance declined even more for cancer survivors living in states that chose to expand Medicaid coverage.[105]

But the ACA also shows the limits of these movements in challenging modern capitalism. Healthcare advocates, President Obama, and Congress were unable (or unwilling) to win passage of a law that included a public option, the right for the federal government to negotiate drug prices, or significant efforts to reduce the market-driven administrative costs of healthcare. And as the 2020 presidential campaign showed, the call for a single-payer health system continued to elicit strong opposition from the healthcare industry, most conservatives, and some liberals but also support from many voters.

According to historians Kevin Young and Michael Schwartz, health-related industries spent abundantly in several categories to shape the final law.[106] In campaign finance, the key players in creating the ACA were dependent on health industry corporations for election and re-election. In 2008, the health sector was Barack Obama's third-most-important source of corporate donors, with health industry donations thirty-two times greater than the combined labor union contributions to Obama. The twenty-three members of the Senate Finance Committee (SFC) received nearly $16 million in 2008 and $20 million in 2010 from health-related companies. Committee members' opposition to a "public option" that would compete with private insurers correlated with donations from the healthcare industry over the previous two decades. During the ACA debates, the healthcare industry spent more money on lobbying than any other industry, including nearly $1 million dollars a day on lobbying and campaign contributions during the 2009 debate. Many elements of the legislation were written directly by lobbyists.[107] According to a 2009 report, almost thirty key lawmakers involved in drafting the legislation "have financial holdings in the industry, totaling nearly $11 million worth of personal investments."[108]

SFC members epitomized the "revolving door" between government and industry. Elizabeth Fowler, senior counsel to the committee, was a key architect of the legislation on the government side.[109] The file of the original bill draft indicates that it was written on her computer. Fowler had been a vice president at WellPoint, one of the nation's largest private health insurance corporations. After the reform became law, she was appointed by President Obama to oversee its implementation. Fowler and other key players moved back and forth between government service and the healthcare industry.[110]

In the decade since the passage of the ACA, President Trump and a Republican Congress have so far unsuccessfully tried to repeal or decimate Obamacare, although they have been able to maintain the uncertainty about its future that can be so frightening to those living with cancer. Even after the COVID-19 pandemic caused millions of Americans to lose employer-provided health insurance, Republicans continued seeking to undo the ACA. In the 2020 primaries and national election, several Democratic candidates for president and Congress advocated for single-payer or "Medicare-for-all" plans, evidently believing that such universal proposals would help them win votes.

Public-interest lawyers have also challenged the industries that dominate cancer care. The American Civil Liberties Union's successful lawsuit against Myriad Genetics stopped the company's effort to patent the BRCA1 and BRCA2 genes that increase the risk for certain forms of breast and ovarian cancer.[111] Similarly, the decisions by Indian courts in 2007 and 2013 to allow Indian companies to make and sell a generic version of Gleevec, a treatment for chronic myeloid leukemia, enabled cancer patients with CML in India to get treatment, even as the prices that Novartis charged for Gleevec in the United States continued to rise.[112]

Industry power limited each of these legal victories: the US Supreme Court did allow the patenting of genes or gene fragments created by companies, enabling industry to modify, patent, and sell for high prices naturally occurring biological materials that could treat cancer. Novartis was able to use its power in international circles to prevent other countries from following India's lead in making generics more available. But these legal victories opened doors for governments, advocates, and social movements to contest the use of intellectual property law to withhold cancer treatments, forced drug companies to take action to attempt to restore their damaged credibility, and highlighted the differences between what's good for business and what's good for protecting health, a distinction corporations seek to hide.

CANCER CARE AND CAPITALISM

The history of cancer treatment in the United States from radical mastectomies, intensity-modulated radiation therapy, megadose drug therapies, and bone marrow transplants to precision medicine often lurched from one promising fad to another. It is understandable that such a terrible disease encouraged doctors and scientists to value hope over evidence. But the choice of innovations depended heavily on new investments from wealthy individuals and companies that hoped to profit. As its scientific enterprise and health-care system became captive institutions ready to shift directions based on the whims of investors, the United States lost key opportunities to reduce the burdens of cancer. By giving corporations a powerful voice in setting science and medical policy, the nation sacrificed a rational evidence-based approach for a casino mentality where the promise of profit decides which medical avenues are pursued and which ignored.

The power of pharmaceutical, health insurance, and the hospital industries to exploit changes in the United States and global economies for their own benefit has often undermined systemic reforms that could improve access to affordable quality care. For example, after the 2008 economic crisis, the 2010 Affordable Care Act, and the continuing public debate about high drug prices, small biotech companies have remained profitable by creating hard-to-copy biologics for niche subsets of privileged populations such as insured or wealthy people with terminal cancers. In addition, big pharmaceutical companies have begun to buy biotech firms with prospects for new niche busters. Had the pharmaceutical industry supported policies to allow Medicare to negotiate for drug prices, they could have saved Americans billions of dollars in healthcare costs and helped to improve access to essential medicines. Because it is now unthinkable for private industries to sacrifice private gain for public good, they chose instead the path that they believed would provide quicker and higher returns for their investors, thus depriving millions of people around the world of essential medicines.

In today's economy, as one analyst observed, "The pay structure at present does not provide financial incentives to find a cure for cancer."[113] Drug companies profit by selling exorbitantly expensive drugs to the few who can pay for a round or two of treatment. Despite the fact that 80 percent of cancers seem to be caused by extrinsic factors,[114] relatively little research has focused on the biological, social, or political interventions that could reduce such exposures, in part because such strategies both offer limited opportunities for profit and threaten the profitability of the many industries that sell carcinogenic commodities or create carcinogens in their production processes.

Instead, government and industry invest billions of dollars in poorly conceived wars on cancer. Researchers and the National Institutes of Health endorse several Big Ideas such as that common diseases will be explained largely by a few DNA variants and that this knowledge will lead to improved diagnosis and treatment. In fact, as three prominent physician-researchers observed in the *Journal of the American Medical Association*, for the most part these ideas have failed to lead to meaningful improvements in health or healthcare in the last two decades.[115]

The costs of increasing corporate control of cancer care are high. By pursuing prevention and treatment options that are the most profitable rather than the most effective for the largest number of people with cancer, the medical enterprise misses opportunities to make progress. Although the various battle plans for the war on cancer mention the goal of reducing gaps in access to and quality of cancer care, progress has been slow and limited. As a result, African Americans, low-income Americans, and women continue to experience worse survival rates, less access to the most-effective treatments, and more inappropriate cancer screening tests. In fact, many of the recent real advances in cancer care have widened rather than closed these gaps.

In a rational and humane system, government, medicine, and science would have the dominant voice in setting national cancer-control policies that lead to more effective and equitable strategies to reduce the burdens of cancer. Instead, modern capitalism has delegated this voice to the corporate sectors who profit from cancer care, ensuring that its priorities will distort and compromise this crucial task.

CHAPTER 5

Work

The Growth of Low-Wage and Precarious Labor

Work gives you meaning, and purpose and life is empty without it.
—*Stephen Hawking*

Work gives people dignity, income, an identity, peer support, and a path to claiming a political voice. Work can also put people at risk of premature death or preventable illnesses or injury, jeopardize self-sufficiency, dignity, or independence, or consume so much time and energy that little is left for the rest of life. How a person experiences work profoundly influences well-being, happiness, and lifetime success. How a society organizes work opportunities shapes public health, economic growth, fairness, and democracy.

Over human history, the impact of work on well-being has varied, with each era and population group experiencing a distinct and dynamic pattern of work experiences and occupational health and disease rooted in the economic and political arrangements of the time and place.

Over the twentieth century, the United States developed an approach to worker health and safety that was shaped by both Fordist principles of mass production and mass consumption,[1] and by Keynesian welfare economic and social policies.[2] This approach led to significant improvements in the well-being of workers but also left big gaps for some populations. A brief review of these advances and inequities sets the stage for examining how twenty-first-century capitalism has changed three key features of work: work organization, including pay, benefits, and voice in the workplace; worker exposures to toxic social and physical environments; and how workers balance work and family responsibilities. Together, these work characteristics are primary determinants of the well-being of workers and their families.

Immigration, industrialization, and urbanization forged both the work arrangements and the occupational safety and health problems of the twentieth century; modifying these processes led to dramatic improvements in worker well-being.[3] Over the twentieth century, more workers came to work for large corporations or the smaller businesses that supplied these corporations. Many of these workers had fixed hours of work, regular pay, and, over time, increasing social benefits such as health insurance and pensions, characteristics that came to be considered "standard work arrangements." Many joined labor unions. Of course, some major groups—Blacks and Latinxs, women, recent immigrants, and others—lacked some or all of these standard arrangements, leading to a highly stratified workforce and disparate burdens of work-related injuries and diseases.

During this period, occupational injuries and deaths in mining and other high-risk industries fell significantly,[4] leading the US Centers for Disease Control to call these improvements one of the ten great triumphs of twentieth-century public health. A study by the National Safety Council showed that between 1933 and 1997 deaths from unintentional work-related injuries declined 90 percent, from 37 per 100,000 workers to 4 per 100,000.[5]

Improvements in worker health resulted from a spate of laws and regulations approved over the century as a result of vigorous advocacy and mobilization by labor unions, reformers, health professionals, and progressive elected representatives. The Employers Liability Acts of 1906 and 1908, for example, reduced worker liability for their injuries through what employers called "contributory negligence," the alleged failure of an injured plaintiff to act prudently. Workers' compensation is an insurance that provides cash benefits and medical care for workers who are injured or become ill as a direct result of their jobs.

In 1911, New York was the first state to pass a workers' compensation law but on March 24, 1911, the New York State Court of Appeals declared this law unconstitutional. The next day, 146 workers were killed in a fire at the Triangle Shirtwaist Factory in New York City, many of whom died jumping from the ninth or tenth floor to the street below to escape the flames and bypass the locked exits. Two years later, New York passed a workers' compensation law that did pass court review. By 1949, every state had enacted a workers' compensation program.[6] These laws acknowledged employers' financial responsibility for work-related injuries but made it difficult for workers to win benefits for many work-related illnesses and prohibited workers from suing their employers. For employers, it creates a "no fault" system that keeps their costs predictable.

The Fair Labor Standards Act of 1938 set minimum wages, mandated overtime pay, and added child labor protections. The Occupational Safety and Health Act of 1970 gave the federal government expanded power to protect the health and safety of workers. Passed because of the mobilization of labor and other social movements, these laws established the capacity and right of the federal governments and, in some limited cases, state governments to improve working conditions, limit hours, set pay, protect rights to organize, and work in safe and healthy settings.

Labor rights emerged from popular responses to industrialization and urbanization and reflected the deep stratifications of twentieth-century America. Some groups such as farmworkers and domestic workers were excluded from these protections. A review of the impact of policy on occupational health disparities concluded that "the historical legacies of racism and discrimination in the United States have contributed to the exclusion of certain workers from protections provided by labor, economic, and social laws and policies, and the concentration of minority workers in more hazardous occupations."[7] Throughout US history, systemic racism led to public policies and business practices that put Black workers at higher risk of occupational illness and death.

Women, farmworkers, recent immigrants, and service and household workers were also often inadequately shielded from the hazards that characterized their places of work.[8] In the 1960s and beyond, these populations fought to gain the protection of the laws that had initially protected mainly white men.

In response to the successes, starting in the last two decades of the twentieth century and continuing today, corporations launched a counteroffensive against the successes of the labor, women's, environmental, and civil rights movements seeking to roll back earlier worker protections. In 1995, the Heritage Foundation, a right-wing think tank funded in part by Joseph Coors, of the Coors beer empire, and Richard Mellon Scaife, heir of the Mellon industrial and banking fortune, recommended closing the Department of Labor. The Heritage Foundation, an architect of Reagan-era deregulation campaigns, called the Department of Labor "one of the most pervasive regulatory agencies in the federal government" that presents "a barrier to the formation of firms and their ability to create jobs."[9]

Also, in 1995 Congress ended a budget conflict that had triggered the first of recurring federal government shutdowns. The approved budget closed the Bureau of Mines and transferred some of its functions to other federal agencies. Federal spending on mine safety was cut by almost $100 million, or 66 percent, and one thousand of its employees were dismissed. Some mining health and safety programs were transferred to the Department of Energy but inadequately funded.[10]

In 2017, with the inauguration of Donald Trump and a Republican Congress, the effort to deregulate workplace health and safety went into high gear. Trump appointed former corporate executives with pro-business track records and several positions, such as the administrator for the Occupational Safety and Health Administration, went unfilled for years. When Trump had to replace his secretary of labor, Alex Acosta, in 2019, he nominated Eugene Scalia (a son of the late Supreme Court justice) who had been a lawyer for Walmart and other companies in their fights against unions. *New York Times* columnist Nicholas Kristof compared the appointment of the anti-union Scalia as secretary of labor to nominating Typhoid Mary to be health secretary.[11]

Toward the end of his first year in office, President Trump announced he had "cancelled or delayed over 1,500 planned regulatory actions—more than any previous President by far" and "instead of eliminating two old regulations, for every one new regulation we have eliminated 22. . . . We aimed for two for one, and, in 2017, we hit twenty-two for one."[12] This dismantling of federal workplace health and safety protections puts workers at risk and removes pressure on employers to improve health and safety conditions in their workplaces.

THE CHANGING FACE OF WORK IN THREE PROFILES

To explain how recent changes in capitalism have led to transformations of how people experience their work lives, I briefly describe three companies that exemplify emerging patterns of work. Walmart, described for its role in changing American diets in chapter 2, is a global megacorporation that has set the pattern for low-wage retail sector jobs and vigorous anti-unionism. KinderCare, the largest for-profit child care chain in the United States, illustrates how sectoral disruptions can disrupt the lives of workers via the privatization of jobs in the growing "care economy," jobs that had been previously nonprofit and public sector. Uber tells its workers, "Drive with us and earn on your schedule" and illustrates the benefits and costs of working in the gig or platform economy.

WALMART

Walmart is the nation's largest private employer, with 1.5 million workers in the United States, and a total of 2.2 million around the world. In the United States, Walmart employs one in ten retail workers. Its annual revenues in 2019 were $514 billion. Despite its size, Walmart faces many of the same pressures as other giant retailers. As new competitors such as dollar stores, Amazon, and chains such as Kroger and Target emerged, annual revenues at Walmart's discount stores fell from $142.5 billion in 2009 to $98 billion in 2018, leading to the closure of 2,214 of these outlets. In the same period, however, Walmart opened even more supercenters, larger stores that sell food and many other items.[13] Although fast-growing Amazon took business away from most retailers, Walmart's low prices allowed it to continue to dominate the retail food market in the United States.

Walmart calls its hourly workers "associates," a term with multiple connotations. Founder Sam Walton used it to evoke the camaraderie he felt on sports teams as a boy. "Associate" also implies that these workers are partners in global multinational business, able to share its profits and success. In fact, the term reveals that these workers are not employees in the traditional sense: they have no contract, no job security, and are not protected by many of the labor laws enacted to protect industrial workers and their unions in an earlier era. According to Walmart, 43 percent of its US associates are people of color, and 55 percent are women.[14] In comparison, only 21 percent of its more senior officers are people of color and 30 percent are women.

In recent years, Walmart has shifted more of its workers to part-time status. In 2005, 80 percent of Walmart workers were full-time; by 2018, an estimated 50 percent were part-time.[15] In an internal memo from that year, a Walmart executive noted that "increasing the percentage of part-time Associates at stores" is a "major cost-savings opportunity."[16] Now, more than five hundred thousand of Walmart's workers are part-time, often with fluctuating shifts and hours to meet the company's changing customer patterns. A 2018 survey of 6,176 Walmart associates found that 69 percent reported that they would prefer to work full-time, suggesting that the heavy reliance on part-time work is a company choice, not a worker choice.[17]

Walmartism. In the twentieth century, the auto maker Henry Ford pioneered an approach to capitalism that combined technological and managerial efficiency of production with worker pay and benefits that enabled employees to buy what they made. By promoting both mass production and mass consumption, Fordism, as it came to be known, served as a foundation for the economic growth and rising standards of living of the last century.[18]

In this century, Walmartism has replaced Fordism, propose Adam Reich and Peter Bearman, two Columbia University sociologists who study Walmart. The key elements of Walmartism are "arbitrary authority of managers coupled with a penetrative system of measurement, observation and feedback," low wages and modest benefits, "flexible specialization" in which workers are assigned a single task but expected to fill in on many tasks as needed, and unstable work schedules that are often changed to match the ebb and flow of consumer demand. Walmartism also asks customers to monitor and rate worker behavior, creates an ethos of a workplace community, and vigorously discourages unions, three sometimes contradictory elements of the Walmart work culture.[19]

In many ways, Walmartism embodies the changing face of low-wage, nonstandard employment, especially as it plays out in the multinational corporations that dominate the growing retail sector of the United States and global economies. Disturbingly, as one scholar noted, through its surveillance of workers, its systems of rewards and sanctions, and its opposition to unions, Walmartism "serves to undermine the structural power of workers to challenge these unfavorable conditions through collective action," making it a major obstacle to improved working conditions in this era.[20]

Investor expectations that quarterly returns remain high and savings be invested in stock buybacks rather than better pay and benefits for workers require Walmart and other service-sector employers to impose constant pressure on their workers, with the threat that in today's economy, workers can be replaced with more willing hands—or robots—if these expectations are not met.

Reich and Bearman have called Walmartism "Fordism in reverse." To stoke consumer demand, rather than paying workers enough to buy the car they are producing, Walmart pays so little that workers are compelled to shop there.[21] In addition, as other scholars have noted, Walmart lowers labor standards, "not just for its workers, but for employees of all competitors and potential competitors."[22] By its size and market share, Walmart sets the standard for how to profit in today's economy by offering everyday low prices sustained by low wages.

Like Fordism, Walmartism also has a consumer face. Walmart's goal is to hire the minimum staff that maximizes profit, selling the most products possible with the least labor. While poor services can deter some customers, Walmart's business model depends not on the quality of service but on the low costs of its merchandise. Walmart has learned that in this economy, most customers are willing to put up with cash register waiting lines, occasionally dirty stores, and limited services if they can save some money.[23] And with their low wages, the only place Walmart workers can afford to buy groceries is at Walmart.

How Workers Rate Walmart

Walmart succeeds in part because many customers and many workers like what it has to offer. Only by understanding what makes the company attractive in today's economy can critics suggest alternatives to the business and political practices that define Walmartism. For women seeking escape from an abusive partner, for retired people who want income and social contact, for people leaving prison who can't find employment elsewhere, for young people juggling college and work, for workers who lost well-paying union jobs in the manufacturing sector, and for others with marginal or underemployment, Walmart offers a path to survival.

As Reich and Bearman observe:

> For many people, Walmart is a new home, a place where they can find friends and build community. For them, the family that they found at Walmart was, like all families, full of problems. But for many of them, the problems at Walmart were less harmful psychologically and physically than the problems that they had left behind. . . . When the choice was between working at Walmart and making a few bucks or sitting on a front porch watching nothing happen, Walmart looked pretty good. [24]

One former Walmart worker interviewed by Reich and Bearman compared the employer to an abusive spouse you know you need to leave, "but you can't find a way out." He said he would "never recommend Walmart to anyone" except for those who did not have other options. Thus, he had suggested that his cousin who dropped out of high school, his ex-girlfriend, and a friend with a criminal record look for work at the company.[25] As the economist Joan Robinson once observed, "The misery of being exploited by capitalists is nothing compared to the misery of not being exploited at all."[26]

But the comparative benefits that Walmart offers come at a cost. Informed by an extensive body of academic and journalistic investigations, further examination of how workers experience working at Walmart spells out some of the costs of low-wage and nonstandard employment.

Compensation. In 2019, Walmart reported that starting wages had increased more than 50 percent in the last three years. A 2018 survey of Walmart workers found that an astonishing 55 percent of the responding Walmart workers were food insecure. Only 14 percent of part-time associates say their earnings are enough to support themselves and their families.[27] In 2005, 46 percent of the children of Wal-Mart's 1.33 million US employees were uninsured or on Medicaid.[28] Walmart's business model is built on low wages. Its competitive edge is price and while market power and integrated supply chains help, its low wages and ability to hire and shed workers as demand waxes and wanes is what enables Walmart to offer the prices that keep customers coming.

In part in response to criticism of its low-wage policies and in part out of necessity to attract workers as the economy improved when the 2008 economic crisis abated, Walmart began to raise wages of many of its full-time workers. In 2015, Walmart CEO Doug McMillon told a meeting of Walmart workers, "It's clear to me that one of the highest priorities today must be an investment in you, our associates."[29] Walmart increased average weekly starting pay to $9 an hour in 2015, $10 in 2016, and $11 in 2018. Illustrating investors' preferences for low wages, the 2015 increase led to a 10 percent drop in the price of a Walmart share the next day and earnings per share were expected to fall by 6 to 12 percent.[30] About the same time Walmart lifted wages, it cut merit

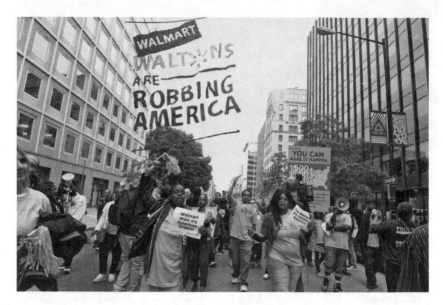

Fig. 5.1 Walmart workers in Washington, DC, call on Walmart's owners to pay a fair wage so workers do not need to use Medicaid and SNAP to get by. "My grandkids go hungry because of low pay at Walmart," said one Walmart worker.
Photo: "WALMART WORKERS, TAXPAYERS ARRESTED CALLING FOR WALMART OWNERS TO STOP ROBBING AMERICA," by UFCW International Union, licensed under CC BY-NC 2.0

increases and launched a training program that could keep workers' hourly pay at $9 for up to 18 months (See Figure 5.1).[31]

The pay increases did help to boost the wages of full-time workers. But if Walmart had chosen to invest the additional $20 billion they returned to shareholders after the 2017 Trump tax cuts instead to worker wages, the increase could have been $5.66 per hour higher, lifting many more workers above the federal poverty line.[32]

To further reduce its payroll after the pay increases, Walmart moved many workers from full-time to part-time hours. According to the 2018 survey of Walmart workers, 59 percent reported that their hours declined after the pay increases.[33] When hours worked declines, the net benefit of a pay raise is of course lost.

By 2019, Walmart reported that starting wages had increased more than 50 percent in the last three years. The average hourly pay for Walmart associates was $14.26 an hour, which at Walmart's definition of full-time as thirty-four hours per week yields an annual salary of $25,200, which is below the national poverty line for a family of four.[34] Part-time workers earn much less. Only 14 percent of part-time associates say their earnings are enough to support themselves and their families.[35]

While low wages characterize employment at Walmart, in their analysis of thousands of interviews and online complaints from Walmart workers, Reich and Bearman observe that the lack of dignity and respect associates experience at Walmart is a more salient problem than low pay. "Getting mad at Walmart's for low wages when low wages are everywhere is like getting mad at the rain," they write.[36] Moreover, as one Walmart worker from a Chicago store put it, "People are so desperate to have a job they'll work for almost anything just to have food on their table."[37] Walmart's pay policies reflect a wider trend across the retail sector. Between 1987 and 2014, labor productivity across the retail sector doubled but average real wages were flat, showing that companies, not workers, were gaining the rewards of their increased productivity.[38]

Supervision and Scheduling. In the 1980s and 1990s, Walmart pioneered the use of information technologies in order to harness its supply chains, distribution system, and retail operations to maximize revenues and profits.[39] More recently, it has adopted these technologies to monitor worker performance, giving the company, managers, and workers the evidence they need to design incentives and penalties to encourage desired behavior. Workers are watched by cameras, scanners, supervisors, and customers.

Managers use the surveillance data to shape workers' behavior. One worker from a Walmart in California described her experiences to Reich and Bearman. At first, she liked the job, but soon managers criticized her for not being able to speak Spanish with the Spanish-speaking customers, then for working the registers too slowly. "They really humiliated me, and they always made you feel that you weren't worthy. . . . Always." She soon realized that managers were making all workers feel bad, criticizing the Spanish-speaking workers for their bad English as they chided her for her bad Spanish.[40]

To enforce its rules, Walmart assigns disciplinary points for unexcused absences and other infractions. Workers get a point for every absence; a no-call/no show is four points; being more than ten minutes late to work is half a point. If associates who have been employed for more than six months accrue more than nine points in a six-month period, they are fired. New employees can be fired for accruing four points in their first six months.[41]

While this system provides ostensible transparency, in fact the many levels of supervision, from corporate to store manager to line supervisor, often result in confusion. A woman who worked at a Walmart in Dayton, Ohio, explained

> You have your immediate manager, who tells you something and you go off and do it. And then another manager sees you doing something . . . and thinking you are not busy, will give you something else to do. And your immediate manager will be, like "where are you at? Where have you been?" . . . It feels like you're getting jerked in 18 different directions, and you can't complain, because you do what the highest level manager tells you to do.[42]

Walmart's worker health policies have also attracted complaints. Based on a survey of more than one thousand Walmart workers, a 2017 report by A Better Balance, a group that advocates for fair work-family policies, found that Walmart routinely refuses to accept doctors' notes, penalizes workers who need to take care of a sick family member, and punishes employees for lawful absences.[43] The group accused Walmart of violating the Americans with Disabilities Act and the Family and Medical Leave Act.

"Walmart should fully comply with the law so that no one is illegally punished for a disability-related absence or for taking care of themselves or a loved one with a serious medical condition," said Dina Bakst, president of A Better Balance.[44] These demeaning and burdensome supervision practices make work more stressful and workers more disgruntled, contributing to Walmart's high turnover rates.

Training. Walmart has made a number of commitments to the education of its workers. In 2018, Walmart launched a new program called Live Better U that offered workers the opportunity to enroll in online degree programs in business, technology, and supply chain management. Available first at three and then six more universities with additional degree programs, the program costs participating workers $1 a day.[45] Walmart covers the additional costs— beyond financial aid—of tuition, fees, and books. In the first year, Walmart reported that seventy-five hundred employees enrolled in this program. Data are not yet available on program completion, a goal that online degree programs often struggle to achieve.

Live Better U and other programs offer some Walmart workers new opportunities to pursue their education. But as Matthew Yglesias observed in *Vox*:

> Unlike higher cash wages (which of course can be used for online college tuition as well as rent, gasoline, movie tickets, medical expenses, etc.), the tuition benefit is likely to be disproportionately appealing to people who are on the more ambitious end of the distribution. It's an effort, in other words, to make Walmart more attractive specifically to the most appealing set of potential workers, a strategy other companies have pursued in recent years.[46]

Yglesias also noted that as the labor market gets stronger, employers search for new ways to recruit and retain employees. But corporate America continues to resist increasing wages above the poverty level across the board, preferring instead to recruit and retain more desirable workers, leaving unaddressed the class and racial/ethnic gaps in access to higher education as well as healthcare, food, and housing that their wage policies have exacerbated.

Discrimination. Over the years, Walmart workers have complained of many sorts of discrimination. Part-time workers report that company policies favor full-time workers and make it difficult for those who want to work more to get the hours they need to support themselves. This contributes to a turnover rate of about 40 percent every year, a reality that puts pressures on the company to improve pay and working conditions to reduce the cost of replacing and training departing associates, especially when unemployment rates are low. In this way, an improving economy gives workers more bargaining power, although without a union it is hard for workers to accrue the power needed to overcome Walmart's opposition to what used to be standard worker rights.

Black and Latinx workers at Walmart are much more likely to report that they are involuntary part-timers and thus locked out of benefits and opportunities that go only to full-timers. In 2009, forty-five hundred Black truck drivers who applied to work for Walmart between 2001 and 2008 filed a class action lawsuit against the corporation for racial discrimination. They said Walmart turned them away in disproportionate numbers. The company denied any wrongdoing but agreed to settle for $17.5 million.[47] According to the lawsuit, a Walmart human resources director told one of the plaintiffs that he would be hired as a lower-paid laborer, rather than a truck driver, because of his "gut feeling" that the applicant had falsified his credit and driving records.

Women working at Walmart report several problems. Walmart's requirement that workers maintain open availability for changing shifts often excludes mothers of young children, who need to balance work and child care. Walmart's point system for automatic dismissal can make that balance difficult. A Latina working at a Walmart in Fort Worth, Texas, explained:

Walmart required me to have "open availability," i.e., to be ready to work 24/7, in order to qualify for full-time hours. I relied on my older children to take care of the younger ones when I worked late into the night. One afternoon at work my daughter called saying that my 10-year-old son never made it home from school. Because Walmart wouldn't let me leave without an automatic "point" on my record (and reaching nine "points" would result in immediate termination), I waited until I got off work to search for him. After the police found my son and returned him home late that night, I knew I had to restrict my availability at Walmart so I could be more present with my kid—even if it meant losing hours and income to support my family. My supervisor punished me by cutting my hours down to an average of 15 per week . . . I'm currently on food stamps, and I clean a house in my spare time for extra cash. At Walmart, you work as hard as you can and it's always the same. . . .You work and you work, but you can't get ahead.[48]

In 2018, the US Equal Employment Opportunity Commission (EEOC) filed a class action lawsuit alleging that Walmart violated the law when it refused to accommodate pregnant employees' requests for a lighter workload, a charge

Walmart denied.[49] Walmart had faced previous suits on pregnancy discrimination in 2014 and 2017.

In part as a result of these patterns of discrimination, Reich and Bearman report that Black and Latinx workers and those from poorer communities experience fewer of the benefits of working at Walmart than their better-off peers. They report fewer friends at work, talk to their managers less, and ask for help with problems less.[50]

Anti-union. Like other giant corporations that control today's economy, Walmart vigorously opposes unionization of its workers. As Lee Scott put it when he was Walmart CEO, "We like driving the car, and we're not going to give the steering wheel to anyone but us."[51] When the meat cutters at a Walmart Supercenter in Texas won a National Labor Relations Board union election in 2000, Walmart announced plans two weeks later to use prepackaged meat and eliminate butchers at that store and 179 others.[52] In 2015, Walmart abruptly announced it was closing its store in Pico Rivera, California, for six months because of "ongoing plumbing issues." That store had the country's most militant chapter of Organization United for Respect at Walmart (OUR Walmart), a group that sought to organize Walmart workers, and had staged a sit-in and several other protests.[53] When the store reopened, none of the activists were rehired.

Walmart also fires associates if they are perceived as being sympathetic toward the labor movement. Using its store video surveillance system, managers claim to have evidence of work violations without any necessity of disclosing what they "found" to the accused associate.[54]

Most workers at Walmart do not have experience with unions and may have trouble recognizing the benefits. In contrast, a worker who had worked for $20 an hour at a steel plant and now earns $9 an hour at Walmart told Reich and Bearman how her Walmart position differed from her previous job. At the steel plant, "there's union contracts, union rules, union representatives. Things that you had to go by, that the workers and the employers all had to go by." At Walmart, however, "managers feel like they can step on anybody they want. . . . They can make you do anything they want. They can make you do 20 jobs and give you your nine dollars."[55]

Walmart helped to write the anti-union playbook that characterizes Walmartism, but it is not alone in deploying this strategy. A 2009 study of over one thousand union election campaigns found that employers regularly fire union supporters (in 34 percent of union election campaigns), threaten to close the business (57 percent), threaten to reduce wages and benefits (47 percent), use mandatory one-on-one meetings with employees to interrogate them about the union (63 percent), and threaten union supporters with disciplinary action (54 percent).[56] These practices reveal that in the twenty-first-century, the labor gains of the twentieth century are under attack. Virulent anti-unionism is both a cause and consequence of low unionization rates. In the past, many employers have also opposed unionization but what seems new is the extent to which many legislators, especially those elected in the conservative waves of the last three decades, are changing the law to abrogate labor rights that had become standard.

Lack of Respect. For many Walmart workers, the cumulative impact of their interactions with the company, store managers, unit supervisors, and customers is a feeling of being disrespected. Two worker testimonials illustrate. A Walmart worker in Ohio had her hours cut so drastically that her normal life fell apart. "I had to burden my parents and ask for help," she said. "And I felt so small. I felt I couldn't do it myself. I felt like less of a person."[57] A worker in California told a similar story. "I heard the company was a good place to work. Instead, I was met with disrespect, favoritism, and lack of empathy. . . .I went from working more than 40 hours a week at $11 an hour to being scheduled for only 16 to 24 hours each week. I regularly watch other employees receive priority scheduling over me. Walmart cut my hours for one pay period and that was all it took for me to fall into debt. Right now, I just can't make ends meet."[58]

The disrespect that these workers experienced was not simply the result of a unique organizational culture or the authoritarian personalities of Walmart's executives, managers, and supervisors. Rather, it reflects the essential characteristics of many types of work in the low-wage economy, an economy structured by the imperatives of twenty-first-century capitalism. And as I show in the next section, this perception of disrespect, of being the victim of discrimination, and of having many paths to seeking a better life shut down has profound effects on worker, family, and community well-being.

KINDERCARE

KinderCare, described in chapter 3, is the largest for-profit company providing early childhood education in the United States. It operates almost two thousand early learning centers and afterschool programs at elementary schools and manages child care programs and benefits for more than four hundred corporations. It educates 185,000 children each day and employs 32,000 people of whom about 30,000 are teachers.[59] In 2015, KinderCare was acquired by the private equity firm Partners Group, a Switzerland-based private markets investment manager with $83 billion in assets under management and serving more than 850 institutional investors.[60]

Working at KinderCare demonstrates some of the distinct features of employment in the fast-growing care economy, jobs that require looking after the physical, psychological, emotional, and developmental needs of other people.

Child care workers, home care attendants, nurses' aides, nannies—these and other job titles are part of this sector of largely female, disproportionately Black, Latinx,or immigrant workers in low-wage, often precarious jobs.

Unlike Walmart and Uber workers, whose experiences have been studied and documented by academics, journalists, and activists, few such accounts are available for workers at the much smaller KinderCare. To understand what KinderCare staff valued and disliked about their work, I reviewed more than forty-two hundred staff ratings posted on five online employer rating platforms.[61] An examination of these posts shows a kaleidoscope of reactions to working at KinderCare, a range that mirrors some of the opinions of Walmart workers.

I have had the best experience of my life working here. . . . I love coming to work every morning. I have a great relationship with my coworkers and direct supervisors. The center director always checks in to make sure we are happy and she's quick to resolve any issues that come about. The families are very appreciative of the work we do for their children and they are genuinely nice to their teachers. It is an environment filled with professionalism, respect, integrity, and honesty. *An experienced employee*

KinderCare is a horrible place to work. They pay practically nothing, and they expect you to go above and beyond for everyone else there. The management is terrible, they don't care about you and they don't care about the families that go there. *Former assistant teacher, Wisconsin*

KinderCare is a great employer in my opinion especially for a mom trying to get back in the workforce after having a child. They offer you to bring your child to the center you work at for a fraction of the fee. They are very focused on training employees and giving second chances as well. *Current director of a KinderCare center*

Working in this company set my life to an all-time low. The managers never pulled their weight. It was a very negative place and being that I spent 40 hours or more a week there, I could no longer function without going home in tears, angry and or shut down emotionally. . . . This "cattle call" of a place is just a large, run for the money, business. . . . Please be aware that the miserable workers there are the ones with a passion for children, but don't get the appreciation or money they deserve. *A former teacher from Connecticut*

While any workplace with hundreds of sites and tens of thousands of workers will get mixed reviews, what might explain these wildly different reactions? Like Walmart, working conditions at KinderCare are the product of corporate culture; the personalities and skills of the site managers and frontline supervisors; and the class, racial, and gender composition of the site's staff.

Thus, the experience of working varies considerably across sites. In addition, experiences vary over time. As KinderCare struggled to respond to the 2008 recession, when demand for child care fell but not investors' expectations for regular returns, the company closed sites, laid off workers, and changed pay and hours. Later, with the influx of private capital, it was able to expand again.

Despite these variations, certain worker reactions seemed more consistent. Far more workers complained on the rating sites about low pay than praised generous salaries. "Benefits and raises are promised but never given," alleged a former assistant teacher in Connecticut. "Regardless of how much I love what I do that does not pay my bills," wrote a current teacher. "I can't afford rent let alone mortgage where I live making under $14 an hour. It is ridiculous."

According to Indeed, the job rating site, based on reports from 1,735 KinderCare employees, average hourly pay for teachers was $12.24 and $11.89 for assistant teachers, about $20,000 a year for full-time workers and well below the federal poverty line for a family of four. Center directors earned on average $45,670 per year.[62] Customer care specialists, charged with enrolling and serving parents and business customers, earn an average of $30 an hour, more than twice as much as teachers, perhaps reflecting KinderCare's roots in the retail sector and its leaders' beliefs that establishing emotional connections to customers is as important for keeping customers as the quality of classroom teaching and learning.

Another recurrent issue for KinderCare workers was the quality of supervision and site management. A former assistant teacher form Indiana wrote, "Barely any training, no sense of urgency in management, no room for growth." Long or irregular hours was a common complaint. "You're expected to work ridiculous shifts with long hours, yet if you get close to overtime all of a sudden, they'll give you a long break or cut hours, so you don't get that extra pay. Many times, I was forced to work 8+ hour shifts with either no break or a very short one," wrote one teacher.

Like at Walmart, KinderCare workers perceived a lack of respect from their employer. An experienced teacher wrote, "Management sucks and they don't care about anyone but themselves. . . .They just forget we are working with little children every day and need respect." A former teacher from Maryland wrote, "If you didn't bow down to management, you will get the least respect."

Despite these complaints, many workers wrote about what they loved about their job. A few quotes illustrate how working at KinderCare could be fulfilling:

I love the diversity of the staff and families.
I loved my kids and for the most part my parents.
Your classroom co-workers are the only thing that helps to keep you sane.
It gets very chaotic at times but once you realize you are shaping (the kids') future, it gives you a great feeling. I don't only change diapers I make lesson plans that give kids the opportunities to learn and grow.

Of note, not a single worker of the forty-two hundred who posted comments on the job rating sites mentioned that KinderCare workers were not unionized and had no organized voice in managing the corporation. KinderCare has a long history of opposing unionization. When service sector unions such as the Service Employees International Union (SEIU) convinced the legislature in Washington and other states to allow low-wage service sector workers to unionize in 2008, KinderCare successfully lobbied Washington legislators to exempt child care workers from this law.[63]

In 2016, an SEIU local succeeded in organizing child care workers at a KinderCare-sponsored center at the University of Southern California. A month later, KinderCare closed the center. Gina Sandoval, a teacher who helped to organize the union, assessed the long-term consequences of their unionization:

> If I was working in another KinderCare center and I heard about this center being unionized, and there were bad things happening at my center, I would gather up my teachers and say, "if they can do it, we can do it too." It's pretty scary for KinderCare to hear that.[64]

A spokesperson for the SEIU local gave a more pessimistic view. "Employees are also feeling very discouraged. They risked standing up to the boss to bring urgently necessary improvements for the kids and families. They have said repeatedly that their struggle to form a union was never about making more money. It was about having a voice."[65] But giving workers a voice is precisely what most owners of low-wage businesses do not want. Such a move could threaten their ability to control their major cost, their workers, especially in a volatile economy, highly competitive markets, and privatizing sectors.

KinderCare and other employers in the care economy also use the emotional bonds their workers feel to clients to engage their allegiance and discourage worker actions that jeopardize corporate control. The teacher who observed that the most "miserable workers there are the ones with a passion for children" recognized the implicit threat that KinderCare posed to its workers. "If you love your children," as another worker put it, "and want to give your kids the opportunities to learn and grow," then "don't challenge our way of doing business because the kids will suffer."[66] Home care and nursing home attendants, nannies, and hospital workers will recognize this all-too-common threat to low-wage care economy workers. By exploiting workers' connections to those they care for, companies shift workers' calculus of the costs and benefits of resistance, leading to benefits for their students or patients but growing burdens on the workers' physical and mental health.

UBER

Uber is the world's largest transportation network company, defined as businesses that use mobile apps to enable people to secure rides from drivers who use their own vehicles and GPS smartphones to identify pick-up locations and inform customers of the precise time the car will arrive. By 2017, Uber operated in 64 countries and 630 cities worldwide and had provided 5 billion rides to passengers. By early 2018, it had 3 million active drivers worldwide, more than 500,000 in the United States.[67] In 2019, Uber reported global revenue of $14.1 billion, up 28 percent from the prior year, but the company was still deep in the red. Uber's origin story states the idea was born on a cold winter evening in Paris, when Travis Kalanick and Garrett Camp, its founders, could not get a ride.

Uber, also known as a ride-sharing company, says its mission is to "ignite opportunity by setting the world in motion." Uber uses the four key components of gig (or platform) economy businesses: online platforms or mobile apps to facilitate transactions among the company, workers, and customers; a user-based rating system; flexibility for workers in choosing hours; and the expectation that workers provide the tools or assets needed to complete their job, in this case a car.[68]

Two deep trends enabled the rise of companies like Uber. First, the development and dissemination of digital and cell phone technologies permitted Uber to create a platform for swift, simple communication between customers, workers, and companies. Second, the Great Recession put so many people out of work or cut their incomes that a ready supply of labor was available. Gig companies like Airbnb and Uber offered the bonus of allowing those with too little income to monetize the assets they had been able to acquire—their homes and cars.

Like other workers, Uber drivers report both positive and negative characteristics of their working conditions. Workers report such well-liked features as:

- "I'm my own boss basically. And people like that feeling. People love that feeling. To be able to work whenever you want, there's no beating that."
- "I drive like 30 hours or so per week, not really full-time. Not really part-time either. I pick whenever I want. It's nice."
- "I have a business I run during the day and this is just extra income. I just do it at night for a few hours usually. . . . So I'm trying to just supplement my income."[69]

For other drivers, social interactions with customers provided an antidote to loneliness or boredom, an easy way to have low-risk human contact and pass the time at work.

But the autonomy, flexibility, and control that Uber offers its drivers has some costs, some inherent in the gig economy and others the consequence of Uber's profit-maximization strategies. Again, some quotes from Uber drivers illustrate these concerns:

> They have their own policies and sometimes they change their policies. Last year it was very good . . . but this year they rode down the rates and they raised some other expenses. . . . No matter what (Uber) gets their percentage.
>
> I tried Uber because back then you can easily in a weekend make 300 or 400 dollars. Now it's up and down, it is not something you can trust. If you want to make money with UberX (a discount version of the service), you have to make 80 hours working and yet you barely make the same as taxi. It's too much.
>
> They have this rating thing some people might misunderstand. I've seen a lot of people that have very new cars, stuck in the middle. . . . If their rating goes down, they might get suspended for a little bit. Imagine you deactivate his account, but he has a new car he has to pay for![70]

What accounts for these different perceptions? A key factor is the heterogeneity of drivers' work experience. According to one 2015 study, 51 percent of Uber's drivers work fifteen hours a week or less, 30 percent work sixteen to thirty-four hours, 12 percent work thirty-five to forty-nine hours a week and 7 percent work fifty hours or more.[71] Strikingly, more than half quit within a year,[72] bringing to drivers' lives all the stress that leaving one job and looking for another imposes.

How much do Uber drivers make? A Buzzfeed investigation in 2016 found that Uber drivers make on average $10.87 an hour. At forty hours per week, this translates into an annual salary of less than $23,000.[73] In 2017, the Federal Trade Commission fined Uber $20 million for deception based on its recruitment ads for drivers that claimed they could make $90,000 a year.[74]

Some drivers use Uber as a career transition after losing a job or moving to a new place. But the majority of full-time drivers depend on Uber for their livelihood. And it is these drivers who are most exploited by Uber's algorithms. In this way the gig economy perpetuates, even exacerbates, the class and racial/ethnic stratifications of the economy. Moreover, drivers who work the most hours and serve low-income communities are at higher risk of robbery, sexual assault, or other crimes, an occasional but recurring experience of Uber drivers.[75]

In its marketing to recruit drivers, Uber masks the complexity of these experiences. For her book on Uber, Alex Rosenblat interviewed 125 drivers, took 400 of her own rides with Uber, and analyzed online discussion boards that Uber drivers use. She observes that Uber "promises drivers freedom, flexibility, and independence," but "for legal purposes classifies them as independent contractors, meaning they are largely excluded from the employment and labor law protections to which employees are entitled."[76] In a 2015 court case in California, Uber's lawyer explained, "Fundamentally, the commercial relationship between these drivers and transportation providers and Uber is one where they are our customer, where we license to them our software, and we receive a fee for doing that."[77] By labeling its drivers as customers, Uber sidesteps the legal and moral obligations of an employer.

Rosenblat also notes that Uber replaces human bosses with algorithms that serve as a "virtual automated manager."[78] While algorithms may be less nasty or bossy than humans, they are even more relentless in ensuring that Uber maximizes revenues from its drivers and maintains control of key parts of the work experience. A driver from Raleigh, North Carolina, told her, "They keep bonking around with the rates and different terms of service. You gotta log in, and all of a sudden there's new terms and conditions; and if you don't sign, you can't drive."[79] In general, Uber takes for itself 20 to 28 percent of the drivers' revenues but constantly changing rules and rates make it difficult for drivers to predict their income.

Rosenblat asked drivers if they would advise a friend to quit their job to work for Uber. One New York driver said, "I wouldn't recommend the driving industry to anyone anymore. It used to be very good. Now you kill yourself. You have to work thirteen, fourteen hours. Usually if you have family you cannot work that long. Now you have to work six or seven days, twelve to fourteen hours. . . . Uber, Lyft, they take too much." Another driver observed, "That all depends on the job you are quitting."

Walmart, KinderCare, and Uber illustrate the changing working conditions that characterize the twenty-first-century workforce. While they differ in important aspects, they also share common characteristics. All three pay low wages and offer few benefits to many of their workers. All use independent contractor or contracted-out status to keep labor costs low. The working conditions and desirability of work in all three is set by complex interactions among workers, on-site managers, and corporate leaders, requiring workers to constantly juggle competing demands. In the retail side of these three businesses, interactions with customers give workers some of the human interactions they crave but also provide employers with an added tool to manage and control their workers. In all three, intrusive and changeable systems of supervision aggravate workers and cause considerable distress. All three employers aggressively counter any efforts to unionize but in each, workers are seeking to create other forms of collective organizations that can protect and advance their rights. All three employers have high turnover rates, a characteristic that profoundly disrupts individual and family physical and mental health.

These company profiles show some of the ways that changes in modern capitalism transformed how jobs influence the well-being of workers, their families, and their communities. Once again, globalization, financialization, deregulation, privatization, and new technologies are triggers for these alterations.

As a result of globalization, if one country changes its wage, benefit, or worker protection rules, Walmart and other transnational corporations can move their operations to a more favorable climate or, better yet, use its economic power to persuade that country to revise or withdraw the problematic changes. While both capital and labor move around the world much more rapidly and easily than they did a century ago, money seeking new profits encounters fewer obstacles in its journeys than do workers seeking better jobs. Global business and political elites have enacted trade, migration, and labor policies that put them in control of who can move when and where, choosing approaches that give them the workers they need at a price they can afford.

Whether US companies need call center operators in India, autoworkers in Mexico or Vietnam, nurses from South Korea or Ireland, or foreign-born engineers for tech start-ups in in Silicon Valley or Seattle, they search the world for workers they need and develop employment practices that enable them to hire those they need. American businesses have always depended on imported labor; what globalization has changed is the scope of their reach and the ease with which they can move either work or workers to best meet their employment needs at the lowest possible cost. As a result, any national allegiance that companies felt to their home country has been diminished, making them ready to move factories, jobs, capital, and tax responsibilities to whatever site will help jack up their return on investment.

Although the specific dynamics vary by industry, the world's economy now has global supply chains, global labor forces, global trade rules, and a global banking system. If workers, regulations, or government in one country become unsatisfactory, corporations can and do move operations to another. For workers, this reality requires that aspirations for better pay, benefits, or working conditions always need to be balanced against the fear that such demands will lead their employer to another, more accommodating nation, a dynamic that has been called a "race to the bottom."[80]

As manufacturing declines, profits from speculation exceed those from making things. As the financial sector grows in importance and power, investors move capital into financial ventures. Since their primary goal is higher returns, pressure to cut costs is high, contributing to lower wages for workers, who are often seen as an adjustable expenditure, rather than an asset worthy of investment through higher pay, benefits, or training. For managers, the pressure is to grow profits, with higher pay or bonuses the incentive. Together these trends increase income inequality.

In its SEC filing to become a public company, Uber told investors, "As we aim to reduce driver incentives to improve our financial performance, we expect driver dissatisfaction will generally increase,"[81] leading Uber to increase its investment in driverless vehicle technologies, a key way to cut labor costs and counter driver demands for pay increases. Taxi and rideshare drivers in the United States, Australia, Great Britain, France, Nigeria, Kenya, Chile, Brazil, and other countries organized a global protest in advance of Uber's initial public offering (IPO), [82] perhaps highlighting one more factor contributing to the investor skepticism that led to the disappointing demand for Uber shares.[83]

How are financialization and globalization connected? As investors are able to find opportunities around the world, they move their capital to wherever the returns are highest. One metric captures the relative importance of financial transactions in the global economy. According to the Bank for International Settlements, in 2016 foreign exchange trading—financial transaction—totaled $5.1 trillion a day compared to only $80 billion a day in trades of goods and services, a ratio of more than sixty to one.[84] In general, moving money is more profitable than making goods or delivering services. As profits from moving money increased, investments that created jobs decreased, and many of those jobs that were created were nontraditional ones with low wages.

The combination of financialization and globalization also makes the world's economy more unstable. The bursting of the housing speculation bubble in 2008 sparked financial crises around the world, leading to loss of jobs and financial insecurity. For the individual worker, as President Harry Truman once observed, "It's a recession when your neighbor loses his job; it's a depression when you lose your own."

Walmart participates in the financialization of the economy in various ways. Although it does not offer its associates pensions, it does offer them the opportunity to save for retirement in a company-organized fund, in which it invests the saving of more than 1.2 million employees in a fund managed by Merrill, a subsidiary of Bank of America. This option offers Walmart one more opportunity to extract additional revenues and to transfer the risk of losing their savings from the employer back to the workers themselves.

Walmart also uses financial markets for other business transactions. For example, the company created its own line of credit cards, proprietary prepaid debit cards, wire transfers, check-cashing services, and other low-fee financial products, in order to ensure that its customers, including its workers, can buy everything they need at Walmart without fear of running out of cash. In these and other ways, Walmart shows that even a company that makes and sells tangible products is tied to the financial sector and uses its reach to find additional ways to make money and transfer risk.[85]

For investors, economic and innovation disruptions can create new opportunities for profit. For workers, however, these disruptions can put a home, a job, pension, healthcare access, or food security at risk, one more way that the costs and benefits of modern capitalism are inequitably distributed. At KinderCare, increases and declines in private equity investments and changes in the economy led the company to open and close child care centers, creating and ending jobs. In the 1980s, the company sold millions of dollars' worth of junk bonds to diversify into fields other than day care.[86] When the 2008 financial crisis led these speculative ventures to fail, KinderCare was forced to close its less profitable centers. The job insecurity contributed to an annual staff turnover rate of 48 percent, a quantitative measure of the disrupted lives of both the children in these classrooms and the teachers who taught them. As one KinderCare teacher posted on the Indeed employer ranking site, "Be careful of this company, known in the industry for hiring and firing quickly. Does not spend time and money to invest and train employees. Use and abuse you."[87]

Deregulation also changes the status of workers. Deregulation of antitrust rules facilitates monopoly concentration, which reduces worker bargaining power. Both Walmart and Uber use the market power from their dominant share of their markets to resist their employees' efforts to increase pay and benefits and improve working conditions. Deregulation of worker protections jeopardizes the health and safety gains of previous decades and compromises the capacity of government agencies to meet emerging threats or identify populations at risk of emerging work hazards.

Privatization of functions that had been mainly public and the growing encroachment of market mechanisms and thinking into previously public spaces also contributed to changes in work. For workers in healthcare, education, sanitation, and public safety, privatization led to weakening of labor unions; erosion of salaries, benefits, and job security; and higher unemployment.[88] Whereas teachers in public schools and preschools often have strong unions or are seeking to unionize, private companies like KinderCare or the companies that operate charter schools rarely tolerate unions.

In places where transportation, public utilities, telephone services or water were privatized, workers in these sectors lost pay and a voice in their workplace. When the person sitting across the table in labor negotiations is the representative of a global corporation rather than a public official, issues like pay and gender equity, work-family balance, or living wages often fall off the agenda.

Proponents of privatization argue that it maximizes efficiency, even if it may reduce equity. Since more efficient delivery of education, healthcare, electricity, or water could in theory reduce the costs and improve the quality of these services, low- and middle-income workers could benefit in their roles as consumers. In practice, however, increases in access appear to be accompanied by increases in price, negating any potential equity-enhancing benefit.[89] In human services, such as the child care that KinderCare provides, privatization seems to contribute to widening gaps in access to these services.[90]

Advances in information technology, artificial intelligence, and robotics are also leading to dramatic changes in work. New technologies have always changed work and in the past century, mechanization and computerization dramatically reduced the number of people growing food, producing cars, and working as secretaries. Today, the pace of change is even more rapid. The McKinsey Global Institute has predicted that by 2030, automation will destroy more than 37 million jobs in the United States and 375 million worldwide.[91] Based on a modeling exercise, researchers at Oxford University estimated that machine learning, artificial intelligence, and robotics place about 47 percent of the jobs in the United States in 2010 at "high risk" of automation in the coming years.[92]

In the twentieth century, flipping burgers at a fast-food outlet symbolized low-wage work but in the twenty-first century this is one of hundreds of tasks that has been targeted for automation. Andrew Puzder, the former CEO of fast-food chains Hardee's and Carl's Jr., and President Trump's initial choice as secretary of labor, explained an employer's rationale for replacing fast-food service workers with robots: "They're always polite, they always upsell, they never take a vacation, they never show up late, there's never a slip-and-fall, or an age, sex or race discrimination case."[93] And at Walmart, robots are replacing workers to shelve and barcode food, gather products for home delivery, and run the checkout aisles.

Another recent change in work has been the growth of service-sector jobs. This results from three trends: technologies that reduce the demand for labor in the manufacturing sector, overproduction of consumer goods that led to declining profits in manufacturing, and capital's search for new profit centers. Workers in this sector provide a service rather than make a product, including jobs in retail, banks, hotels, real estate, education, healthcare, social services, computer services, and other industries. Between 1980 and 2005, the share of labor hours in service occupations in the United States grew by 30 percent after having been flat or declining in the three prior decades.[94] Service jobs generally pay lower wages than manufacturing jobs. As public-sector jobs in healthcare, education, social services, and other municipal functions were privatized beginning in the 1980s, the wages for these transferred jobs also fell and many previously public workers lost the protection of unions that some government jobs had provided. In this and other ways, privatization contributes to rising inequality.[95]

NEW TYPES OF WORK

These changes in the dynamics of capitalism have led to the emergence of several new types of work. Together, these alterations have exacerbated some old occupational health problems and created new threats. Understanding the common social and economic causes of these changes and their impact on health and equity is an essential first step toward reversing these adverse consequences on the well-being of workers.

Precarious employment describes jobs of limited duration with limited protection from labor-market uncertainties and often oppressive treatment at work and limited worker control over wages, benefits, and working conditions.[96] It has blossomed as employers sought wage flexibility, fewer constraints on hiring and firing, and relaxed employment protection policies.[97] Business owners needed this freedom, they said, to respond to the increased competition of globalized and deregulated markets. Precarious jobs usually fail to offer the higher pay, more generous benefits, job security, and unionization that some manufacturing-sector jobs in high-income countries provided in the mid-twentieth century. Both globalization and automation have contributed to the rise of precarious jobs. Part-time work at Walmart or Uber is an example of a precarious job.

While precarious employment has always been part of capitalism, the economist Guy Standing has postulated the emergence of a new class he calls "the precariat." He writes that the growing number of precarious workers have "no secure occupational identity; no occupational narrative they can give to their lives . . . have to do a lot of work-for-labor relative to labor . . . that is not remunerated; they have to retrain constantly, network, apply for new jobs, and fill out forms of one sort or another." He also notes that the precariat is the "first working class in history that, as a norm, is expected to have a level of education that is greater than the labor they are expected to perform or expect to obtain . . . the source of intense status frustration."[98]

Contingent labor has been defined by the US Department of Labor as workers who do not expect their jobs to last or who report that their jobs are temporary. They have no implicit or explicit contract for ongoing employment. In 2017, BLS estimated that 3.8 percent of workers—5.9 million people in 2017—are contingent workers, a decrease from 2005.[99] This category includes consultants, independent contractors, on-call workers, and workers provided by contract firms. Studies show that contingent workers earn less, are more likely to live in poverty, receive fewer benefits, and are more likely to be young or Hispanic than workers in standard worker arrangements.[100] The pressures that lead employers to hire contingent workers are similar to those encouraging precarious labor but contingent workers include a wider range of job titles, including highly paid consultants or contract workers. Contingent labor gives employers the flexibility to respond quickly to the changing demands of financialization—getting rid of one thousand contingent workers to boost quarterly returns is a much simpler task than laying off one thousand permanent employees. For Walmart and Uber, one of the advantages of having "associates" or "partners" as their labor force is these just-in-time workers can be hired, fired, or rehired as the need arises. In 2020, the COVID-19 pandemic and its economic consequences reinforced the value of contingent workers to employers—and the costs to workers.

One way that big corporations control their labor costs is by contracting out tasks that can be done less expensively or more efficiently by other, cheaper workers. A list of some of the tasks that have been contracted out reads like an ad for the jobs of the twenty-first century: human resources, research and development, building services, recycling, regulation and compliance, accounting, credit card collections, call centers, mortgage and check processing, information technology and data processing, logistics and transportation, machine maintenance, cable installation, food services and food processing, parts manufacturing and assembly, laundry, housekeeping, diagnostic labs and MRI scans, and clinical research trials.[101]

The gig economy describes contingent work in the digital economy. Some of the largest gig economy employers in the United States are Uber and Lyft, transportation services; TaskRabbit, a platform that connects freelance workers with customers who want help with everyday tasks such as cleaning, moving, delivery, and handyman work; and Care.com, which provides child care, adult and senior care, pet care, and home care to customers who are seeking caregivers. Other services such as Airbnb allow individuals to rent their homes. In 2016, 24 percent of Americans reported earning some pay from the gig economy but it served as the main source of income for only 2 percent of the workforce. While the gig economy offers workers expanded autonomy on work hours, employers can terminate gig workers simply by deactivating them from the platform. One analyst observed that for gig workers, "uncertainty and insecurity are the price for extreme flexibility."[102] Gig jobs also provide fewer protections to both workers and customers.

Earlier online businesses such as Craigslist and eBay set the stage for the gig economy, but it was the later introduction of new digital technologies that enabled the peer-to-peer interactions that now characterize the "sharing economy." Unlike other forms of nonstandard employment, the gig economy attracts younger and more educated workers; most gig economy workers are between the ages of eighteen and thirty-four, and many are college educated. In 2009, journalist Tina Brown wrote, "To people I know in the bottom income brackets, living paycheck to paycheck, the Gig Economy has been old news for years. What's new is the way it's hit the demographic that used to assume that a college degree from an elite school was the passport to job security."[103] As growth of middle- and high-income jobs continued to stagnate after the recovery from the Great Recession, the gig economy sometimes serves as a social safety net for workers with high income volatility or gaps in employment.[104]

The label of sharing economy implies carpooling, workers cooperatives, and couch-surfing, alternatives to capitalism. But in reality, for many gig economy workers the experience is similar to the early days of industrialization, when no laws set limits on working hours, overtime pay, or benefits. In this way, the tech moguls who promote the sharing economy have done more to change how people think about work than they have changed the conditions of work for those they employ. By making the need for extra work a normal experience, they have obscured the reality that it has become increasingly difficult for one worker working one job to earn enough to support a reasonable life.

Low-wage labor, another broad category, is the fastest-growing job sector in the United States, accounting for most new jobs created since the 2008 recession. According to a recent report from the Brookings Institution:

> More than 53 million people, or 44% of all workers ages 18 to 64 in the United States, earn low hourly wages. More than half (56%) are in their prime working years of 25–50, and this age group is also the most likely to be raising children (43%). They are concentrated in a relatively small number of occupations, and many face economic hardship and difficult roads to higher-paying jobs. Slightly more than half are the sole earners in their families or make major contributions to family income. Nearly one-third live below 150% of the federal poverty line (about $36,000 for a family of four), and almost half have a high school diploma or less.[105]

Low-wage workers are concentrated in the food service, home care, cleaning services, and agricultural sectors. Many are involuntary part-time workers and they are disproportionally female, Black and Latinx. Low-wage workers often struggle with unpredictable and unstable work schedules, disrupting their families and their finances. In 2017, 78 percent of very low-wage workers lacked healthcare through their jobs.[106] Some low-wage workers are in the gig economy and some, but not all, have precarious jobs. They work in both traditional and nonstandard employment categories.

The informal economy is considered "a separate marginal economy not directly tied to the formal economy, providing income or a safety net to the poor," as defined in 1972 by the International Labour Office.[107] Another definition describes informal economy workers as those who engage in productive activities that are not taxed or registered by the government.[108] The informal sector includes some care workers such as nannies and maids, construction, and others working "off the books" and clearly illegal jobs such as procuring sex workers or selling drugs or guns.

In the last century, most scholars considered the informal economy as a phenomenon of low- and middle-income countries. More recently, however, some have emphasized the connections between formal- and informal-economy jobs in high-income countries as well.[109] As global clothing corporations based in wealthy nations contract out work to home-based sewers, street drug dealers sell the excess opioid painkillers manufactured by major drug companies, and street vendors in South Africa buy supersized food packages from the nearest global supermarket outlet to sell at a discount in smaller sizes in their townships, the boundary between formal and informal economies becomes blurred.

As the United States and Western Europe have tightened immigration and safety net policies, the informal economy becomes the default employment choice for many immigrants, especially those who are undocumented. It is estimated that 75 percent of day laborers in the United States are undocumented immigrants, consigned to the informal economy because of lack of papers and therefore unprotected from wage theft, safety hazards, and low pay.[110] For discouraged and underemployed workers, the informal economy offers opportunities for earning income. While enumerating the size of the informal economy—sometimes called the shadow economy—is complex, one study comparing its size in 143 countries between 1996 and 2014 estimated that in the United States in that period, the informal economy accounted for just over 8 percent of gross domestic product.[111] A 2015 survey found that about 20 percent of non-retired adults at least twenty-one years old in the US generated some income informally that year.[112]

How many workers are employed in these sometime overlapping sectors? While differences in definitions preclude a definitive answer, a 2018 report by the Bureau of Labor Statistics of the US Department of Labor estimated that 15.5 million US workers—about 10 percent of all workers—have "alternative arrangements" for their primary employment, including independent contractors, on-call workers, temporary help agency workers, and workers provided by contract firms. Notably, this count does not include workers who have a traditional main job but engage in some alternative work on the side (e.g., a Lyft driver who works occasionally on weekends but has a full-time job during the week).[113]

In 2015, 42 percent of American workers—more than 33 million workers— earned hourly wages of less than $15 an hour, and these low-wage workers were more likely to be women, Blacks, or Latinxs and more likely to work in the service sector.[114] Workers making the minimum wage today ($7.25 at the federal level) make 25 percent less than they did in 1968, after adjusting for inflation.

The National Employment Law Project calculates that by 2024, workers in all fifty states will need at least $15 per hour to afford the basic needs of food, education, and shelter.[115] Others make the case that even $15 an hour already makes it hard to survive in many places in the United States. Moreover, six of the ten largest occupations with median wages less than $15 are also among the jobs projected to grow the most by 2022, including retail salespersons, food service workers, janitors and cleaners, nursing assistants, and personal care aides, suggesting that in this economy, low-wage jobs will continue to grow more rapidly than better-paid positions.

Scholars of work and labor history struggle diligently to accurately characterize the complex ecology of the twenty-first-century workforce and enumerate its constituents. But these sometimes overlapping categories can obscure the shared characteristics and common causes for growth of nonstandard, contingent, gig, low-wage, and informal jobs. Work influences health via three pathways—work arrangements such as pay, benefits, and rights to organize; workplace exposures to toxic physical and social conditions; and workers' capacities to balance home and work responsibilities. Examining how each of these pathways influences the well-being of workers and their families can yield insights into the changes needed to improve worker health.

CHANGES IN THREATS TO WELL-BEING

In the second half of the twentieth-century United States, compared to the past and future, workers in the manufacturing sector and increasingly the service sector were more likely to be organized, more likely to be able to stay in one job for many years, and more likely to enjoy the benefits of regularly enforced health and safety rules and other worker-protection policies. Women, recent immigrants, and Black and Latinx workers were less likely to receive these benefits, making working conditions and work arrangements an important cause of gender, race, and other inequities in health.

WORK ORGANIZATION AND HEALTH

In this century, as a result of the growth of precarious, contingent, low–wage, and informal employment, more workers in the United States end up with less income than they need to support themselves and their families; fewer social benefits such as healthcare, pensions, and sick leave; less ability to join and benefit from unions; and a diminished voice to influence their daily lives in the workplace. Each of these characteristics of work has influences on one's health.

Low wages. Low wages jeopardize health in obvious and not-so-obvious ways. Insufficient income makes it more difficult to get necessities of life such as adequate housing, healthy food, and medical care. Low-wage workers are employed in riskier settings, and thus experience higher rates of injuries and stress and have less access to the resources that can restore health or prevent deterioration, a gap that puts them at further disadvantage. As Samuel

Broder, former director of the National Cancer Institute, has observed, poverty has been shown to be a carcinogen,[116] thus elevating the cancer risks of low-wage workers who cannot afford protection against many carcinogens such as living in polluted neighborhoods, eating unhealthy diets, or working with asbestos. Low wages often force both parents to work to bring home an income to support the family or take a second or even a third job. These added work obligations give less time to sleep, an activity essential to well-being, and give parents less time to spend with their children and fewer resources to protect them, putting the physical and mental health of their children at risk.

The cumulative burdens of long working hours, child care, and the time needed to allocate limited resources to ensure the survival of the household often impose a sense of time urgency on low-wage workers, a feeling associated with mental and physical health problems.[117] Both the rich and poor experience time poverty but the wealthy can buy back time in the market. They can, for example, pay maids to clean their houses, nannies to care for their children, and accountants to file their tax returns. For low-wage workers, the added burden of time poverty further depletes their capacity to protect their health. In these ways, low wages contribute to added health burdens via all three pathways discussed here.

Mental Health. Most employed adults spend more waking time at work than in any other single place, making workplaces a powerful influence on mental and psychological well-being. In the industrial age, occupational health researchers focused their attention on work's impact on physical health through toxic exposures, workplace injuries, and cardiovascular risks. Of course, these hazards still exist and continue to endanger workers. But changes in the characteristics of work and new insights into the complex and intimate relationships between physical and mental health have focused recent attention on the psychological impact of work.

Work affects psychological well-being directly by eliciting biological, neurological, and emotional responses that can trigger or exacerbate depression, anxiety, and other common psychological disorders. Work organization also influences psychological well-being indirectly by creating conflicts between work and family demands, encouraging unhealthy coping behaviors such as tobacco, alcohol, and drug use, or by exposing workers to repeated gender, racial, or other forms of discrimination and hostility from supervisors, coworkers, and customers. Most profoundly, working conditions can undermine an individual's sense of dignity and self-respect, essential foundations for health and mental health.[118]

Depression and anxiety exact a growing burden on personal and public health. Mental and substance-use disorders are consistently the leading causes of years of life lived with disability worldwide and also contribute to premature mortality.[119] Depression is a leading cause of suicide, which accounts for eight hundred thousand deaths around the world each year. Rates of depression and anxiety appear to be increasing and rates of depression are increased by poverty, unemployment, life events such as the death of a family member or friend or a relationship breakup, physical illness, and problems caused by alcohol and drug use.[120] Globally, the number of people with anxiety disorders, characterized by feelings of anxiety and fear, increased 15 percent between 2005 and 2015, primarily because of population growth and aging.

Suicide is associated with a variety of working arrangements including low wages, unemployment, irregular schedules, and stressful exposures.[121] One study comparing suicide rates in states with different levels of minimum wages found that a one-dollar increase in the real minimum wage was associated on average with a 1.9 percent decrease in the annual state suicide rate in adjusted analyses. The authors concluded that a one-dollar increase in the hourly minimum wage nationally would result in about eight thousand fewer deaths by suicide each year.[122]

Unlike most health conditions, which follow a consistent social gradient in which people with lower socioeconomic positions and more disadvantages experience higher rates of illness, depressive and anxiety disorders present a more complex picture. For these conditions, individuals in the middle strata seem to have higher rates than those in lower and upper positions.[123] Understanding the causes of this discrepancy may help to provide insights into how recent changes in workplace organization influence the psychological well-being of workers.

One explanation of the unusual pattern of depression and anxiety is that workers who experience what sociologists call "contradictory class locations,"[124] defined as work roles that are neither wholly wage laborers nor fully owners of the means of production, are subject to unique pressures and conflicts. Seth Prins, a psychiatric epidemiologist, and his colleagues at Columbia University and the University of Toronto, analyzed data from a national study of 21,859 individuals and found that compared to workers and owners, managers and supervisors had significantly higher rates of depressive and anxiety disorders. They concluded that "contradictory class locations may entail greater exposure to exogenous exposures" such as experiencing responsibility for failure at work, being the target for complaints from both workers and owners, and having chronic conflicts with those above and below them in the work hierarchy.[125]

While prior work on "contradictory class positions" has focused mostly on standard forms of work and well-defined job categories such as worker, supervisor, manager, and owner, new work forms in twenty-first-century capitalism explode these categories. For many workers in growing nonstandard sectors, these contradictory roles define the jobs. At Walmart, KinderCare, and Uber, as at other large workplaces, the complex interactions among different levels of supervisors, workers, and customers and the sometime-arbitrary delegation of authority and responsibility put many staff in these contradictory locations. Independent contractors may work for many employers, giving the appearance of autonomy. But their tasks are set by the business that contracts with them, making some dependent on the sometime-changing whims of their employers, the emotional experiences associated with depression and anxiety.

While more empirical research is needed, nonstandard forms of work generated by modern capitalism may be exposing millions of workers to more frequent psychological experiences that contribute to depression and anxiety. Emotions like loneliness, isolation, alienation, conflict-induced anger at work or at home, fear of losing needed work, and low self-esteem from failing to meet competing demands of co-workers, supervisors, and family—and how people cope with these emotions—can trigger or exacerbate depressive and anxiety disorders.

The alternation of stress and boredom, a common experience in retail workplaces like Walmart and Uber, is a direct consequence of hiring practices that balance minimal staffing with maximal customer service. And it may also be a recipe for exacerbating depression and anxiety, the two most common psychological complaints in the United States today.

Psychiatry has reacted to the evidence on the role of work in mental health in a few ways. Within work settings, the usual prescription for depression and anxiety is to promote mental health counseling, which is often hard to find, expensive, or of such short duration as to have limited impact.[126] On the clinical side, modern psychiatry views mental illness as a biochemical imbalance and recommends drugs to correct these imbalances. In some cases, these medications provide significant relief for some patients with depressive or anxiety disorders, but their effect can be short lived or accompanied with side effects. Still another response has been to emphasize the value of accepting negative emotions and employ cognitive and behavioral strategies to cope with them.[127] None of these approaches changes the underlying work conditions that provoke the stress.

Prevention is seldom considered. One obvious solution to the rise of negative and harmful emotions and organizational cultures that trigger anxiety or depression is to reorganize workplaces to minimize these experiences and environments. But reorganizing work relationships and structures that have emerged from recent changes in capitalism is a task as appealing to most business owners as rolling in poison ivy. In chapter 8, I describe worker cooperatives, one effort that does seek to transform the organization of work.

How do mental health disorders affect the lives of workers? Firstly, their influence extends over decades. "Unlike other chronic conditions that usually don't start in workers until their 40s, 50s or even 60s," explained L. Casey Chosewood, director of the Office for Total Worker Health at the National Institute for Occupational Safety and Health, "mental health concerns typically present in a worker's 20s or 30s and can last throughout almost the entire working career."[128] Depression and anxiety can lead to unemployment and lost wages for workers and reduced productivity for employers.

Depression and anxiety can also contribute to substance use, which can be both a cause and consequence of these disorders. Many workers cope with their mental health problems with self-medication, using tobacco, alcohol, or other legal or illegal drugs. One study found that work stressors contributed to alcohol and illicit drug use before work, during the workday, and after work,[129] suggesting that workplace problems spill over into home life—and vice versa.

Shift work, a characteristic of many low-wage and nonstandard jobs, contributes to insomnia, both a trigger and a consequence of depression and anxiety,[130] as well as to chronic diseases, accidents, higher levels of substance use, and unhealthy eating patterns.[131] It too influences well-being both at work and at home. In the dynamic profit-maximizing global economy, some workplaces stay open twenty-four hours a day while others change shifts in response to recessions or expansions.

External events such as the COVID-19 pandemic or the police murder of George Floyd can also trigger anxiety and depression, further exacerbating workplace influences and adding to the feeling of loss of control.

Heart Diseases. Cardiovascular disease (CVD) is the leading cause of premature death and preventable illness in the United States and globally. It accounts for about 30 percent of deaths around the world and in the United States shortens life spans by an average of seven years.[132] Diabetes, hypertension, stroke, coronary artery disease, and obesity are either causes, consequences, or both of CVD, demonstrating its giant shadow on global health.

Public health campaigns against smoking, unhealthy diets, and physical inactivity—leading causes of CVD—have contributed to reductions in CVD deaths in the United States and other high-income countries. Changes in clinical practices have also contributed. However, the potential for modifying workplaces to reduce CVD has been less recognized and less tackled. An expert panel of cardiovascular and occupational health specialists concluded in 2013 that between 10 and 20 percent of all CVD deaths among working-age populations can be attributed to work exposures, suggesting the potential public health benefits of job redesign.[133]

Recent research has suggested that several work characteristics can elevate the risk for CVD. Jobs that strain workers by limiting their latitude over work processes, jobs that minimize job security and opportunities for advancement (categorized as "effort reward imbalance"), and jobs that require "threat avoidance vigilance," a high degree of alertness to avoid accident or injury, set in motion biological processes that contribute to CVD.[134]

Do these findings suggest a way to lower the toll from the world's leading killer? On the one hand, new understanding of the work characteristics that lead to CVD could guide restructuring of jobs to reduce exposures that damage human hearts. On the other hand, in the twenty-first century, the fastest-growing job sectors are the nonstandard jobs that reduce worker control, lower job security, require high degrees of vigilance, and weaken the cultures, laws, and values that in the past offered workers some health protection. Of course, earlier jobs also had risks, but in the twentieth century the labor movement and occupational health specialists sought (with varying levels of success) to apply new science on workplace disease to improving conditions. In this century, despite a growing body of evidence on the hazards of low-wage, precarious, and nonstandard forms of work, current social and economic policies are increasing the work arrangements that put workers at risk.

To date, most clinicians and public health experts have been unable or unwilling to take on the pathogenic features of current work environments. Part of this reluctance may be explained by their lack of training in this area; another by the biomedical mindset that changing the rules of capitalism is not the job of health professionals, or, as I have described previously, the belief that there is no alternative to the current arrangements.

WORK EXPOSURES AND HEALTH

Each of the work sectors expanding in recent decades exposes workers to settings with distinct patterns of health and disease. Often these exposures are different from those experienced by manufacturing workers in the last half of the twentieth century when more workers were unionized, jobs were more secure, and health and safety regulations were more regularly enforced.

Despite sectoral differences, nonstandard workers, including precarious, contingent, gig economy, low-wage, and informal sector employees, face some similar exposures. Some groups such as immigrant workers who lack documentation, workers in the informal economy who lack legal protection, and very low-wage workers who cannot risk losing a job, are forced to accept jobs that better-off workers reject because of low pay or safety hazards.

For younger workers, job instability, low wages, and other characteristics of nonstandard jobs, combined with high prices for housing and college, also led to higher levels of stress and increased appetite for alcohol, opioids, and other drugs, again with a negative impact on premature death and preventable illness.

Because they seldom belong to unions, nonstandard workers lack the health and safety and other protections that these organizations offer. These two factors also make nonstandard workers less likely to complain or pursue remedies when their rights are violated. Since many nonstandard workplaces are privatized, deregulated, or outside the formal economy, the occupational health and safety and wage regulations that protect standard workers do not exist or go unenforced. In addition, many nonstandard workers have two or more jobs, compounding their exposures to risk. Finally, undocumented immigrants, women, Blacks, and Latinxs are disproportionately represented in nonstandard jobs, exposing them to the double or triple burdens of dangerous exposures, workplace sexual harassment, racism, and immigration bias.

Physical Exposures. Nonstandard and low-wage workers are concentrated in riskier industries: construction, food services, agriculture and transportation, sectors with higher than average accident and injury rates. Those jobs based in the informal economy, such as construction day labor, often lack any formal health and safety protection or assured access to workers compensation, an insurance system that provides medical benefits and wage replacement to workers who are injured on the job.[135] For example, day laborers in the construction industry or off-the-books restaurant workers have among the highest accident rates of any type of worker—and the most precarious lives.[136]

A forty-six-year-old Latina who had worked in a factory through a temp agency for five years told researchers about her experiences:

> Many injustices happened here. OSHA would come and they would fix things for just a while. . . . I injured my back by carrying 45 pounds of candy. They made me wait 4 to 5 hours to take me to their clinic because I was working the night shift. The main office told me I had to say that I injured myself because I picked up something in the wrong position and I had to say that to the clinic people.[137]

Agricultural workers are often regularly exposed to pesticides or herbicides. Such exposures have been linked to cancer, reproductive problems, kidney diseases, and other health problems.[138] One recent review found that chronic occupational exposure to organophosphate pesticides was associated with neuropsychological problems such as difficulties in executive functions, psychomotor speed, verbal skills, memory, attention, processing speed, and coordination.[139] Workers can also bring these toxic products home on their clothes, and migrant farm workers and their families also live near sprayed fields, putting their families at risk of harm.[140] As the production of processed food became industrialized and ultra-processed foods become the mainstay of the global diet, global agricultural producers have increasingly relied on pesticides and herbicides to increase production, reduce labor costs, and increase profits, thus further endangering farm workers.

These physical exposures add to the cumulative adverse impact of the previously described work environments that contribute to psychological problems associated with emerging work organizations. While Walmart, KinderCare, and Uber may be safer places to work than coal mines or garment sweatshops, the new workplaces that now employ tens of millions of Americans contribute to the most serious, expensive, and burdensome health problems facing the nation and the world.

WORK-FAMILY CONFLICT

Workers have always struggled to balance the demands of work with those of family life, but the growth of low-wage and nonstandard employment has amplified these conflicts, increasing both the number of workers exposed and the intensity and diversity of competing demands. Other changes in modern capitalism—the erosion of safety-net programs, the privatization of public services, and stagnating wages—have further aggravated the problem. Work-family conflicts affect people of all classes and incomes, but like other work-related health conditions in the United States, the burden of these conflicts falls most heavily on those more represented in low-wage and nonstandard jobs—women, Blacks and Latinxs, and recent immigrants.

Work-family conflicts destabilize psychological well-being in several ways. In most American families, all adults in the household work, and most children live with working parents.[141] This requires parents—most often mothers—to find affordable child care, get their children to care in time to be able to be at work, and fill in the gaps when their child is sick or school is closed. Many parents working without job security or paid family sick leave regularly must choose between sending sick children to school or leaving them home alone or risking losing their job through too many absences.

Work-family conflict also contributes to the wage gender gap. According to the Pew Research Center, in 2018 women earned 85 percent of what men earned. While the women's movement helped to narrow the gap, which was 64 percent of men's wages in 1980, gender discrimination persists. Pew Surveys also show that 42 percent of working women report gender discrimination at work, and 25 percent of working women said they make less than a man doing the same job.[142]

Gender segregation also contributes to the gaps. Women, and especially women of color, are overrepresented in low-paying but fast-growing service jobs such as child care, home healthcare, and food service. The nation's failure to establish paid and parental leave policies—in large part because of employer opposition to such policies—further disadvantages women. About four in ten mothers report that they have taken a significant amount of time off or reduced their work hours to take care of family responsibilities. These decisions often lead to lower pay or missed opportunities for promotion.

Sexual harassment and sexual violence have long been part of many workplace cultures and their adverse impact on the physical and mental health of women has been amply documented.[143] The #MeToo movement focused public attention on the problem but only recently have labor and women's organizations begun to document and act against sexual violence against women in low-wage and precarious occupations.

Employer unwillingness to take responsibility for the burdens that their work arrangements impose on women reinforces old-fashioned gender roles—women spend more time taking care of children, preparing food, and doing household work. These responsibilities contribute to the stress, time pressure and family conflicts that exacerbate depression, anxiety, and other psychological problems. Many companies have leave policies that exacerbate inequitable work experiences. Walmart, for example, offers paid leave only to their salaried employees and not to hourly workers.[144] In addition, lack of gender=equitable benefits leads some women to delay childbearing so as not to fall behind at work, a decision that elevates risk for adverse birth outcomes associated with later childbearing.[145]

Once again, the United States is an outlier among high-income market economies in failing to establish national policies that assist workers in balancing family and work life. In Finland, for example, new parents get a full year of paid parental leave, which they can share between them. As a couple who moved from the United States to Finland explained:

> We've now been living in Finland for more than a year. The difference between our lives here and in the States has been tremendous, but perhaps not in the way many Americans might imagine. What we've experienced is an increase in personal freedom. Our lives are just much more manageable. To be sure, our days are still full of challenges—raising a child, helping elderly parents, juggling the demands of daily logistics and work.[146]

While a variety of historical and cultural factors contribute to the United States' low ranking on this issue, the determined opposition of business groups and their power in the political system are important causes.[147] The broad evidence that worker and family-friendly policies contribute to improved individual and community health make overcoming this opposition a priority.[148]

DEATHS OF DESPAIR—A NEW OCCUPATIONAL HAZARD?

In 2015, Princeton economists Anne Case and Angus Deaton proposed that the increase in mid-life mortality among white Americans between 2000 and 2014 is the result of cumulative disadvantages that occurred over decades. They attribute these deaths—caused in large part by drug overdoses, suicide, and liver disease—to deterioration in economic and social conditions and labeled them "deaths of despair."[149]

In some ways, this new pattern of illnesses and deaths is the flip side of the rising burden of nonstandard and low-wage work. Those most affected by the so-called deaths of despair are the white working-class men who benefited most from the twentieth-century economy. These men have lost many of these benefits—better wages, regular work, union protection—leaving them vulnerable to drug abuse, alcohol, suicide, and other conditions. For this population, loss of earlier privilege was the cost paid as a result of changes wrought by twenty-first-century capitalism

In 2017, more than 152,000 Americans died from alcohol and drug-related fatalities and suicide, the highest number ever and more than twice as many as in 1999.[150] In the fifteen years between 2000 and 2014, white non-Hispanic mortality rose by thirty-four deaths per one thousand. In contrast, in the same period, death rates for Blacks and Hispanics declined substantially.[151]

In subsequent studies, Case and Deaton reported that the mortality rate for men aged fifty to fifty-four with less than a bachelor's degree increased by 14 percent while the rate for men with a bachelor's degree or more fell by 30 percent.[152] Another analysis found that between 2007 and 2017, drug-related deaths increased by 108 percent among adults of all races aged eighteen to thirty-four, by 69 percent for alcohol-related deaths, and by 35 percent for suicides.[153]

What does all this have to do with work? Of course, many factors contribute to so-called deaths of despair. The aggressive marketing of OxyContin and other opioids by the Sackler family–owned Purdue Pharma, and other companies played a major role in more than seven hundred thousand drug overdose deaths reported in the United States between 1999 and 2017.[154] But changes in work triggered by twenty-first-century capitalism are a key driver. For older rural whites, especially men without college, the loss of decently paid manufacturing jobs and the burdens of musculoskeletal injuries that persist after jobs end led to increased alcohol, tobacco, and opioid use. These behavioral responses to loss and pain in turn lead to higher rates of suicide, overdose, liver disease, and tobacco-related illnesses.

Recent declines in Black and Latinx death rates result in part from successful public health campaigns against HIV infection, homicide, and tobacco-related diseases. Another less positive reason for the shrinking gap is the increase in white death rates from overdose, suicide, and alcohol. In a cruel irony, in an economy driven by profit rather than human need, the unintended strategy for closing the racial and class gaps in health is to increase the death rates for the better-off groups.

Some scholars have rightly warned that the "deaths of despair" focus on white workers overlooks the persistently higher death and illness rates among Blacks and Latinx. Workers of color have long experienced higher rates of deaths from most causes including work-related illnesses and injuries, often the result of social and economic policies and enforcement practices that reinforce racial inequality.[155] But by viewing the increasing burden of ill health attributable to the rise of low-wage and nonstandard work and the rise in "deaths of despair" as the result of the loss of better jobs, these two phenomena are both consequences of changes in work in modern capitalism.

The COVID-19 pandemic highlighted yet another threat to low-wage workers and yet another failure of existing worker-protection policies. Workers in such diverse sectors as nursing homes, healthcare, meat packing, shipping centers, and agricultural work faced higher than average rates of COVID-19 infection and death. For these workers, living in poverty, often in crowded housing, with limited health insurance coverage or sick leave, and lack of unions, combined with the failure of industries to enforce health and safety rules created a cascade of risk that burdened these low-wage workers, especially Black and Latinx ones.

RESISTANCE AND ALTERNATIVES

In the twentieth century, workers in the United States and elsewhere won new rights to organize and set legal standards on pay, overtime, child labor, and health and safety. While these victories were partial and often failed to protect workers at highest risk—women, recent immigrants, Blacks and Latinxs, and those in the informal economy—workers claimed a voice in setting working conditions and engaged in ongoing battles to protect and expand that voice.

Beginning in the 1970s and especially in the last two decades, business leaders and their allies in government sought to roll back these advances. Current low unionization rates, low wages, shrinking benefits, deregulation of health and safety rules, and new business-friendly interpretations of labor and employment law illustrate how much workers have lost.

But even as workers lost some their earlier gains, they have found new ways to organize and win concessions from corporations. My examination of several victories and partial victories seeks to identify how corporations respond to such campaigns and the strategies that might enable workers to better protect their well-being now and in the future.

When meat cutters at a Texas Walmart Supercenter organized a union, Walmart switched to prepackaged meat and fired the workers. When the Service Employees International Union organized child care workers at a KinderCare center at the University of Southern California, KinderCare closed the center a month later. Uber chose a different route: it formed a partnership with a New York regional branch of the International Association of Machinists and Aerospace Workers to fund and create the Independent Drivers Guild. The guild won some concessions from Uber, but many Uber drivers and some labor scholars regarded it as a company union, an effort to deter an organization that genuinely represented workers.[156]

Workers who were unable or unwilling to strike found other ways to act. At Walmart, current and former associates organized a large online discussion group. The group grew exponentially in its first four years, reaching almost fifty thousand members by 2018. Reich and Bearman described this online community as "a beehive of activity, vibrant to the point of being overwhelming. . . . The group provides a sense of what can happen online, good and bad."

The challenge for such an online community, they note, is "to channel belonging into a sense of common purpose sufficient for collective power."[157] At Uber, drivers use an online platform to monitor company application of its many rules and to share news on how Uber uses its algorithms to change compensation. In Cleveland, Lyft and Uber drivers created their own radio channel to provide an alternative way to exchange information and provide support to each other.

In 2017, a livery driver posted his suicide note on Facebook, accusing Uber of wrecking his job. His searing indictment soon went viral. Douglas Shifter, the driver, wrote:

> I have been financially ruined because three politicians destroyed my industry and livelihood and Corporate NY stole my services at rates far below fair levels. . . . I am not a new driver and I was the most skilled and experienced driver to my knowledge in the business. . . . We are being shaken down by politicians who sell out to the biggest contributors to their greed and power. . . . I hope with the public sacrifice I make now that some attention to the plight of the drivers and the people will be done to save them." [158]

Schifter's heartbreaking plea was answered in part in 2019. After six taxi driver suicides, the New York City Council and State Legislature took up measures to give taxi drivers, including those at Uber and Lyft, added protections.

Another response to declining unionization and union organizations was the creation of worker centers and independent worker organizations. Many low-wage occupations have traditionally lacked unions—day laborers, agricultural workers, food service workers, laundry workers, domestic workers, and others. To help these disenfranchised workers gain a voice, labor activists, civil rights groups, and community organizations, sometimes with the support of mainstream unions, created worker centers and independent labor organizations. These have educated, mobilized, and organized workers, offering legal representation, hiring halls, health and safety workshops, and workforce training programs.[159]

A 2006 survey found 139 worker centers in the United States.[160] By 2018, there were 260.[161] Many got significant financial support from foundations. In 2017, the US Chamber of Commerce reported that 68 US workers centers had received philanthropic support between 2013 and 2016 totaling $50.8 million, with grants ranging from $5,000 to $14.3 million in that period.[162]

Centro Humanitario, a worker center located in a gentrifying neighborhood in Denver, Colorado, illustrates this approach.[163] A banner in front reads "Day Laborers Available Here," a notice of the hiring hall that offers day laborers a safe place to get work that pays minimum wage and employers an opportunity to get screened candidates for their jobs. The center offers ESL classes, computer classes, leadership trainings, and "Know Your Rights" workshops. It has helped start worker collectives. Members (who pay dues of $15 a year) are provided with a picture ID card, the only form of identification some possess. The center rents members lockers to store documents and food.

In 2014, Centro Humanitario helped to win passage of the Wage Protection Act, a law that seeks to prevent wage theft in Colorado. It also refers victims of wage theft to Denver lawyers who handle these cases. With a local professor, the center completed a study of the working conditions of Colorado domestic workers. It is also an affiliate of the National Day Laborers Organization Network and the National Domestic Workers Association (NDWA), showing how worker centers can operate at both local and national levels.

The National Domestic Workers Association works for respect, recognition, and inclusion in labor protections for domestic workers, the majority of whom are immigrants and women of color. It has more than sixty affiliate organizations and local chapters and thousands of members. Domestic workers in all fifty states can join NDWA and gain access to member benefits, connection with other workers, and opportunities to get involved in the domestic worker movement. NDWA shows how worker organizations can begin to organize new categories of low-wage and precarious workers that traditional unions have sometimes been unable or unwilling to engage.

In 2019, NDWA worked with Senator Kamala Harris and Representative Pramila Jayapal to introduce in Congress the Domestic Workers Bill of Rights Act. This law would require employers to provide a written agreement that spells out pay, duties, schedules, and time-off policies. It would also make sure that employers use fair scheduling practices, so workers do not lose pay because of last-minute scheduling changes. As Ai-jen Poo, founder of the NDWA explained, "It makes sense that domestic workers, who often work alone with no human resources departments, would pave the way for policies that could help other workers who would otherwise fall through the cracks."[164]

Centro Humanitario, NDWA, and other worker organizations have helped low-wage workers to improve their working conditions and gain power, but they struggle with two tensions. First, on the one hand, they seek to address the daily working and living conditions of their constituents, a time-consuming task that can seem like a bottomless pit. On the other hand, these groups want to change the structural conditions and policies that jeopardize their constituents, another seemingly overwhelming task. While some observers encourage worker centers to make one or the other of these goals the priority, their success seems to come from blending the two, helping individuals to improve their jobs and lives and taking on building power and challenging corporate control.

A second dilemma is finding the right balance between becoming a national presence with a voice in Washington and relationships with employers, versus being an authentic voice for workers themselves. Some academic observers, for example, have criticized the national workers organizations for embracing market-based approaches and taking on the "logic of finance, replacing organizing campaigns with market-based projects."[165] They claim that these organizations' partnerships with employers and their financial dependence on major national foundations illustrate this transformation. The coalitions respond that policy change is a more effective way to protect more workers and if they want to have an influence, then Washington-based legislative lobbying is the name of the game.

Bringing authentic worker voices into the national discussion on work arrangements and work policies that would better protect workers is a key goal. To do so, advocates will need to integrate grass-roots organizing with what some activists call grass tops advocacy designed to reach opinion leaders and elected officials.[166]

While the central goals of labor unions have traditionally been to win contracts that improved pay and working conditions and to represent workers in their grievances against their employers, unions have also always had political and policy objectives. As the proportion of workers represented by unions has declined, worker organizations have forged new alliances and tested new strategies to win legislative and political victories. In some cases, unions have enthusiastically endorsed these broader political goals; in other cases they have emphasized the narrower goal of representing only their dues-paying members.

Fast Food Forward, a labor organization seeking to organize workers in fast-food chains, led a successful campaign to raise the minimum wage to $15 an hour in New York City and New York State, victories that were later picked up by several other cities and states.[167] Since 2011, Fast Food Forward and its allies have won wage increases for 22 million Americans.

Other coalitions mobilized civil rights, labor, and women's organizations to pass state and local sick leave and family leave laws (See Figure 5.2).[168] More than 90 percent of low-wage and part-time workers lack access to paid family leave.[169] California passed a law in 2002 after an intense battle led by the California Federation of Labor, the state association of mainstream labor unions, and many state and national women's organizations. After the victory,

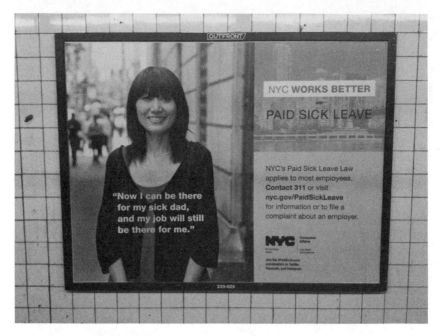

Fig. 5.2 A subway poster promoting New York City's paid sick leave law.
Photo: [permissions and high-resolution image to come by 7 Sept 2020]

Karen Nussbaum, a long-time labor and women's activist at the AFL-CIO told a reporter:

> Advocates can go to other states and make the case that if a state as concerned as California was about balancing its budget can do this, other states can do it as well. The ability to take time off when your family really needs you is so meaningful that I never found it easier to ask people to weigh in, to make phone calls to put this one over the edge. But the employer community fought this one very, very hard.[170]

Labor and women's activists heeded Nussbaum's advice and by 2020, 13 states and Washington, DC, had enacted paid family leave laws, providing four to twelve weeks of paid leave.[171] A study in California showed that after the law was passed, more women with new children took leaves, especially more women who were less educated, unmarried, or nonwhite.[172] Men also took additional leave, although at much lower rates.

Other campaigns have encouraged state attorneys general to increase enforcement and penalties against wage theft and state and federal agencies to more vigorously enforce occupational safety and health laws for low-wage, nonstandard, and immigrant workers.[173] Wage theft describes the practice of employers failing to pay workers their full salary, a common problem facing low-wage and immigrant workers. In New York and California, Uber and Lyft drivers have organized to require their employers to recognize them as workers, rather than independent contractors, thus giving them the protection of minimum-wage laws, overtime pay, and unemployment compensation.[174] In 2019, California approved such a law.

In these and other ways, nonstandard workers won some of the protections that safeguard workers in more standard jobs. Mainstream labor unions, worker centers, and other civil society groups have joined to pass laws and strengthen enforcement that made tangible improvements in the lives of millions of workers. By acting directly in the political arena, these mobilizations have been able to overcome some of the weaknesses of traditional labor unions and suggest new directions for expanding labor rights and power in the coming decades.

Often, these efforts challenge profits and corporate control. Corporations have responded to these new forms of worker organizing in various ways. A common response is to make concessions. After 2015, Walmart increased the wages of its workers several times. Several factors probably contributed to this decision, including negative media coverage of Walmart as a low-wage employer, growing national attention to economic inequality, and an improving economy, which made it harder for Walmart to attract workers with its low wages. This experience suggests that by connecting activism and public education to deeper economic trends, labor activists can win more victories than by either strategy alone.

Another rationale for corporate concessions is to deter or delay more transformative changes or tougher government regulation. Walmart's first pay increases to an average of $11 an hour came after a groundswell of national activism around the $15 an hour minimum wage. Later raises came after President Trump's tax cut lowered Walmart's taxes by more than $1 billion a year, refocusing national attention on inequitable taxes.[175] By raising wages on its own, Walmart preserved its own power to grant, withhold, or roll back subsequent pay increases. In 2019, Walmart's CEO endorsed raising the $7.25 an hour federal minimum wage, but recommended regional variation, again limiting the impact on the company's bottom line.[176]

Divide and conquer is another tried and true tactic that corporations use. Uber funded its own union, the Independent Drivers Guild, to divide its workers from other taxi drivers led by the National Taxi Workers' Alliance, a labor organization that sought to unite paid drivers of all categories.

Corporations also use their lobbying and legal muscle to counteract workers' or government efforts to improve working conditions. Preemption is a legal strategy that seeks to stop one level of government from acting in an arena allegedly assigned to another level. By 2019, corporate lobbyists had persuaded twenty-five states to enact statutes preempting local minimum wage laws. As the National Employment Law Project reported, by 2019, twelve cities and counties in six states (Alabama, Iowa, Florida, Kentucky, Missouri, and Wisconsin) had approved local minimum wage laws only to see them invalidated by state statute, harming hundreds of thousands of workers in the process, many of whom face high levels of poverty. The preemption strategy was led by the American Legislative Exchange Council (ALEC), a powerful business-friendly national lobbying group supported by the US Chamber of Commerce and big corporate lobbying groups.[177]

The rise in low-wage and nonstandard labor, declining rates of unionization, and increasing corporate political power have required workers and their organizations to change the ways they seek to improve working conditions. In the last few decades, workers have evolved several promising strategies for lifting wages, adding benefits, and creating new forms of organization. As always, employers also modify their strategies to protect their bottom lines and their capacity to control their workforce without interference. How labor and owners manage these changing dynamics in the years to come will have a decisive influence on the well-being of workers, their communities, the economy, and the health of the planet.

CHAPTER 6

The Future of Transportation

Uber and Autonomous Vehicles or Mass Transit?

The . . . right to travel . . . occupies a position fundamental to the concept of our Federal Union.

—*Justice William Brennan, Shapiro v. Thompson, 394 U.S. 618 (1969)*

Mobility, the capacity to move from one place to another, constitutes an essential condition for human freedom and well-being. People travel to visit friends and family, go to work, get medical care, find food, attend school, seek adventure, and flee violence, discrimination, and poverty. How a society organizes transportation shapes opportunities for achieving life, liberty, and the pursuit of happiness.

In the twentieth century, the automobile industry had a dominant role in shaping transportation options and also daily living conditions in wealthy nations. The growth of the auto industry brought numerous benefits to hundreds of millions of Americans. It enabled more people to find work, live where they wanted, take vacations, enjoy wider food and medical care choices, and define new cultural identities as adventure-loving explorers, family chauffeurs, or rebels without a cause.

The choices of the auto industry also imposed costs on people in the United States and around the world. In the twentieth century, motor vehicle collisions caused the deaths of about 60 million people globally.[1] The growing death and illness toll from air pollution results in part from the products and practices of the auto industry and its opposition to tighter emissions controls.[2] In the United States, cars and trucks account for 20 percent of the carbon emissions responsible for global warming, making it a leading cause of human-induced climate change.[3] Suburbanization, the twentieth-century process that led to urban sprawl, more segregated housing and schools, and more isolated family life, relied on the millions of autos the industry churned out and its active political support and lobbying for autocentric public policies.[4]

To understand the role of modern capitalism in shaping transportation options and well-being in this century, I consider three stories: the efforts by Uber, Lyft, and other transportation network companies to take over urban mass transit markets; the evasion of regulation and cover-ups of dangerous defects in motor vehicles by General Motors, Volkswagen, Takata, and other auto and auto-supplier companies; and the involvement of tech, auto, and transportation network companies in shaping the development of autonomous vehicles and policies to reduce their risks. These stories illustrate how twenty-first-century capitalism influences the national transportation system and the impact of their choices on individual, community, and planetary health.

PUBLIC TRANSIT AND RIDE HAILING COMPANIES

In 2019, 82 percent of the 329 million people in the United States lived in urban areas and by 2030, 60 percent of the world's population will be urban. How people in cities travel will shape both the daily lives of the majority of the world's population and the architecture of the world's transportation system. For several decades, most health and urban planning experts have agreed that affordable, widely available, and efficiently run mass transit—a system of transport for passengers by group travel on buses, trains, ferries, or other vehicles and available for use by the general public—offers the best opportunities for health, sustainability, and equity for city dwellers.[5]

Mass transit reduces traffic deaths, pollutes less than private cars, takes up less space, costs less, encourages physical activity, and offers other social, economic, and health benefits.[6] When integrated with opportunities for active transportation—walking and biking—mass transit systems also reduce obesity and chronic diseases and improve mental health.[7] While the COVID-19 pandemic highlights the infectious disease risks of crowded mass transit, the overall health and environmental benefits of mass transit versus individual auto travel are clear and transmission of COVID-19 on mass transit appears to be limited.

Cities are complex ecosystems and it is rare to achieve scientific consensus that a single intervention—strengthening mass transit—offers multiple benefits and relatively few disadvantages. Despite this consensus, however, progress on making mass transit the default choices for getting around in cities has been slow. Opposition to mass transit from the automobile industry and its allies is not new. In the first half of the twentieth century, the industry promoted urban and suburban design and development that discouraged mass transit and active transportation, opposed tax or environmental policies that discouraged car use, and lobbied against public spending on mass transit.[8]

But as evidence on the health, environmental, and equity benefits of mass transit accumulate, current efforts by Uber, Lyft, and other transportation network companies to replace mass transit are especially disturbing. In its 2019 filing with the Securities and Exchange Commission prior to going public, Uber notes that in the sixty-three countries and seven hundred cities in which it operates, people travel 4.4 trillion miles per year on mass transit, 37 percent of the total annual market of 11.9 trillion miles.[9] With the new capital it raises from its public offering, Uber plans "to better compete with personal vehicle ownership and usage and public transportation."[10] The benefit of wooing customers away from "well-established and low-cost public transportation options," notes Uber in its filing, is that the total value of the mass transit market in the countries in which it operates is $1 trillion a year. This becomes a tempting target for a company that has yet to make a profit and reported a $5 billion quarterly loss in late 2019 and declining revenue growth.[11] The disappointing response to Uber's 2019 IPO and investor insistence that the company move to profitability will increase the pressure to find new sources for profit.

While the long-term goal of Uber and Lyft is to replace mass transit for as many riders as possible, in the shorter term, making deals with public transit systems is another way to bring in new revenue streams and attract new customers. Since 2015, Uber has negotiated more than twenty deals with transit systems in Denver, Dallas, Tampa-St. Petersburg, and elsewhere. For cities, in the short-term—the way elections and budgets encourage politicians to think—these deals offer a less expensive way to make it easier for residents to reach places not served by public transit than to build new subway or light rail lines or buy a fleet of busses.

In Tampa-St. Petersburg and Dallas, for example, the city subsidizes the cost of an Uber ride, using taxpayer dollars to pay for the ride between the bus stop and the passenger's final destination.[12] In Denver, customers can use the Uber app to buy their transit ticket. Uber does not make money on the transaction but benefits when the customer stays in the app to book an Uber ride from the train station to their final destination.[13]

In theory, a public mass transit system that included vans and cars could take the place of these partnerships with Uber and Lyft, which has its own deals—fifty by mid-2020—with urban transit systems. Governments seeking to expand mass transit, however, face a number of obstacles. Most public officials are reluctant to raise taxes to pay for transit improvements. Expanding lines to less densely populated areas can be expensive, as revenues are lower. Using mass transit to cover that "last mile" between the bus or train stop and the passenger's home is also expensive and operationally challenging. Moreover, most mass transit systems have trouble serving people with disabilities or the growing population of older Americans who may have trouble getting to the rail stop or onto the bus.

So Uber and Lyft just happen to have solutions that can overcome these difficulties. As CEO Dara Khosrowshahi put it, Uber wants to become the "Amazon of transportation." "Cars are to us what books were to Amazon," Khosrowshahi said at a tech conference in 2018. "Just like Amazon was able to build this extraordinary infrastructure on the back of books and go into additional categories, you are going to see the same from Uber."[14] Already Uber delivers meals (Uber Eats), distributes bicycles and scooters (Jump Bikes), and sells mapping apps (daCarta) and artificial intelligence training programs (Mighty AI).

So what is the problem with Uber becoming a city's transportation hub? Aren't these partnerships a triple win for customers, governments, and companies like Uber and Lyft? Four problems complicate that optimistic interpretation.

First, the deals introduce Uber to desirable new customers, potentially removing these riders from both mass transit and traditional taxi systems, putting drivers out of work, and reducing public support for mass transit. Like the privatized charter schools that skim proficient students (with parents who can pay) from public school systems, ride-hailing companies weaken public transit systems that are already underfunded.

Second, these deals can make governments dependent on Uber, which can then raise prices or change the terms of the agreements as it chooses. In Innisfil, Ontario, an exurb of Toronto, Uber charged a reduced $1 flat fare when it started driving residents to replace traditional bus lines. But when the program proved popular, Uber hiked the flat fares and slashed multi-trip discounts.[15] "With public agencies, there's a protocol for how to hold them responsible, whereas with private companies, their bottom line is profit," explained Naomi Iwasaki, a transportation planner and advocate in Los Angeles. "They look at their users as customers, not constituents."[16]

Third, these arrangements often increase air pollution and other adverse impacts. While ride hailing can reduce private car trips, as riders shift from busses and subways to Uber cars and SUVs, they contribute to increased congestion and pollution. The net effect, studies suggest, is more vehicles on the road, not fewer. "It's taking us back to a city where there's less and less space for public transit," noted Jared Walker, an Oregon-based transportation consultant. "It may make sense to pursue that (business) strategy, but it may also be a strategy that's destroying the world. It's certainly destroying the urban world."[17] Ride-hailing can also lead to increases in traffic miles traveled as a result of "deadheading," drivers traveling in search of fares. And more cars on the road lead to more carbon and other greenhouse gas emissions, contributing to climate change, an existential threat to cities and the planet.

The growth of transportation network companies can also lead to a fourth problem, reductions in transportation equity. Equitable transportation systems are affordable, and bring benefits to and enable full participation in society for all sectors of the population.[18] A study by the economist Raj Chetty found that geographic isolation—measured by commute times—influenced people's ability to escape poverty.[19] When low-income urban or rural families can't reach schools, jobs, or medical care if they lack a car, their capacity to thrive is diminished.[20] When Uber and Lyft avoid isolated or poor communities, raise fares, and undermine or disparage mass transit, they contribute to transportation inequity, raising one more obstacle for those living in poverty. Moreover, Uber's growth jeopardizes the jobs of transit workers and traditional taxi drivers, pushing more workers into the gig economy with its low wages and meager benefits.

Already, Uber, Lyft, and their competitors have contributed to a crisis facing mass transit. Even before the COVID-19 pandemic, transit ridership was declining across the United States. If strong gains in use of mass transit in the New York area are excluded, transit ridership in the top fifty cities nationally declined by 7 percent over the past decade.[21] Annual ridership in 2017 was the lowest since 2005. These drops make it harder for systems to pay for the $90 billion maintenance backlog a 2015 Department of Transportation study found.[22] In 2018, Uber logged 5 billion trips and Lyft 619 million.[23] A 2018 study of ride-hailing users in Boston found that almost half would have used public transit if ride-hailing had not been available.[24]

Even New York City—with its flat fare, twenty-four-hour service, and coverage of most city neighborhoods—in some ways the paradigm of a transit-friendly city, is having trouble maintaining its mass transit system. A tax-averse governor is unwilling to pay for needed infrastructure improvements, a president hostile to New York City has withheld federal funding for transit improvements, and the aggressive lobbying campaigns of Uber and Lyft seek to ensure its ability to make a profit. In these ways, the capitalist credos of low taxes, privatization, and deregulation have the cumulative impact of jeopardizing the maintenance of a more equitable but rapidly aging public transit system.

And COVID-19 has amplified these problems, slashing ridership on mass transit and highlighting the societal costs of a deteriorated infrastructure, crowded subways and busses, and inadequate maintenance and cleaning.[25]

In a capitalist society, if a private business can offer a service that some people want, they can do so, even if the costs to society as a whole of the new venture are unknown or they are known to exceed the value of the benefits to select customers. Turning partial or full responsibility for transportation planning to companies like Uber and Lyft undercuts any pressure to create a more sustainable, equitable, and efficient public transit system. It usually makes profitability and increased revenues, rather than more livable communities, the bottom line. And it reinforces the inequitable access to transportation by class, race, and ethnicity that now characterize urban transportation systems.

In cities around the nation, public officials are developing commercial partnerships with Uber and Lyft, but also enacting regulations to limit their autonomy, or suing them. As private transportation companies like Uber, Lyft, Taxify, and other transportation network companies consolidate, will the power of this transit conglomerate overwhelm the ability of cities to make urban transportation more affordable, healthier, more sustainable, and less burdensome? How city and state governments, elected officials, advocates, and community residents interact with transportation network companies in the coming decade will determine the future of urban transportation.

AUTO INDUSTRY EVASION OF REGULATION AND COVER-UP OF DEFECTS

For better or worse, most Americans still depend on automobiles for most of their travel. In the last several years, the combination of globalization, financialization, and deregulation have created a volatile market for motor vehicles that led the automobile industry to make decisions that put drivers, passengers, pedestrians, and the planet's health at increased risk. A few examples show how this process plays out at some of the largest automobile companies in the world.

General Motors. In 2001, General Motors (GM) detected a defect in an ignition switch during preproduction testing of the Saturn Ion, a compact car sold between 2003 and 2007. The defect led to unintentional shut down of the car's motor and, as was later discovered, disabled the deployment of airbags. Three years later, GM found the same problem on the Chevrolet Cobalt, a subcompact to be released in 2005. GM rejected a proposal to fix the problem because it would be too costly and take too long. That same year, a sixteen-year-old Maryland resident, Amber Marie Rose, died when her 2005 Cobalt crashed into a tree after the ignition switch shut down the car's electrical system and the airbags failed to deploy.[26] The unfortunate young woman served as the canary in the coal mine that showed the extent of GM's risky practices.

Over the next thirteen years, General Motors struggled to explain its actions and limit the damage to its auto sales, stock prices, and reputation. Its own internal report on the scandal, known as the Valukas Report, after its lead author, concluded:

> From the switch's inception to approximately 2006, various engineering groups and committees considered ways to resolve the problem. However, those individuals tasked with fixing the problem—sophisticated engineers with responsibility to provide consumers with safe and reliable automobiles—did not understand one of the most fundamental consequences of the switch failing and

the car stalling: the airbags would not deploy. . . . This failure, combined with others . . . led to devastating consequences. . . . The . . . switch approved in 2002 made its way into a variety of vehicles, including the Chevrolet Cobalt. Yet GM did not issue a recall for the Cobalt and other cars until 2014, and even then, the initial recall was incomplete. GM personnel's inability to address the ignition switch problem for over 11 years is a history of failures.[27]

As a result of the Valukas report, fifteen GM employees were fired and five were disciplined.

In 2014, GM issued seventy-eight recalls of 28 million vehicles, 12 percent of which were related to ignition switch problems. By 2015, the ignition switch defect was found to have caused an estimated 124 deaths and 275 injuries. Two years later, General Motors paid $120 million to settle claims from dozens of states, resolving one part of its legal battles. In the settlement, GM conceded that "certain employees of GM and General Motors Corporation knew as early as 2004 that the ignition switch posed a safety defect because it could cause airbag non-deployment."[28]

In 2018, a federal judge in New York approved a motion filed by prosecutors to dismiss the federal case against GM, after determining that GM had fulfilled the terms of its settlement with the government on the ignition switch defect. The settlement included a $900 million fine and three years of monitoring by the federal government.[29] GM continues to fight—and negotiate—individual and class-action claims in various courts.

GM left it to its new CEO, Mary Barra, a long-time GM insider, to make its apologies and seek to restore credibility and consumer trust. Barra apologized publicly and copiously, visited the families of victims, and created a compensation fund before legal liability had been established. At the announcement of the federal settlement in 2015, she said, "The mistakes that led to the ignition-switch recall should never have happened. We have apologized and we do so again today," she said. "I believe that our response has been unprecedented in terms of candor, cooperation, transparency, and compassion." *Fortune* credited Barra with changing the culture of GM and then–US prosecutor Preet Bharara observed that the cooperation by GM executives had been "fairly extraordinary. . . . It's the reason we're here after 18 months rather than four years."[30]

But GM's settlements of the ignition switch problems did not satisfy everyone. The $900 million fine GM paid as part of its 2015 deferred prosecution agreement with the federal government represented less than 6 percent of GM's revenue for the year, making it a cost of doing business rather than a powerful deterrent to future criminality.[31] Similarly, the Department of Justice's frequent use of deferred prosecution agreements in corporate—but not individual—prosecutions undercuts the deterrent effect of criminal convictions. Since these agreements usually do not require defendants to admit wrongdoing, they miss an opportunity to de-normalize corporate cover ups and deceptions.

GM's failure to correct a lethal problem it had recognized and its decision to ask for a federal bailout from taxpayers in 2010 did not lead company executives to change their pro-business mindset. In 2018, GM paid no taxes, in part due to the Trump tax cut, and despite the 2010 federal bailout. And since 2015, GM has spent $10 billion on stock buybacks while closing plants in Ohio and elsewhere. Finally, no GM employee faced criminal charges for the ignition switch cover-up. As Clarence Ditlow of the Center for Auto Safety put it:

> GM killed over 100 people by knowingly putting a defective ignition switch into over one million vehicles. Yet no one from GM went to jail or was even charged with criminal homicide. This shows a weakness in the law not a weakness in the facts. GM killed innocent consumers. GM has paid millions of dollars to its lobbyists to keep criminal penalties out of the Vehicle Safety Act since 1966. Today thanks to its lobbyists, GM officials walk off scot free while its customers are six feet under.[32]

Takata. Massive recalls affected suppliers of automobile parts as well as auto makers. Takata Corporation was a Japanese automotive parts company with production facilities on four continents. The company rose to prominence in the early 1990s by designing and selling an airbag less expensive than those produced by more experienced companies.[33] A few years later, when Takata offered General Motors a much cheaper airbag and GM asked its current supplier, Autoliv, another global supplier, to use this design and match the price, the company declined. "No we can't do it. We're not going to use it," Autoliv's head chemist told GM.[34] GM switched to Takata, seeing an opportunity to cut costs. As the auto industry globalized and consolidated, automakers chose to develop supply chains that relied on a single or a few producers of key parts, enabling the companies to bargain down prices and outsource expensive expertise. But this dependence on a single supplier also created vulnerabilities.

Takata became the supplier of airbags to nineteen carmakers around the world, including BMW, Volkswagen, Mercedes-Benz, Ford, Chrysler, and Honda. Airbags are designed to inflate at the time of a collision, protecting the passengers inside. Takata used a metal cartridge filled with propellant wafers to inflate its airbags. Unfortunately, due to differences in temperature and humidity in different regions of Takata's global markets, in some places the airbags exploded, hurling shrapnel at drivers and passengers.[35] By early 2019, according to the National Highway Traffic Safety Administration (NHTSA), exploding airbags had caused sixteen deaths in the US and twenty-four deaths and three hundred injuries worldwide. About 10 million inflators were recalled in the US in 2019 with as many as 70 million to be recalled by the time recalls are set to end in late 2020, by far the largest recall ever.[36]

In 2017, Takata pleaded guilty to falsifying test data and reports to auto-makers. It was fined $25 million and required to establish restitution funds of $125 million for individual victims and $850 million for damages caused to auto companies. Replacing the defective airbags proved to be difficult, forcing the NHTSA to establish a triage system that sent replacement airbags to the geographic regions at highest risk of explosions due to temperature and humidity. "It was not possible for all replacement parts to be available right away, and some vehicles were at much higher risk of a dangerous airbag explosion than others," explained an NHTSA spokesperson.[37]

In 2017, Takata filed for bankruptcy protection in the United States and Japan, selling its assets—and liabilities—to an American company, Key Safety Systems. Takata's president, Shigehisa Takada, explained that with the company losing value, filing for bankruptcy protection was the only way it could survive. "We're in a very difficult situation, and we had to find ways to keep supplying our products. As a maker of safety parts for the automobile industry, our failure to maintain a stable supply would have a major impact across the industry."[38]

Volkswagen. GM and Takata chose less expensive design options to solve technical problems and later discovered their solution had inadvertently created safety hazards, which they then covered up and lied about. Volkswagen crossed an additional ethical boundary by deliberately designing software that controlled its vehicles' emissions to deceive government regulators by making its emissions of nitrogen oxides and small particles appear to meet environmental standards when in fact they did not. By designing software that could detect the testing process, it reduced the emissions during the test, then reverted to the normal combustion process. The EPA found that VWs equipped with the cheat device emitted up to forty times the legal limit of nitrogen oxides.[39]

While VW's deception was not a safety issue for the driver, it certainly created health problems. Automobiles, especially diesel vehicles, emit two harmful pollutants: particulate matter and nitrogen oxides. Particles smaller than 2.5 micrometers (about 3 percent of the width of a human hair) are small enough to penetrate deep into the lungs and thus pose significant health risks, while nitrous oxides have been shown to cause or exacerbate respiratory and cardiovascular diseases as well as premature deaths.[40]

Researchers in the Netherlands studied the value of the heath damage caused by VW's emissions cheat and concluded:

From 2009 to 2015, approximately nine million fraudulent Volkswagen cars, as sold in Europe and the US, emitted a cumulative amount of 526 kilotonnes of nitrogen oxides more than was legally allowed. These fraudulent emissions are associated with 45 thousand disability-adjusted life years (DALYs) and a value of life lost of at least 39 billion US dollars, which is approximately 5.3 times larger than the 7.3 billion US dollars that Volkswagen Group has set aside to cover worldwide costs related to the diesel emissions scandal.[41]

Most of these burdens were experienced in Europe, which had more VW diesel vehicles on the road than did the US. Two *New York Times* analysts estimated that the excess pollutants in the affected VWs sold in the United States between 2008 and 2015 could be expected to cause 106 deaths but they did not calculate other harms.[42]

Of note, the initial discovery of VW's defeat devices came not from government regulators in Germany or the United States but from three engineering students studying at West Virginia University. The three, two from India and one from Switzerland, were completing placements at the university's Center for Alternative Fuels Engines and Emissions in 2013. With a small grant from an international nonprofit, they rented three VWs and used the center's mobile testing equipment to test the cars in an emission laboratory and on the road. They noticed dramatically different results when they tested VW emissions in the laboratory and on the road. Their report on their findings is what alerted government regulators to the problem.[43]

AN EPIDEMIC OF DEFECTS

Some journalists' investigations of the outbreaks of auto defects have attributed the problem to the greed of auto companies or their CEOs or the "anything goes" culture at these businesses. But these explanations do not explain why problems arose across three continents and unfolded in the years after the 2008 financial crisis. To gain insights into the why now and here questions requires examining how recent changes in capitalism played out in the auto industry.

First, a globalized auto industry and increasing competition among a handful of giant corporations put intense pressure on each company to win new markets and revenues. The emergence of successful global auto companies in Europe, Japan, and elsewhere in the 1970s and beyond and the international trade agreements of the 1980s and 1990s, which made it possible for US and other national automakers to sell around the world, created new competition for the global market. After World War II, the United States dominated the global auto market, in part because so many Americans could afford to buy cars. But as wealthier middle classes arose in Europe and middle-income countries, more people bought cars in those nations, opening new sales opportunities for many carmakers.

At the turn of this century, the six largest global auto companies accounted for more than two-thirds of industry revenue but by 2017 that had fallen to little more than one-third.[44] In 2008, GM was surpassed by Toyota Motor Corporation as the world's largest automaker, losing a lead it had held for decades. In 2016, Volkswagen squeezed ahead of Toyota in annual number of autos produced, but the next year Renault-Nissan-Mitsubishi Alliance took the lead. Companies that missed opportunities to secure a place in the game of musical chairs orchestrated by a volatile global economy found themselves sitting on the floor.

Economic downturns, unstable currency exchange rates, changing trade rules—all defining characteristics of twenty-first-century capitalism—made long-term planning difficult. The rise of autonomous vehicles, discussed in the next section, and the resulting growing interest of tech companies in the auto industry further complicated planning and stability. Choosing to acknowledge and correct a defect that may or may not end up threating sales and profits was risky, but so was failing to anticipate the potential liability. This "damned if you do" and "damned if you don't" climate may have led some auto executives and their staffs to risk the "don't" strategy.

Second, changing and volatile consumer demand made longer-term planning difficult. By the late 1990s, fewer young people and fewer urbanites wanted to drive or own a car. American customers preferred first sports utility vehicles (SUVs), then compact sedans, and then SUVs and pickup trucks again, with some brief interest in hybrid and electric cars. Of course, auto industry advertising and promotional campaigns played a role in these choices, but fickle car buyers provoked deep anxiety among auto industry executives, who feared that today's choices may not please tomorrow's buyers. Absent some external pressure, investing money in fixing last year's cars instead of meeting tomorrow's demands seemed risky.

Third, the disaggregation of global supply chains became increasingly complex and threatened the autonomy of major car companies that had previously made most parts themselves. At the 2016 Detroit Auto Show, Sergio Marchionne, the CEO of Fiat Chrysler, warned that contracting out production of electric powertrains to third-party suppliers risked carmakers losing control over elements of a vehicle's contents to suppliers. "If we start losing any of that," Marchionne said, "we will not be able to hang on to any proprietary knowledge and control of that business."[45] Takata's exploding airbags illustrated the damage that supplier decisions can impose on carmakers.

Another reason the number of automobiles with defects increased was the changing regulatory approaches of the National Traffic and Motor Vehicle Safety Act, the main US regulator of car safety. Spurred by consumer, health, and environmental activism and Ralph Nader's 1965 expose of the car industry, *Unsafe at Any Speed*, Congress unanimously passed and President Lyndon B. Johnson in 1966 signed a law to create a new agency charged with keeping people safe on America's roadways.

The National Highway Traffic Safety Administration was designed to create an "engineering utopia" in which cars would be safe despite their drivers. Reflecting congressional and public faith in technology, one participant in the congressional auto safety hearings asked, "If we can send a man to the moon and back, why can't we design a safe automobile here on Earth?"[46] But that ambitious aspiration soon encountered opposition from the economic and political system that was emerging to challenge the consumer and health protection advances won by the social movements of the 1960s.

As Yale legal scholars Jerry Mashaw and David Harfst describe in their comprehensive review of the legal history of NHTSA, the agency was unable to fulfill the vision of its proponents.[47] Moreover, by 1974, the NHTSA was encountering significant pushback to its efforts to mandate passive seatbelts, airbags, and ignition interlocks. Challenges came from the auto industry, the courts, and even the Congress that had passed the new law. Between 1966 and 1986, seventeen of NHTSA's safety rules were challenged in court with twelve of these suits coming from industry groups. The agency lost half these challenges, decisions that weakened its authority to make rules and raised the bar on the evidence needed to justify regulatory action.

In 1981, President Reagan claimed that "strangling regulation," including safety regulation, was the root cause of the auto industry's economic troubles and withdrew previously approved safety rules and offered additional regulatory relief measures.[48] Congress did not provide much support either. It adopted the cost-benefit mindset of the Reagan Administration and failed to clarify legislatively what type of evidence was needed to warrant safety regulations.

Throughout its battles with regulators, the auto industry found a powerful political ally, Representative John Dingell from Detroit, who viewed representing the auto industry as a key constituent service. Two of Dingell's sons worked for the automobile industry and his second wife, Deborah Dingell, now a congresswoman herself, was a lobbyist for General Motors.

For nearly six decades, Dingell championed the auto industry in Congress. He fought mandatory airbags in the late 1970s, played a key role in providing federal funding to bail out Chrysler and General Motors after the 2008 financial crisis, and in 2014 helped automakers stave off a proposed bill that would have boosted maximum fines for delaying recalls to $250 million—up from $17 million.[49] Justifying his action, he said, "This is still a free nation, where people buy what they want and where the government doesn't tell them what they can buy." One auto safety advocacy group estimated that one hundred thousand lives could have been saved had all the safety measures Dingell opposed gone into effect when they were first put on the table.[50]

Not surprisingly, given the opposition, the NHTSA soon stopped using its authority to mandate new technologies. Between 1987 and 2002, according to Mashaw and Harfst, "significant rulemaking at NHTSA atrophied nearly to the point of extinction."[51] The measures passed in the earlier era continued to save lives but the agency no longer acted as an independent watchdog mandated to anticipate and prevent emerging threats. Instead, Congress and the NHTSA created a new system of co-regulation that focused on recalls of defective cars.

In this approach, the auto industry would develop new safety technologies, and test them by selling to high-end customers, limiting its financial risk by using its small cohort of customers willing to pay more for safety as the guinea pigs for the new technology. Once the auto industry had shown it could master these technologies, Congress passed new laws mandating their installation on many or all vehicles. Examples of problems addressed by this approach included improving side-impact protection, preventing rollover of cars and SUVs, improving seats belts for children and small people, and installing anti-lock brakes.

These measures helped to bring the benefits of protection to a wider population, contributing to a more equitable distribution of the benefits of new technologies. But by leaving innovation to the industry, government willingness to co-regulate allowed the automobile makers themselves to determine which safety measures could pass their cost-benefit calculations, abdicating government responsibility to make protecting health a higher goal than protecting profits.

Between 1991 and 2005, Congress passed three omnibus directives, mandating the NHTSA to require auto companies to meet these standards. Adverse court decisions declined, in part because congressional intent was clear and in part because the rules used only technologies already developed and tested by the industry.

The NHTSA also responded to the industry by opposing the development of new, tougher regulation and instead focusing on its authority to recall cars with defects. Recalls required a lower standard of evidence than regulations and generally generated public support rather than criticism. Who could be against fixing defective cars? In 2018, automakers in the United States issued 914 recalls, affecting 29 million vehicles, more than 10 percent of all the vehicles registered in the United States that year.[52] Between 2011 and 2015, 147 million vehicles were recalled, about 57 percent of all vehicles registered in 2015.

Owners of defective cars certainly expect to be notified if their vehicles are defective and for the defect to be expeditiously repaired. But waiting to act until people are killed or injured, as happened with recalls for the General Motors faulty ignition switch, leaves consumers to be the canaries in the coal mine. According to an investigation by *The Wall Street Journal*, in about one in four major recalls since 2015, less than half the vehicles recalled have been fixed within eighteen months, leaving about 70 million unrepaired cars on the road.[53] Most disturbing, it is not known whether recalls actually protect lives since few studies evaluate their impact on deaths and injuries.[54] As Mashaw and Harfst observe, recalls are "coercive with respect to the disclosures manu-facturers must make and the corrective action they must take" but that elec-tion is entirely up to the consumer.[55]

Recalls reinforce the notion of individual responsibility for safety, the long-standing mantra of the industry, which asserts that most injuries and deaths are the fault of drivers, not automakers. It also limits the responsibility of automakers to ensure that their products are safe before they sell them. In short, NHTSA has abandoned its watchdog role to become "a provider of con-sumer safety information, an enforcer of implied warranties (product recalls), a codifier of industry practice, a broker of voluntary agreements, and a pro-moter of best practices and guidelines."[56] In this way, NHTSA aptly illustrates a common transformation of regulatory agencies in twenty-first-century capitalism.

Between 1966, the year that the National Traffic and Motor Vehicle Safety Act passed, and 2018, more than 2.2 million people in the United States have died in motor vehicle collisions. Since 1990, more than 79 mil-lion people have been injured in automobile collisions. In a 2015 report, NHTSA estimated that since 1960 motor vehicle safety technologies in-cluding seat belts, airbags, child safety seats, and electronic stability control have saved 613,501 lives, about 25 percent of the total automobile crash deaths in that period.

While deaths per million miles traveled have declined sharply through 2010, for the last decade the number of deaths has remained stuck at about thirty thousand to forty thousand deaths per year, with about seventy times as many annual injuries as deaths. Moreover, deaths per million miles trav-eled in the United States are more than twice as high as the rates in Sweden, Switzerland, and the United Kingdom. These statistics show the success of the auto industry and its allies in getting Americans to drive more, but the nation's limited progress in creating a regulatory system that makes auto safety a priority.

BIG TECH, BIG AUTO, AND BIG RIDE HAIL AND AUTONOMOUS VEHICLES

In the nineteenth century, horses dominated individual transportation and railroads and trollies moved people within and between cities, and in the twen-tieth century it was automobiles. Most observers agree that in the twenty-first century, autonomous vehicles (AVs) or driverless cars will become a dominant form of human transportation. AVs have the potential to bring health, envi-ronmental, equity, and economic benefits to users and society as a whole but they also pose grave risks. How will the United States and other nations decide how to balance these benefits and risks? And how will recent changes in capitalism influence how the costs and benefits of AVs are distributed and how this new technology is deployed and managed?

Autonomous vehicles are defined as vehicles that can make decisions independent of human action and in the face of uncertainty.[57] They rely on new technologies such as artificial intelligence, global positioning systems, lidar (light detection and ranging sensors), thermal and infrared imaging, and vehicle-to-vehicle and vehicle-to-infrastructure communications systems. All these technologies collect and analyze data to inform real-time driving decisions (See Figure 6.1).[58]

The Society of Automotive Engineers International defines several levels of automation, from partial automation, where human drivers can choose to use tools like automated cruise control, to full automation, where the vehicle fully controls all dynamic tasks.[59] Currently, transportation planners have no standard approach for testing and approving AVs. However, most observers conclude that AVs will spread rapidly in the coming decades. One analyst predicts that by 2050 half of the world's vehicle fleet will be autonomous and by 2070 more than 90 percent.[60] Strategy Analytics, a business research group, estimates that autonomous driving technology will enable a new "Passenger Economy" worth $7 trillion by 2050.[61]

Like moths to light, these predictions have attracted a wide cross section of global corporations to the AV market. Google started its AV program in 2009 and by 2017, Waymo, the Google AV spin-off, had accumulated 3 million miles on its AV cars in four US states. Already all Tesla models have some self-driving capacity and by 2020, Audi, BMW, Mercedes-Benz, and Nissan had AVs on the market. General Motors is partnering with Lyft and Volvo with Uber to create AV taxi systems.[62] IBM is creating plug-and-play automated driving tech systems for existing car companies.[63]

AVs have the potential to bring several significant social benefits. First, they could reduce the global toll from automobile crashes, which now account for nearly 1.25 million deaths and 20 to 50 million injuries or disabilities each year.[64] By automating control, some deaths attributable to drunken or distracted driving, vision problems, or risky aggressive driving could be prevented.

But experts disagree about how big a reduction is likely.[65] Based on the widely cited statistic that 90 percent of auto deaths are caused by human error, some AV advocates claim that fully autonomous vehicles could reduce deaths by 90 percent. But this ignores key experiences with other technologies. The complex software and hardware used by AVs can fail with catastrophic results, as shown by the handful of deaths in experiments in the past decade. Some drivers may take more risks, such as not using seat belts, and some pedestrians may assume AVs will not hit them, crossing roads with less caution. In

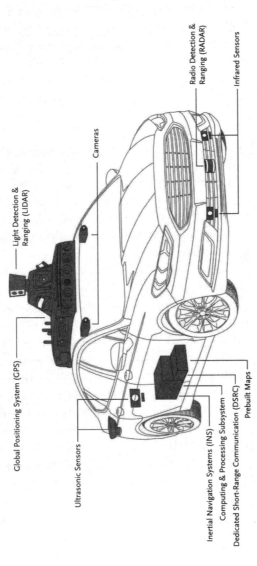

Global Positioning System (GPS)

Light Detection & Ranging (LIDAR)

Cameras

Radio Detection & Ranging (RADAR)

Infrared Sensors

Ultrasonic Sensors

Inertial Navigation Systems (INS)

Computing & Processing Subsystem

Dedicated Short-Range Communication (DSRC)

Prebuilt Maps

Fig. 6.1 Autonomous vehicles—driverless cars—use a variety of technologies to replace human senses and judgments. Each has its own capacities and vulnerabilities, and most have not been tested in field conditions.

Photo: Key technologies and additional ICT devices in a generic CAV for navigation and communication, 2018, in Morteza Taiebat, Austin L. Brown, Hannah R. Safford, Shen Qu, and Ming Xu, *Environmental Science & Technology* 2018 52, no. 20: 11449–65, https://pubs.acs.org/doi/10.1021/acs.est.8b00127. Please contact the American Chemical Society for further permissions.

order to achieve reductions in congestion and travel time it will be necessary to allow vehicles to operate at high speeds and to travel close together in dedicated lanes, increasing the risk of serious crashes.[66]

AVs can also reduce congestion and pollution, including harmful toxics and greenhouse gasses. The level of declines will depend on the proportion of AVs that are electric rather than fossil-fueled, and whether AV-shared taxi services replace personal auto use. Some studies conclude that under some circumstances, AVs can significantly reduce miles traveled, emissions, and greenhouse gases (GHG). One study found that electric AV taxis would cut per-mile GHG emissions by more than 90 percent compared to conventional vehicles.[67] A simulation study found that if New York City's entire taxi fleet were electric AVs, the fleet would generate 73 percent fewer GHG emissions and consume 58 percent less energy than a non-electrified automated fleet.[68] Alternatively, lower costs and shorter travel time could increase demand for these vehicles, and lead to increases in miles traveled and decreases in walking, and bicycle and mass transit use.

AVs can potentially lower costs for users, government, and society as a whole. Private AV taxi services are expected to cost less than traditional taxis and less than personal vehicles. Mass transit, however, is far less expensive than either of these options.[69]

However, the AV industrial complex has embraced a prior auto industry goal to justify its proposed solutions to mobility. For more than a century, industry-influenced transport planners have made the uninterrupted flow of traffic the holy grail rather than seeking to design transportation systems that make it easier, safer, and less polluting to move around. A centralized corporate-controlled AV system may in fact lead to improved traffic flow but not reduce pedestrian injuries and deaths, air pollution, or transport encroachment on public space. Solving the technological problem of improving traffic flow fits within the industry wheelhouse and is likely to be profitable. Making healthier, more livable communities may not. The 2020 decision by Sidewalk Labs, a Google affiliate, to close its Toronto "smart cities" project to redesign that city's downtown, citing the economic turmoil from the COVID-19 pandemic, shows this hesitation.[70]

AVs can also have an impact on transportation equity. They can make it easier for the 30 percent of the population who do not drive—adolescents, older people, those with disabilities—to move around.[71] Policies of AV companies and governments could make the ability to get to work, food, healthcare, and education more accessible and affordable.

However, if AVs are mostly privately owned and managed, costs could increase and have the opposite effect, making mobility less accessible for low-income groups and rural residents. The growth of private AVs could diminish public support and financing for public mass transit, with the harm concentrated on the low-income populations that benefit most from mass transit. As one transit planner put it:

> I could easily see a situation in which we get the regulatory framework for AVs wrong, that we're too laissez-faire, too deregulatory about it and effectively that the vulnerable parties . . . the older, non tech-savvy people are unable to access the benefits and that the 16 to 25 demographic is priced out of being able to access it and in effect becomes a luxury urban transport for yuppies.[72]

At worst, the growth of AVs could accelerate and exacerbate transport apartheid, in which wealthier individuals have access to multiple safe, comfortable travel options while less advantaged groups are forced to use unsafe, crowded, and time-consuming modes of travel.[73] The poorest households in the country spend up to 40 percent of their net income on transportation, compared with the 20 percent the average American spends. Furthermore, the growth of household expenditures on transportation is increasing much faster for the poor, African Americans, and Latinxs than for whites and the middle class as whole.[74]

Already transportation systems in rural Mississippi, urban South Africa, Mexico City, and elsewhere illustrate the human and economic costs of inequitable and segregated transportation systems. A related concern is that differential access to AVs could contribute to further suburbanization and urban sprawl,[75] just as taxpayer and policy support for the automobile industry in the post–World War II period led to the growth of racially segregated suburbs.

Finally, the growth of AVs will have employment consequences. Some new jobs will be created to service and maintain AVs and their infrastructure and produce the software and hardware needed to control AVs. But many jobs will be lost, including in the automobile and transportation industries. About 3.8 million workers operate motor vehicles such as trucks or taxis; truck drivers are the most vulnerable to automation because they drive mainly on highways, with navigation that is easier to automate than urban driving.[76] Truck driving is one of the few jobs where workers without a college degree can still make more than twice the federal minimum wage. A 2017 report by Goldman Sachs found that when AVs reach peak saturation, loss of driver jobs could reach three hundred thousand a year.[77]

What will determine which of the potential benefits and costs of AVs are actually realized and how they will be allocated among different population groups? Currently, policy makers and voters lack the evidence needed to make informed decisions. Despite burgeoning academic, government, and business studies of AVs, most authors emphasize the complexity of studying AV impact and the uncertainty and variability of available data.[78] In general, studies commissioned by industry and investors emphasize the positive impact of AVs while those by independent researchers highlight possible risks. How policy makers use this evidence and assess the validity of conclusions will influence their decisions.

Policy analyses of options for AVs consider the role of local, state, or regional and national governments in regulating safety, sustainability, pricing, and other outcomes. Strikingly absent from these analyses, however, is any assessment of the role of industry in shaping these decisions.

The track record of corporate transport companies in protecting public well-being raises serious concerns. The automobile industry has consistently minimized the safety and environmental problems of its products, covered up defects, and used its political power to defeat, delay, or weaken regulation.[79] Tech companies like Google and Microsoft have also resisted government regulation, defended their rights to keep the data they collect private, and used their concentrated control of mass and social media to frame policy debates in terms favorable to their interests.[80] Transportation network companies like Uber and Lyft have lobbied to preempt local governments from regulating them, made campaign contributions to sway politicians, and threatened to leave jurisdictions that impose unwanted rules.[81]

The previous practices of these industries, the impact of recent additional constitutional protections for corporate speech and financial contributions, and local and state government's reluctance to regulate private transport or make new investments in public mass transit suggest that Big Auto, Big Tech, and Big Transport Networks will exert powerful influence on AV policies in the years to come.

Policy makers will need to make difficult and technically complex decisions about how to balance the individual benefits of AVs—shorter travel times, lower costs, more convenient access—with its potential public benefits such as less pollution, fewer collisions, and more transport equity. In some cases, pursuing the former conflicts with achieving the latter.

As British transportation researchers Tom Cohen and Clemence Cavoli observe, the public and politicians must decide whether to regulate AVs mainly with what they call "anticipatory governance" or with the more traditional laissez-faire approach in which markets determine the direction of AV public policy.[82] Anticipatory governance acknowledges uncertainty, avoids technological determinism, and values the precautionary principle, each of which can lead to conflict with corporate actors.

If corporations seeking to harvest some of the $7 trillion that the AV economy is predicted to generate by 2050 put their powerful thumbs on the policy scale to ensure that politicians approve only those solutions that increase their revenues and profits, the prospect for achieving the potential social benefits from AVs seem dim.

The challenge facing those seeking alternatives to a corporate-imposed autonomous vehicle future is to bring together the many now-separate constituencies who will pay the costs of this approach. Urban residents seeking more accessible and affordable mobility, the many workers now dependent on our fossil fuel–dependent transportation system, the hundreds of millions of people sickened by air pollution and displaced by climate change, all these and more will benefit from advancing people-centered rather than profit-driven transportation systems.

HOW MODERN CAPITALISM HAS CHANGED TRANSPORTATION

As these profiles of various sectors of the auto industry show, recent changes in capitalism have precipitated transformations in transportation, as they have changed how individuals encounter other pillars of health. The globalization of the automobile industry and its supply chains has reduced the capacity of national governments to regulate emissions, safety, and working conditions and increased the power of concentrated, multinational auto companies to influence trade, regulatory, and tax policies that favor their interests.[83] As the Takata exploding airbags story shows, the global auto industry's reliance on a single or a few suppliers for key parts leaves both companies and drivers vulnerable to defects that can have a global impact.

These adverse consequences of globalization are both a cause and a consequence of the deregulatory imperative of modern capitalism. In both the United States and Europe, auto companies are gaining a bigger voice in shaping regulatory policies. NHTSA has redefined its mission from fostering the use of new technologies to make cars safer to allowing the industry to develop and test new safety systems, then mandating the use of those that are practical and cost-effective for industry.[84] In the European Union, lax enforcement allowed Volkswagen to cheat on its emissions tests for more than a decade.[85]

Technological determinism, the capitalist-inspired belief that new technologies inevitably drive innovation, led governments around the world to support the world's largest corporations to develop AVs, missing the opportunity to use their authority to ensure that the AVs would benefit, rather than harm, human well-being, urban living, and environmental quality. Techno-optimism, the belief that new technologies inescapably benefit humanity,[86] further justified the deployment of AVs and also enabled the corporations developing AV technologies to mask their focused pursuit of their self-interest, whatever the human consequences of their choices.

For auto industry insiders, the presumption that AVs will reduce injuries and deaths is a matter of faith, an illustration of techno-optimism. At a 2016 press event, Elon Musk, the CEO of Tesla, the maker of electric cars, warned journalists with doubts about self-driving cars that "if, in writing something that's negative, you effectively dissuade people from using an autonomous vehicle, you're killing people."[87]

However, researchers who study AVs are skeptical about Musk's faith in the technology. "People in the international road safety community aren't running around incredibly excited about autonomous vehicles," says Ben Welle of World Resource Institute for Sustainable Cities.[88] "We don't know if they are going to work, or when they're going to work. And meanwhile we know what we can do: we can get over this idea that we must engineer unending car flow. And we can do that now." In this and other ways, corporate leaders seek to replace evidence with their faith in technology as the criterion for making policy decisions.

In a 2011 speech to auto executives, Lawrence Burns, former General Motors research and development chief and Google self-driving car adviser, sought to convince his audience to accelerate the development of AVs. "It's within our grasp, and I believe the consumers are going to love what we come up with—and I think there's going to be ways to make some really good money doing it. . . . Why are we waiting?" he asked.[89]

In fact, only a few years later, experience had tempered this giddy enthusiasm as AVs faced technological and political challenges. But by that time techno-optimism had convinced Google, General Motors, Ford, and Uber to invest so much in AVs that private capital's continued pursuit of this avenue for growth and profits was assured. This determination, it appears, was motivated as much by the fear that a global competitor would succeed at solving some critical component of AV technology as by evidence that such vehicles were safe, profitable, or more sustainable than alternatives.

THE HEALTH IMPACT OF TWENTY-FIRST-CENTURY TRANSPORTATION

By the end of the first two decades of the twenty-first century, the established and emerging transportation systems supported by modern capitalism posed a variety of challenges to mobility, well-being, climate, and both urban and rural quality of life. In the United States and other high-income countries, getting from one place to another contributed to premature deaths and preventable injuries, exacerbated class and racial gaps in health and wealth, took time away from more pleasurable pursuits, and aggravated the climate crisis. In low- and middle-income countries, the choices made by global transportation industries had an even greater impact with the burdens falling more heavily on those living in poverty.

Other forms of transportation also pose dangers to health and the environment. Witness the recent failure of both Boeing and the Federal Aviation Administration to detect, prevent, remediate, and disclose to the public what they knew about safety problems in the Boeing 737 MAX aircraft.[90] But the overwhelming dependence on motor vehicles for transportation and commerce makes cars the most significant threat to well-being.

In the United States, motor vehicle crashes are the leading cause of death in the first three decades of Americans' lives and kill about ninety-six people every day. Although the number of deaths has declined in recent years, motor vehicle–related injuries send more than 2.3 million people to hospital emergency departments every year.[91] And pedestrian fatalities in the United States have increased 41 percent since 2008,[92] increases attributed to the rise of SUVs, an innovation that brought huge profits to the automobile industry but more injuries and deaths to pedestrians as well as passengers and drivers.

SUVs also illustrate the vicious cycle of capitalist consumption. In the 1990s, automakers doubled down on SUVs because they were more profitable and at that time faced few foreign competitors. American auto companies spent billions of dollars promoting ever-larger SUVs, misrepresenting their safety record and appealing to, as one Chrysler marketer put it, to the "reptilian brains" of drivers who wanted to experience (even if only in their imagination) the thrill off-road driving or the confidence that comes from being able to flatten any other car.[93] GM, Ford, and Chrysler then insisted they were only seeking to meet customer demand for SUVs, a demand they had worked hard to nurture. When car sales declined after the 2008 fiscal crisis, carmakers continued to promote and sell SUVs by offering generous auto loans to car buyers, thus contributing to more debt, air pollution, and motor vehicle deaths.[94] Auto loans reached a ten year high in 2019.

Another cause of the increase in pedestrian injuries and deaths is distracted driving, a consequence of the tech industry's success in making cell phones ubiquitous and seemingly essential in all settings. Since 2010, deaths of cyclists, which had been declining, started to rise, increasing 25 percent by 2017.[95] Overall, deaths and injuries from traffic cost the nation about $44 billion in medical expenses and work losses every year.

Survivors of motor vehicle crashes—and family members of those killed—experience lower quality of life, higher levels of stress, and much higher medical costs. These costs are disproportionately borne by those with low incomes, people of color, and other vulnerable populations.[96] For some, the experience makes them traffic safety activists. "My 12-year-old son was killed in a crash in front of our home," explained one mother from New York City. "He kissed me goodbye and said, 'I love you Mommy.' I never imagined those would be his last words. [My son] was bright, kind, athletic and had a huge heart. We miss him every day. After his death, I joined with others and helped found Families for Safe Streets in N.Y.C."[97]

Globally, according to the World Health Organization, about 1.35 million people die each year as a result of road traffic crashes, the world's tenth leading cause of death.[98] For children and young adults aged five to twenty-nine years, road traffic injuries are the leading cause of death. In 2015, the "2030 Agenda for Sustainable Development" set the ambitious target of reducing the global number of deaths and injuries from road traffic crashes by 50 percent by 2020, a goal not achieved. More than half of all road traffic deaths are among pedestrians, cyclists, and motorcyclists. More than 90 percent of the world's fatalities on the roads occur in low- and middle-income countries, even though these countries have only 60 percent of the world's vehicles. Although we know how to reduce these burdens—improve vehicle safety, enforce traffic rules, and increase mass transit—a 2018 WHO report on traffic safety concluded, "Drastic action is needed to put these measures in place to meet any future global target that might be set and save lives."[99]

Nor is the lethal impact of motor vehicle transportation limited to those killed in car and truck collisions. In fact, air pollution has overtaken crashes as the primary cause of auto-related preventable deaths. In the twenty-first century, the health, economic, and social costs of air pollution have increased dramatically, despite some improvements in pollution control in previous decades. According to the Lancet Commission on Pollution and Health, air pollution accounted for 9 million premature deaths in 2015, three times the number of deaths from AIDS, tuberculosis, and malaria combined, and fifteen times the number from all wars and other forms of violence.[100] Social and productivity losses due to air pollution are estimated to amount to $4.6 trillion a year, 6.2 percent of global economic output.

Fossil fuel combustion is the primary cause of air pollution, accounting for 85 percent of particulate matter—the most toxic form of air pollution—and for almost all the pollution by nitrogen and sulfur oxides. Seventy percent of the diseases caused by pollution are non-communicable (chronic) diseases such as lung and heart diseases and cancer, the most expensive and burdensome illnesses for individuals, families, and healthcare systems.[101] Emerging research suggests that air pollution can also disrupt endocrine function, contribute to inflammation, increase low birth weight, and have neurotoxic effects on child development—frightening findings that suggest that its harmful effects may be larger than known and likely to grow. Those living in highly polluted areas were also at higher risk of dying from COVID-19 infection.

Many sources including power plants, heating, and manufacturing also contribute to air pollution, but motor vehicle emissions are a primary cause. According to the United States Environment Protection Agency, in 2018 motor vehicles caused 75 percent of carbon monoxide pollution in the US, 61 percent of nitrogen oxides, and 20 percent of volatile organic compounds.[102] Motor vehicles also contribute a stew of air toxins such as benzene, formaldehyde, and diesel particulate matter, compounds that are known or suspected to cause cancer or other health problems and environmental effects.

In 2017, according to the EPA, transportation contributed 29 percent of human-produced greenhouse gas emissions in the United States and were the largest single contributor.[103] Cars and trucks accounted for 82 percent of transportation's contribution. In its 2019 special report for policy makers, the Intergovernmental Panel on Climate Change warned:

> Deferral of GHG emissions reductions from all sectors implies trade-offs including irreversible loss in land ecosystem functions and services required for food, health, habitable settlements, and production, leading to increasingly significant economic impacts on many countries in many regions of the world.[104]

Fortunately, as the Lancet Commission observed, multiple strategies to reduce air pollution have been demonstrated to be effective and cost-effective, especially in high-income countries. Their report concludes that "pollution control provides an extraordinary opportunity to improve the health of the planet. It is a winnable battle."[105]

Current transportation options shape human well-being in other ways. Some urban planners fear that AVs could exacerbate sprawl and suburbanization by making it easier and cheaper to leave cities, where housing, food, and other pillars of health are often more expensive. As one critic of the auto industry's influence on quality of life observed, the worst outcome of the automobile-centered twentieth century may be "the assumption that it's people who need to get out of the way of these lethal machines, instead of the other way around."[106]

Urban sprawl, defined as the diffusion of urban features such as dense or high-rise housing and shopping corridors into less developed land near a city, and suburbanization, the shift of populations from central cities into less dense suburbs, have been linked with adverse effects on physical and mental health, quality of life, and the environment.[107] Compared to urban residents, those living in suburbs or sprawled places drive more, putting them at risk of collisions and episodes of road rage. They also use more energy to heat and cool their homes, contributing to air pollution and climate change. Suburban residents exercise less, elevating risk for chronic diseases and mental health problems, and have higher risks of social isolation and its mental health consequences. Suburban development also facilitates residential segregation, maintaining the high social and health costs of racial stratification.

Of course, many people enjoy the benefits of suburban living such as more space, less crowding, and more outdoor time. The relevant point for this discussion is that the particular elements of suburbanization that were influenced by the auto industry and its allies contributed significantly to its harmful health and environmental consequences.

As communities and nations consider their options for transportation and mobility, the basic questions that confront social decisions on other pillars of health also arise in this sector. Who decides and who reaps the benefits and costs of these decisions? In the twentieth century, the automobile industry and its allies created a transportation system that brought new freedoms and new lifestyles to millions of Americans but also killed and injured millions, polluted the air, worsened climate change, and degraded the quality of life in urban and suburban areas.

What will be the future of transportation in the coming years? Without significant political change, the multinational companies that drive and profit from the transportation sector will continue to play the leading role in setting local, regional, national, and global transportation policies. Thus, the stories of Uber and Lyft's efforts to replace public mass transit; the limited concern for safety and honesty that General Motors, Takata, Volkswagen, and other companies showed when facing defects or competitive pressures; and the aggressive actions by carmakers, Big Tech companies, and transportation network companies to put rapid deployment and profitability from AVs ahead of safety, environment impact, or equity do not provide grounds for optimism.

As in other sectors, however, a deeper and longer-term assessment of the future impact of transportation on well-being and planetary health requires an analysis of the forces resisting corporate influences and testing alternatives to market-driven transportation

RESISTANCE AND ALTERNATIVES

Since the founding of the auto industry, some organizations have always challenged its practices and its right to be the dominant force in creating the nation's transportation options. In the 1920s, city residents and local newspapers often protested the arrival of motor cars, describing them as perils imposed by elites and one more threat to urban survival.[108]

In 1970, on the first Earth Day, college students in Boston trashed a car with sledgehammers, calling cars "killers of people." In New York City, students demonstrated in front of General Motors headquarters, carrying banners that said, "GM Takes Your Breath Away." They accused GM of producing one-third of the nation's air pollution.[109]

In 2002, the Evangelical Environmental Network, a coalition of religious and environmental groups, launched a campaign asking, "Would Jesus Drive an SUV?" They urged Ford, GM, and other automakers to stop producing and marketing gas-guzzling, dangerous, and polluting SUVs and asked their religious followers to set an example by refusing to buy vehicles that endangered the health of the planet. Reverend Jim Ball, the founder of the network explained, "We're asking the basic question: 'what would Jesus drive?' We think Jesus is Lord of our transportation choices, as well as our other choices. When you need a car, you should buy the most fuel-efficient one that truly meets your needs. We believe transportation is a moral issue because it and the pollution it creates have a serious impact on people's lives."[110]

Today, a variety of nongovernmental organizations, community coalitions, and government agencies continue to confront auto dominance and to seek healthier, more sustainable transportation options. I examine a few to assess what they have—and have not—achieved and how the auto industry has responded to their critiques.

The Center for Auto Safety. The Center for Auto Safety was founded in 1970 by Consumers Union and Ralph Nader to serve as a consumer safety group that protects drivers. Fueled by the same environmental, consumer protection, and health and safety movements that led to the passage of the National Traffic and Motor Vehicle Safety Act in 1966 and the establishment of the US Environmental Protection Agency in 1970, the center took on several roles including serving as a watchdog of the NHTSA; educating the public, the media, and policy makers about car safety issues so these constituencies could put additional pressure on carmakers to make safer cars; and advocating for stronger safety laws and more vigorous enforcement. The multiple strategies it used, often in partnership with other groups such as Consumers Union, Public Interest Research Groups, and the Union of Concerned Scientists, magnified its impact, achieving synergies beyond the reach of any single strategy or group.

By creating a national, coordinated, relatively coherent, multilevel, and multi-issue interest group, the center and its partners were able to force one of the world's most powerful industries to make concessions, and to somewhat modify its most harmful practices. They were also able to challenge the industry narrative that it always put safety first and that its technological savvy was the best protector of drivers, pedestrians, and the earth's environment.

In their fifty-year history, the center has an impressive record of achievement. It has instigated the recall of tens of millions of defective automobiles and parts, including the products of GM, Chrysler, Ford, Toyota, Volkswagen, Firestone tires, and Takata; strengthened highway safety laws; protected auto safety consumer and safety laws under attack by industry and the politicians it supported; launched a Safe Climate Campaign to strengthen auto emission standards and fuel efficiency, thus linking auto safety and environmental groups in the effort to reduce fossil fuel use.[111]

The director of the center was Clarence Ditlow, an engineer and lawyer who started his career as one of Nader's Raiders, passionate young activists who came to Washington to work with Nader to pass, then monitor, new laws to protect consumers, health, and the environment. Until his death in 2016, Ditlow and his colleagues sued the auto industry; testified before and lobbied Congress; and wrote op-eds, books, and policy reports. As *The New York Times* observed, Ditlow led the center with a budget less than half of what GM paid for a single Super Bowl commercial. "He was the nightmare of the misbehaving auto industry and the dream of safety-conscious motorists," said Ralph Nader.[112]

The center specialized in using the Freedom of Information Act, and "defect petitions," another consumer tool, to force the NHTSA to investigate a defect and publish its findings in the Federal Record. The center also mined NHTSA's public databases to discover and publicize problems. Through a Freedom of Information request in 1978, for example, Ditlow discovered a secret memo that raised questions about the safety of Firestone 500 steel-belted radial tires. The center's publicity of the findings led to a recall of 15 million tires, albeit only after twelve deaths.[113] Jackie Gillan, another auto safety expert, called Ditlow "the Sherlock Holmes for auto safety when it came to investigating faulty vehicle systems."

By using new rights to obtain corporate information won in the 1960s and 1970s to investigate and publicize auto safety problems over the next forty years, the center helped to fill a regulatory void and create an accountability system that other corporate watchdog groups could emulate when regulators lose the will or resources needed to fulfill their mandates.

After it had collected and analyzed data, the center also developed new ways to communicate with the public. In 1993, the center organized a demonstration outside the annual meeting of GM stockholders in Oklahoma City to urge the company to recall the millions of what it called "rolling firebombs"—pickup trucks with fuel tanks that the NHTSA reported were more likely to burst into flames after side-impact crashes than other brands. GM had resisted the request for a recall.[114] The NHTSA newsletters to its fifteen thousand members created a national network of informed auto safety advocates who could act at the local, state, and national levels.

Both the auto industry and regulators often criticize the center. The NHTSA accused the center of undermining government oversight activities and of working too closely with product liability lawyers, a group Ditlow considered useful allies. Overall, the center contributed to winning billions of dollars in fines and settlements from the auto industry and forcing the recalls of tens of millions of vehicles. Ditlow shrugged off the inevitable criticism from the industry. Asked about his 1991 criticism of defects in Chrysler vehicles, then led by Lee Iacocca, Ditlow said, "He makes 'em; we recall 'em. We have a standing offer to stop our opposition when they stop making bad cars."[115]

In recent years, the center has joined the fight to regulate ride-hailing companies like Uber, and AVs. In a 2019 public letter to Uber's CEO, Dara Khosrowshahi, the center wrote to urge Uber to stop sending out Uber cars that had been recalled but not repaired. "Uber can stop the use of cars with open safety recalls on its platform at the proverbial push of a button," wrote Jason Levine, the new director of the center. "Uber claims to be a sophisticated technology company but, so far, your company has refused to use easy-to-access technology to decrease the danger of unrepaired recalls to your customers and drivers."[116]

Levine also wrote an op-ed on self-driving cars criticizing the NHTSA for rolling back federal safety regulations "in order to accelerate the sale of self-driving cars, despite the lack of evidence that vehicles lacking manual controls are safe. This effort to deregulate, combined with the existing and highly questionable federal policy of allowing the testing of driverless cars anywhere in the U.S., creates risks that go beyond sharing the road with these vehicles."[117]

Today, the center and similar groups play critical roles in educating the public and policy makers; putting pressures on regulators, politicians, and corporations to pay attention to health, safety, and the environment; and using legal and legislative methods to devise solutions to established and emerging problems.

In the long run, groups like the center struggle to find the right balance between being one more player in the complex regulatory system of modern capitalism and a catalyst for more transformative change. On the one hand, civil society watchdogs risk justifying the lax regulatory status quo by serving as a backstop for regulatory failures and inadequacies. If the center is already monitoring NHTSA, ask legislators, why should we spend more taxpayer money on more intensive scrutiny? On the other hand, should groups like the center push for more radical change, for example, for withdrawing the corporate charters of auto companies that have more than three major recalls within three years (the three strikes and you are out corporate death sentence),[118] do they risk credibility and impact in routine regulatory monitoring? A strength of the center is its ability to act both as a part of the regulatory process, using established rules, and acting outside this framework using more disruptive and adversarial strategies.

Alternative urban transportation in New York City. The advocacy organization Transportation Alternatives seeks to reclaim New York City's streets from the automobile and advocate for better bicycling, walking, and public transit for all New Yorkers. The group notes that streets and sidewalks constitute 80 percent of public space in New York City (the equivalent of fifty-eight Central Parks)—but right now, the lives of city residents are polluted, congested, and endangered by car and truck traffic.[119] Informed by the belief that this public space belongs to the people of New York City, Transportation Alternatives organizes demonstrations to urge more bike lanes and better protections for pedestrian and bike riders, analyzes city and state transit proposals, testifies at legislative hearings, and prepares reports and policy briefs.

In 2019, Transportation Alternatives played an important role in convincing New York City to close 14th Street, a major Manhattan thoroughfare, to car traffic for eighteen months, leaving it open only for busses, delivery trucks, and emergency vehicles. After the change, the time it took busses to cross Manhattan at 14th Street, dropped from thirty minutes to twenty-one, a gift to riders to use as they chose.[120]

In response to the COVID-19 pandemic, Transportation Alternatives encouraged an "approach to city building that uses temporary, affordable, and easily-implemented solutions, often starting small and piloting more permanent change." By reclaiming public spaces from automobiles and opening streets for walking and bicycling, cities can support a new kind of public life and demonstrate the benefits of post-auto cities.[121]

Families for Safe Streets is an organization of victims of traffic violence and families whose relatives have been killed or severely injured by aggressive or reckless driving and dangerous conditions on New York City's streets.[122] It grew out of the work of Transportation Alternatives and continues to receive support and guidance from its sponsor.

In a message to its followers after two important legislative victories at the state level, Transportation Alternative leaders explained how its persistent advocacy has started to change New York City's car culture. "In the battle to reclaim New York City's streets, our to-do list is always a mile long, but we're betting that all those tiny advances will add up to a radical transformation.," wrote an organizer. After winning legislation that required the city to install speed safety cameras in 750 school zones around the city, Transportation Alternatives and other activists convinced the state legislature to approve a congestion pricing plan that would encourage New Yorkers to use mass transit rather than cars to travel downtown. In just a few weeks of legislative activity, wrote the activists, the future of transportation in New York City took a big step away from the car.[123] Later, city-level rules to create pedestrian islands, protected bike lanes, signal retiming, and wider sidewalks were also approved.[124]

Two decades of transportation advocacy in New York City have helped to challenge the notion that there is no alternative to a city dominated by car culture. In 2019, Corey Johnson, the speaker of the New York City Council, following the path opened by advocates, introduced legislation designed to "break car culture" in New York City by developing policies that gave priority to pedestrians, cyclists, and mass transit rather than private automobiles.[125] Johnson has also supported "Fair Fares," a program to subsidize mass transit fares for low-income New Yorkers, a move that could reduce inequitable access to public transportation. In 2019, New York City also passed a congestion pricing plan that would charge drivers for entering downtown Manhattan at peak hours, a policy supported by New York's climate action movements.

That Johnson, who says he has never owned a car and rides the subways all the time, believes he can build political support by challenging car culture is one measure of a sea change in city politics, where most elected officials had facilitated rather than challenged auto-centric transportation policies and regarded car critics as out-of-date Luddites. While recent city leaders, including mayors Michael Bloomberg and Bill de Blasio, had also championed mass transit, they generally proposed specific technical plans for dedicated bus lanes, congestion pricing to discourage cars, or more subway repairs, rather than presenting an overall critique and alternative to a car-dominated transit system.

Many forces contributed to the ascendency of car culture, but none was more important than the auto industry itself, long the nation's largest advertiser and one of its most effective lobbying groups. Today the auto industry is facing many disruptive forces and ensuring a stake in the AV market or winning new markets in middle-income countries are higher corporate priorities than promoting car use in big cities. But the persistence of car culture in New York—a city less car dependent than Los Angeles, Phoenix, or Houston—testifies to carmakers' success in capturing streets and minds for their products and the long shadows that corporate-promoted products cast, even as they are replaced by newer ones.

The many organizations and individuals seeking to promote walking, bicycling, and mass transit over cars have not yet transformed the physical and mental spaces that automobiles still dominate in New York and other cities. Moreover, the reduction in use of subways and busses after the COVID-19 pandemic raises new challenges to mass transit.

Activists have, however, created an opening for another vision of urban mobility in which residents, government, and civil society have a voice in shaping urban transportation systems (See Figure 6.2). They have begun to de-normalize the preventable deaths and injuries, pollution, and traffic congestion that automobility imposes. They have promoted the goal of transportation equity, an approach that challenges transportation apartheid, the creation of separate systems of travel for people of color and the poor and the better off. Whether this alternative will be able to create a culture that replaces car culture and car cityscapes in the years to come will require the many groups now working mostly separately on auto safety, urban design, mass transit, bicycling and walking, pollution, climate change, and transportation inequity to forge a common agenda and political alliances that can challenge those who profit from maintaining the auto-dependent status quo.

California Air Resources Board. California Air Resources Board (CARB), the California agency charged since 1967 with protecting the public from the harmful effects of air pollution and developing programs and actions to fight climate change, is an example of a government agency that is committed to and capable of requiring the auto industry to act more in the public interest. Together with civil society groups, government agencies constitute the third leg for the platform that will be needed to develop effective and sustainable alternatives to corporate-dominated automobile transportation.

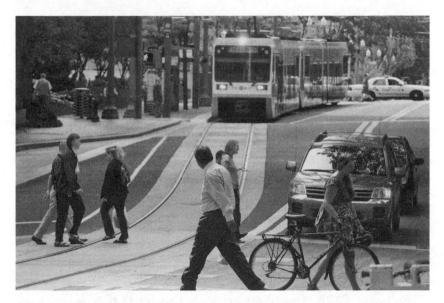

Fig. 6.2 Cities like Portland, Oregon are developing new mass transit systems that encourage more walking and less use of cars.
Photo: TriMet, licensed under CC BY 2.0

Since CARB was created before the US Environmental Protection Agency was established in 1970 and charged with developing and enforcing national standards for clean air, it won the right to continue enforcing the more rigorous California air pollution standards. Congress twice extended this right but in 2019, President Trump revoked this authority, triggering a lawsuit from twenty-two state attorneys general challenging his decision, a case that in 2020 was still working its way through the legal system.

In 2006, CARB won new authority from the California legislature through the Global Warming Solutions Act which assigned the agency a key role in planning how the state would meet its greenhouse gas reduction target of reducing GHG levels by 2020 to the level of 1990. Unlike narrower technocratic approaches to reducing human-induced climate change, California required consideration of multiple causes including fixed sources like power plants, agriculture, and transportation. By considering the co-benefits of GHG reductions, such as declines in other auto pollutants that exacerbate asthma, CARB helped to highlight the broader social benefits of reducing carbon emissions.[126]

CARB was also mandated to ensure that all communities have a voice in shaping climate change policies. "It is critical that communities of color, low-income communities, or both, receive the benefits of a cleaner economy growing in California, including its environmental and economic benefits," proclaimed CARB's 2017 scoping plan.[127] CARB also appointed an Environmental

Justice Advisory Committee (EJAC), a legislatively created advisory body, that organized almost twenty community meetings throughout California to discuss the climate strategy, and held nineteen meetings of its own to provide recommendations on the plan.

While CARB staff did not always accept the suggestions of this group, it was forced to hear its members' concerns and the community meetings created constituencies that were able to monitor implementation of the plan and pursue other advocacy routes to achieve their aims. Some environmentalists criticize CARB's endorsement of cap and trade, a market-based strategy to reduce carbon emissions. They argue that weak emissions caps, volatility in emissions allowance prices, and overly generous allocations of emissions allowances to regulated entities make cap and trade less effective albeit more politically palatable to the fossil fuel industry than, say, carbon taxes.[128] Once again, however, CARB has opened public space for these debates, enabling scientists and advocates to bring evidence to policy makers and the public.

In addition, CARB assessed the impact of California's policies on climate justice, the concept that no population should bear a disproportionate burden from climate change or its remedies. Policies that provided car rebates for electric cars or for installation of solar heating, for example, often benefited the wealthy, leaving the poor unprotected or without access to mitigation tools. California also required CARB to develop a plan to model the impact of proposed climate policies on various populations and to monitor their actual effect, especially on low-income groups and communities of color.

In its interactions with the auto industry, CARB offers a refreshing alternative to the more passive approach that many government agencies take in their interactions with corporations. Yes, CARB staff sit at the same table with auto-industry executives to uncover shared interests. But when the auto industry sued California in 2004 to overturn its clean car laws, CARB lawyers took the case to the US Supreme Court and won on every front.[129] CARB also mounts vigorous communications campaigns to counter industry misrepresentations and educates public officials on the auto industry's role in air pollution.

Since President Trump sought to roll back regulation of auto emissions in 2017, CARB and California have fought back on two fronts. In 2019, Ford, Honda, BMW, and Volkswagen signed an agreement with California to voluntarily follow its standards, rather than the lower standards proposed by President Trump.[130] Executives of these companies determined it was less risky to profits to meet fixed national or international standards that could withstand legal scrutiny and maintain public support than betting that President's Trump's rollbacks would endure.

For global corporations, standards that vary by place and time are usually more expensive than stable rules, even more stringent ones. "We believe as a company in protecting the environment, bringing innovative technology to the market and protecting American jobs," said a Volkswagen spokesman about the California agreement, hoping also perhaps that VW's agreement might help to rehabilitate the company's damaged image from its previous deceptions on emissions control devices.

California state government also played a leading role in organizing a national coalition to oppose Trump's weakening of standards. Twenty-four governors, including three Republicans, urged the president to abandon his plan, joining environmentalists and labor unions in opposing the rollback. "Strong vehicle standards protect our communities from unnecessary air pollution and fuel costs," the governors' group observed, noting that cars are "the largest source of carbon pollution in the United States"[131] CARB scientists played an important role in summarizing the scientific evidence that backed the governor's position.

In 2016, California achieved is 2020 GHG reduction goal of reducing levels to the 1990 level, an impressive accomplishment in an era when many states and nations were failing to achieve goals. CARB played a key role but the threats to continued progress are real. In 2017, vehicle tailpipe emissions increased by almost 1 percent, perhaps a consequence of a growing economy. Thirty-two million Californians breathe ozone or polluted air each year and vehicle emissions are responsible for 40 percent of GHGs and more than 40 percent of smog-forming emissions.[132]

California still has a long way to go to meet its health-based goals and federal air-quality requirements. How CARB, California state government, and the health and environmental activists who have played key roles in cleaning California's air will fare in their continuing battles with politicians like President Trump, anti-regulatory business groups, and the auto industry and its allies will depend on their future ability to mobilize public support for clean air and firm action to counter the human and corporate activities that lead to climate change.

For the last century, the automobile industry has allied with governments in the United States and elsewhere to pursue policies that encouraged more people to buy and drive more automobiles. This alliance was created on the shared belief that cars and trucks promoted economic growth, increased mobility and freedom, and assured growing auto industry profits. While government regulators, often pushed by consumer, health, and environmental activists, sought to limit the adverse impact of cars, only remedies that did not seriously jeopardize economic growth or auto industry profitability could make it through the policy gauntlet that contemporary capitalism had constructed.

Today, the consequences of this approach jeopardize human and planetary health and the quality of city life. To avoid the fate of escalating automobile damage, organizations like the Center for Auto Safety, municipal alliances and social movements that promote mass transit and safe streets over car culture, and smart government regulators like the California Air Resources Board will need to forge new alliances that consolidate their synergistic but now mostly separate impact to overcome the power and control of the auto industry and its growth-at-any-cost partners.

CHAPTER 7

Social Connections

Extracting Profit from Human Relations

Predicting a continuation of the thing that is happening . . . is not simply a bad habit like inaccuracy or exaggeration. . . . It is a major mental illness, and its roots lie partly in cowardice and partly in the worship of power, which is not fully separable from cowardice."
—George Orwell[1]

THE RISE OF GAFAM

The corporate behemoths of Google, Amazon, Facebook, Apple, and Microsoft, often labeled collectively GAFAM, represent the face of twenty-first-century capitalism. In her incisive analysis of what she calls surveillance capitalism, Shoshana Zuboff writes that GAFAM seeks to "extract the dark data continent of your inner life—your intentions and motives, meanings and needs, preferences and desires, moods and emotions, personality and disposition, truth telling or deceit" in order to summon them "into the light for others' profit."[2]

Social connections have always been a foundation for human well-being. How individuals connect to others in their family, tribe, or community; how they find the goods and services they need; and how they engage with others to achieve shared goals determines their opportunities for health, disease, and life success. As people met their most basic needs for food, housing, and safety, they were able to attend to their relationships to others, which became important for establishing self-respect, dignity, and autonomy, prerequisites for psychological well-being.

In the previous two centuries, capitalism had created ingenious methods to extract profit from the labor of workers and the natural resources of the earth. In the twenty-first century, it developed an additional source of revenue—the behavioral data that companies collect from their customers' hardware and digital use. Making these data a commodity to buy and sell has profoundly altered how people live and interact with one another.

GAFAM has taken capitalism's imperative to expand its influence to a new domain. By collecting, monetizing, and selling data that track people's inner consciousness, attention, and daily behaviors, GAFAM and its Big Tech competitors have acquired powerful new tools to document, influence, and predict the decisions of individuals. Increasingly, businesses in all sectors use these tools to shape how people connect to others, interact with the marketplace, and participate in politics, thus defining a significant extension of capitalist power.

In the shift from twentieth- to twenty-first-century capitalism, many transnational corporations aspired to become, as Naomi Klein has put it, weightless—to employ the fewest workers, stretch out supply chains to reduce accountability, contract out as many tasks as possible, and produce images rather than things.[3] No sector offered better opportunities to realize these corporate dreams than the giant tech companies. The copious revenues from the behavioral data they sold enabled them to achieve this desire. In this chapter, I examine how modern capitalism created the soil in which GAFAM could grow and exploit this new resource and describe the impact of this change on human well-being. Inspired by the opening Orwell quote, I ask whether considering the rise of these companies as inevitable and their adverse consequences inescapable is simply a bad habit or intellectual and moral cowardice and the worship of power.

Who are the members of the GAFAM club and what role do they play in the United States and global economies?

Google. Founded in 1998, Google was the pioneer in turning human experience into digital data, mapping the internet for data it could turn into commodities, and creating new businesses to market these products. At its start, Google services were free, hooking people into Gmail as their connection to a new world. A list of just a few of the business ventures Google (and, after 2015, its parent holding company Alphabet) owns or operates show its penetration of daily living.

- Google Maps and Google Earth are geographic information and mapping platforms that enable users to plot directions and visualize three dimensional images of anywhere on the planet on their mobile phone or desktop.
- YouTube is a video-sharing platform that allows users to upload, view, rate, share, and comment on videos, and subscribe to other users' video channels. Its 1.3 billion users watch 5 billion videos a day.[4]
- Android is a mobile operating system (OS), purchased by Google in 2005, and designed primarily for touchscreen mobile devices. Android has been

the best-selling OS worldwide on smartphones and tablets with more than two billion monthly active users in 2017.
- NEST is a smart home products distributor that sells smart speakers, smart displays, streaming devices, thermostats, smoke detectors, and security systems including smart doorbells, cameras, and smart locks. These technologies allow users to control home functions remotely.
- Sidewalk Labs is an "urban innovation business" that seeks to improve urban infrastructure through technological solutions and help cities to use data to tackle issues such as efficient transportation and energy use. Sidewalk was created because Google cofounder Larry Page wanted a city in which his company could experiment.[5]

Each of these Google/Alphabet companies sells products to its customers and also sells user data to marketers, who utilize it to track, reach, advertise to, and influence the decisions of their own potential customers. With these and other companies, Google has eyes on almost every domain of human experience for a substantial portion of the world's population.

Acknowledging the authority of his company, former Google CEO Eric Schmidt observed, "Almost nothing, short of a biological virus, can scale as quickly, efficiently, or aggressively as these technology platforms, and this makes the people who build, control, and use them powerful too."[6] Schmidt also celebrated the lack of meaningful regulation of their turf: "The online world is not truly bound by terrestrial laws . . . it's the world's largest ungoverned space." In 2019, Alphabet/Google reported revenue of $161 billion and 119,000 employees.

Amazon. As the world's largest e-commerce marketplace and now the world's largest retailer, Amazon sells more than 353 million products. Its personal assistant Alexa helps users find what they need on the internet and in the real world. It also sells cloud computing (via Amazon Web Services), digital streaming, and artificial intelligence, likely sources for growing revenues in the decades to come. Founded as on online bookstore in 1994 by Jeff Bezos, Amazon rapidly expanded in several different directions. Bezos is now the wealthiest individual in the world. Some of Amazon's subsidiaries are Twitch, a live streaming video platform; IMDb, an online database for information on films, TV, and streaming productions; Whole Foods, the upscale supermarket chain that Amazon purchased in 2017; Ring, a home security specialty company; Zappos, the leading footwear and apparel website in the world; and PillPack, Inc., an online pharmacy company purchased in 2018 to allow Amazon to move into the lucrative online prescription business.[7]

Of all US online shoppers, 92 percent and close to two-thirds of all Americans, say they have purchased something from Amazon, which is by far the largest online retailer.[8] By 2023, 300 million people in the US are expected to be online shoppers. By harvesting data on consumer choices from these companies and from Alexa, Amazon has a ringside seat in the homes of an expanding portion of most Americans households. Amazon uses these insights to target its own marketing and to sell to other advertisers. Although Amazon trails Google and Facebook in its sales of digital ads, this business is projected to grow 50 percent a year in the next few years. This makes Alexa an important and growing source of profit, derived from what it learns about its customers through their online interactions.[9] In 2020, Amazon's revenue was $322 billion, and by July 2020, it reported one million employees.[10] As for other Big Tech companies, the COVID-19 pandemic created new opportunities for growth for Amazon's online markets.

Facebook. The world's top social media platform, Facebook, was founded in 2004, the origin story of its founding in a Harvard dorm room by Mark Zuckerberg and his friends now spread around the world in works like Aaron Sorkin's film *The Social Network* and Ben Mezrich's book *The Accidental Billionaires.*

Like other Big Tech founders, Zuckerberg portrayed Facebook as a transformative service designed to improve the world. He rejected the strategy of charging users a fee for service as telephone companies had done in an earlier century. "Our mission is to connect every person in the world. You don't do that by having a service people pay for," he insisted,[11] sidestepping the fact that the data Facebook collected from users was the source of its advertising revenues. In 2019, Facebook's worldwide advertising revenue was almost $70 billion, more than quadruple its 2015 ad revenues.[12] Advertising revenue accounted for almost 98 percent of Facebook's income. By the end of 2019, Facebook employed 44,942 people.

In its first fifteen years, Facebook bought more than seventy companies, including Instagram, a fast-growing social medium with more than one billion users. This purchase transformed the company's growth from sagging to flourishing as teens left their mothers to stay as Facebook users, as they switched to Instagram, a brilliant use of targeted marketing.

Apple. Founded in 1976 by Steve Jobs and his partners, Apple is a multinational technology company that designs, develops, and sells consumer electronics, computer software, and online services. Unlike the three GAFAM companies previously described, Apple sells branded physical products to consumers—iPads, iPhones, Mac computers, and watches. These devices enable consumers to bring social media platforms into every corner of their lives and businesses to track their customers. Like the other companies, Apple offered its own personal assistant, Siri, whose exceptional voice recognition software was originally funded as a defense research project by US taxpayers.

Other Apple companies sell the creative content users can consume on its devices: the iTunes Store, the iOS App Store, Apple Music, and Apple TV+. Like other GAFAM companies, Apple extracts data from these interactions to sell to advertisers. In 2020, Apple expects to earn $2 billion from App store ads alone.[13] Apple's 2019 revenues were $260 billion, and it employed 139,000 people that year.[14] By revenue, it is the world's largest technology company. In 2018, Apple became the first public US company to be valued at more than $1 trillion.

Microsoft. The oldest of the GAFAM family, Microsoft was founded in 1975 by Bill Gates and Paul Allen. Over the years it has acquired leading networking sites including LinkedIn, a business and professional social platform; Skype, a global video chat site; Hotmail, a webmail service; and GitHub, a software development and data repository company. By 2019, GitHub reported 37 million users and more than 100 million repositories, the central file storage locations used to store data.[15]

Shortly after becoming the CEO of Microsoft in 2014, Satya Nadella announced that Microsoft too was going into the data acquisition and sales business. A report Microsoft commissioned concluded that "companies taking advantage of their data have the potential to raise an additional $ 1.6 trillion in revenue over companies that don't."[16] "The opportunity we have in this new world is to find a way of catalyzing this data exhaust from ubiquitous computing and converting it into fuel for ambient intelligence," wrote Nadella, succinctly summarizing GAFAM's new business model.[17]

Several other big, well-known companies operate globally in the intersecting technology and social media space: IBM, Netflix, Oracle, Tumblr, Twitter, and Reddit in the United States and Alibaba, Samsung, TikTok, Huawei, WeChat, HonHai (Foxconn), Baidu Tieba in South Korea, Taiwan, and China. In the last decade, a few Chinese tech companies have begun to challenge US domination of this sector, but it is in coming decades that this battle will play out.

I focus here on the five GAFAM companies because of their daily presence in the lives of so many people, their political and economic influence, and the growing body of scholarship on their practices and social impact. Together, these five companies account for about 13 percent of the market capitalization of all S&P 500, the index that measures the stock performance of five hundred large companies listed on stock exchanges in the United States.[18] Even more astonishing, in 2019, a year in which tech companies were under attack in Congress and the media, the 40 percent gain in the S&P benchmark in the tech sector outpaced the 25 percent gain in the overall benchmark. That year, the rise in value of GAFAM companies accounted for more than 20 percent of the returns of all S&P 500 companies.[19]

In addition, GAFAM and its other Big Tech cousins work closely with each of the sectors described in previous chapters. Amazon owns Whole Foods and seeks to use its home delivery platform to become a major deliverer of food to people's homes. Apple and Google are partnering with healthcare industries and research industries to collect, analyze, and eventually sell medical data that can be used to design and market new treatments for cancer and other illnesses.[20] Schools and educational testing companies at all levels have partnered with Apple, Microsoft, and Google to buy and install hardware and software for their learners, sending data back to the companies to refine the next generation of products and conditioning children to depend on these products for lifetime learning. Google's AV spinoff Waymo partnered with Jaguar to develop a fully self-driving Jag and Apple hitched up with Volkswagen to produce an autonomous employee shuttle van while Uber and Facebook partnered to create Messenger, an app that allows users to sign up for Uber and request a ride with one tap.

In his 1901 novel *The Octopus*, Frank Norris described the emerging railroad industry as a predatory octopus that squeezed farmers, consumers, small businesses, and workers to extract profits across the economy. "Every state has its own grievance," Norris wrote. "If it is not a railroad trust, it is a sugar trust, or an oil trust, or an industrial trust, that exploits the People, because the People allow it. The indifference of the People is the opportunity of the despot."[21]

Today, the highly concentrated tech companies have become the new octopus, extracting their own earnings by enabling companies in all sectors to find new ways to squeeze out profit by using the innovations of Big Data and digital technologies to monitor, predict, and influence their customers wherever they go.

THE BENEFITS AND COSTS OF GAFAM

Without a doubt, GAFAM and its cousins have brought significant benefits to billions of people. Thanks to Google, anyone with access to the internet can tap into the world's cumulative knowledge and find in seconds what used to take years or lifetimes to learn. Thanks to Facebook, families and friends can stay in touch across the country or planet, sharing stories, pictures, and news, and providing emotional support in times of need. Thanks to Apple, parents whose children have phones can find their children anywhere, consumers can find and buy what they want in seconds, and patients can transmit medical information to their doctors from their home. Thanks to Zoom, millions of people can work at home, thus reducing their risk of COVID-19 infection. It is almost inconceivable that anyone would willingly give up these advantages of the twenty-first century to go back to an unconnected world.

But as I have shown with ultra-processed food, precision medicines, and autonomous vehicles, new technologies, however wonderful, when deployed by giant corporations for making profit also bring new costs. To barrel into the future without considering and characterizing these costs, weighing the alternatives, and engaging in a national conversation about these options is to risk our children's and grandchildren's future well-being and happiness.

In recent years, public officials, consumer and privacy advocates, and others have tempered the near-universal enthusiasm for the convenience and benefits of GAFAM products and practices with growing concerns about their impact on the social and economic fabric of our nation and the world. Whether the government hearings, litigation, media investigations, and new regulatory and antitrust proposals generated by this scrutiny will lead to meaningful changes in GAFAM practices or political power remains to be seen.

I focus here on the broad adverse health impact of GAFAM practices, a key contributor to the costs these companies externalize to society. These can be classified in several categories: psychological well-being and mental health, consumption of unhealthy products, environmental impact, and privacy. And, according to a growing body of health research, democracy, civic engagement, and equity are also now understood as fundamental influences on well-being, making GAFAM's threats to these values perhaps its greatest cost.[22]

PSYCHOLOGICAL WELL-BEING AND MENTAL HEALTH

Basic foundations of psychological well-being influence the ways individuals perceive themselves, how they interact with others, and how they participate in the social networks and communities that define them. Today, by bombarding people with messages and images that influence these outcomes, social media platforms like Facebook, Instagram, TikTok, Snapchat, and Twitter have joined family, peers, and community as key determinants of mental health.

In some cases, social media help users find like-minded friends, reach across boundaries, and engage more fully in the world. For example, Instagram messages saying "You are strong and beautiful" to those with body image concerns can, according to one study, counteract depression.[23]

But a growing body of evidence also shows powerful harmful effects. And many experts fear that their adverse impact will overshadow potential benefits as the multinational companies that control social media increasingly deploy these technologies in intrusive ways designed to increase corporate profit.

Social isolation refers to a psychological state in which individuals lack a sense of social belonging, authentic engagement with others, and satisfying relationships.[24] Social isolation is as strong a predictor of early death as such well-established risks as smoking, obesity, or elevated blood pressure.[25] Social isolation can also lead to illnesses through a variety of pathways, including anxiety and stress that in turn lead to harmful immune, hormonal, or inflammatory changes. Isolation can also discourage healthy eating, sleeping, and exercise patterns and reduce connections to others who can provide intimacy, social support, and referrals to healthcare, employment, or public benefits.[26]

More than a fifth of adults in the United States (22 percent) say they often or always feel lonely, lacking in companionship, left out, or isolated from others. Many of these individuals say that their loneliness has had a negative impact on their lives.[27] On the positive side, a study that summarized surveys on loneliness of a nationally representative sample of more than 385,000 high school students between 1991 to 2012 found declines in reports of feeling lonely over this time span.[28] However, the actual connections to others fell over this time, suggesting that fewer social connections may not be perceived as loneliness, in effect making heightened isolation the new normal.

How do social media influence loneliness? Based on a national sample of young adults aged nineteen to thirty-two, researchers examined perceptions of social isolation among young people with different levels of social media use.[29] They found that young people with the highest level of use—on average more than two hours a day—were twice as likely to report high levels of social isolation compared to those with the lowest level of use, those who reported on average less than thirty minutes a day.

A study published in 2017 followed the Facebook use of more than five thousand people over three years. It concluded that higher use correlated with self-reported declines in physical health, mental health, and life satisfaction.[30] The authors found that the negative associations of Facebook use were comparable to or greater than the positive impact of offline interactions, suggesting a possible trade-off between offline and online relationships. Conversely, another study found that quitting Facebook for even a week leads to increases in life satisfaction and more positive emotions.[31]

One proposed pathway between high social media use and isolation is the phenomenon known as Fear of Missing Out or FOMO. One group of researchers defined FOMO as "feelings of anxiety that arise from the realization that you may be missing out on rewarding experiences that others are having. FOMO can be identified as an intra-personal trait that drives people to stay up to date of what other people are doing, among others on social media platforms." These researchers found associations between use of private social media platforms such as Facebook and Snapchat and higher levels of problematic social media use.[32] FOMO leads social media users into an anxiety-provoking catch-22: stay off social media and one might miss out on finding out what fun things friends are saying and doing. Spend too much time staring only at the screen and one might miss out on actually having fun with friends. Either choice, however, can lead to new revenues for the platforms or their advertisers seeking to attract fun-loving youth.

Like the creators of gambling casinos, social media companies design their platforms to grab and hold attention, to encourage binging, and to divert users from other pursuits, including face-to-face interactions with others. Facebook users' quest for more "likes" and "friends" lead them to spend ever more time online, encouraging some to develop what some researchers label "Facebook addiction," a risk especially for those seeking a flawless presentation to the world.[33]

For others, negative feedback on their physical appearance or prior posts can lead to lower self-esteem and disengagement from both virtual and face-to-face interactions with others. Of course, some teenagers have always been sensitive and prone to withdrawal from the world. What is different about the new social media is their ubiquity and their penetration of vast segments of the population, characteristics designed by their makers to increase ad revenues and to make them all but impossible to escape.

Between 2007 and 2018, according to surveys of representative samples of young adults enrolled in college, the prevalence of depression and anxiety has doubled, with anxiety increasing by 24 percent and depression by 34 percent in that period, staggering increases.[34] While several factors appear to have contributed to this increase, including financial insecurity and rising college debt, increased isolation due to social media use is another documented contributor.

Several studies show that young adults who use social media more have higher rates of depression. For example, a study of a representative sample of US young adults aged nineteen to thirty-two (both in and out of college) found that those with "problematic social media use"—defined as social media use with characteristics of other addictive behaviors such as mood modification, tolerance, and withdrawal—were significantly more likely to reports symptoms of depression than non-problem users.[35] Researchers hypothesized that problematic social media users neglected more constructive aspects of their lives, internalized online experiences, engaged in excessive self-comparison with others, or got too little sleep, all possible paths to depression (See Figure 7.1).

Social media platforms also create opportunities for bullying, a phenomenon that has attracted the attention of policy makers, activists, and mental health professionals. Children have always bullied other children and parents have always tried to protect their offspring. But modern capitalism has fundamentally altered the context for bullying. First, it has enabled the privatization of the digital public sphere, leaving it to big corporations rather than families or communities to monitor how children treat other children in this new space. Second, corporations have accumulated the capital and technology to make their devices almost universally available. It is now as easy to

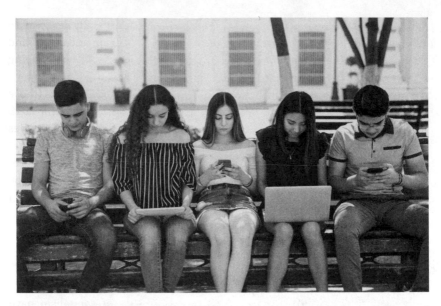

Fig. 7.1 Many young people now spend more time on their devices than speaking to each other. Higher levels of social media use are associated with higher levels of social isolation, depression, and anxiety.
Photo: © AntonioDiaz / Adobe Stock

share bullying messages with a million or a billion others as with the intended victim. Third, the emergence of surveillance capitalism has given social media companies the capacity to document, record, and analyze every act of cyber-bullying and sell what it learns to advertisers, governments, or other interested parties.

Unlike face-to-face bullying, the digital bully is usually anonymous whereas the content of the bullying is often visible to substantial segments of the victim's world. Among the health problems attributed to online bullying are moderate to severe depressive symptoms, substance use, and suicidal thoughts and attempts.[36] Facebook and Twitter executives did not intentionally create platforms to promote bullying. But profit-motivated design features such as Like and Dislike buttons, comments, and calculations of users' reach and influence keep those "hooked" on these media coming back for more. Combined with these companies' active resistance to effective regulation, these trends make the use of social media for harassing and denigrating others all but inevitable.

As one social media activist put it, "The simple fact is, if you go on the internet today and threaten to murder or rape someone, nothing is going to happen. Until we introduce consequences into the equation, the situation is not going to get better."[37]

The bottom line is that whether social media are physiologically addicting, as some researchers posit, or psychologically habituating, their "stickiness," as UK addiction researcher Mark Griffiths writes, is intentionally designed to "get users (many of which are adolescents) coming back again and again" and thus exposing them to higher risk of depression, anxiety, isolation, bullying and other negative experiences.[38]

And despite the conventional wisdom that millennials and Gen Zers (those born between the mid-1990s to the mid-2000s) love social media, a 2019 Deloitte survey of more than 13,400 millennials across forty-two countries and territories and more than 3,000 Gen Zs across ten countries found that 55 percent said that in their view, on balance, social media does more harm than good. Nearly two-thirds (64 percent) of millennials said they would be physically healthier if they reduced the time spent on social media, and six in ten said it would make them happier people.[39]

Consumption of Unhealthy Products

Both the twentieth- and twenty-first-century variants of capitalism have depended for their survival on continued economic growth driven by personal consumption. Personal consumption accounts for about 70 percent of the US Gross Domestic Product, up from 62 percent in 1960. In 2018, US households spent $12.9 trillion on goods and services.[40] When the economy falters, as it did during the Great Recession and after COVID-19, policy makers and businesses urgently strive to encourage American households to spend more.

GAFAM's contribution to this economic imperative has been to make it ever easier to consume more. One or two clicks will bring groceries, clothes, electronics, books, alcohol, tobacco, or medicine to the front door of almost every household in America. Targeted digital marketing of these and other products allows sellers to find just the right time and medium to make the pitch—and the sale. Tech companies create hundreds of new products from iPhones to personal assistants like Alexa and Siri to NEST home security and protection devices to tempt customers to spend more.

By 2023, the global e-commerce market will be worth an estimated $2.8 trillion, an increase of almost 60 percent from 2018.[41] China has the largest e-commerce economy, followed by the United States. In this country, Amazon has the largest share of the sector. In the coming decades, online ordering of food, continuing shifts to online retail purchasing, and digital consumption of entertainment are expected to contribute to continued growth in e-commerce.

The digital economy and expanding e-commerce offer consumers some clear benefits: more choices, less time and travel needed for shopping, and, in some cases, lower prices. But making it easier to buy and spend more has several harmful consequences on individual and public health.

First, the digital economy makes it easier to buy and sell unhealthy products such as tobacco, alcohol, unhealthy food, firearms, and ineffective, inappropriate, or illegal medicine and drugs. E-commerce markets make it easier for sellers and buyers to evade regulation, which is often still focused on the non-digital economy. As elected officials and regulators look to fill these regulatory gaps, corporations seek new ways to evade or delay rules, sanitize their images—or develop more responsible practices that do not jeopardize profits.

Indeed, producers of tobacco and e-cigarettes, unhealthy food and beverages, and alcohol, have developed sophisticated digital marketing strategies to appeal to various populations. Adolescents and young adults, high consumers of these products, are especially important targets as they are promising candidates for becoming lifetime customers and are no longer protected by the regulations that limit marketing to younger children. The digital ad campaigns of these corporations are designed by Marlboro, Coca-Cola, McDonald's, Juul, and Anheuser-Busch InBev, now the leading de facto health educators of America's children and youth.

But the capacity of these producers of unhealthy commodities to reach hundreds of millions of young people around the world depends on the platforms Amazon, Facebook, and Google have created and on the behavioral data they sell these companies to target their messages and nudge customers into buying their products.

A few examples illustrate the scope and impact of digital marketing of unhealthy products. As young people spend less time watching television and more time on other screens, food companies have migrated their marketing to these new media. These ads promote almost exclusively energy-dense, nutrient-poor products such as fast food, sugary beverages, candy, and snacks,[42] and researchers have shown that increased viewing of these ads leads to higher consumption.[43] This effectiveness leads food makers to spend more than $13 billion a year on all forms of food marketing.[44]

Adolescents and young adults are a promising and profitable market for these companies. Carol Kruse, a Coca-Cola marketing executive, explained to a trade magazine, "We're especially targeting a teen or young adult audience. They're always on their mobile phones and they spend an inordinate amount of time on the Internet." Kruse noted that Coke-funded research found that "yes, indeed, an online ad unit can make an emotional connection and encourage consumers to buy more of our products."[45]

Using its MyCokeRewards program, the company enrolls users (using a code from the bottle cap) in contests and giveaways, tracking data from each visitor. A consumer analysis firm explains that this gives Coke "mountains of data" it can use to personalize the look and messaging of a particular web, email, or mobile content, or send an exclusive offer. By 2009, some 285,000 Coke drinkers were entering on average seven codes per second on the MyCokeRewards page.[46] Teens and young adults have the highest rates of soda consumption and sugary beverages are the product most associated with global increases in obesity and diabetes.[47]

Other strategies food companies use to reach children and young people with digital ads are creating immersive environments that engage young people in product-related fantasies; infiltrating social networks to enlist young people, often unwittingly, as "brand ambassadors" in their own social media use; utilizing location-based and mobile marketing designed to target customers as they pass or enter food outlets; and studying and triggering subconscious reactions to food that will increase desire and consumption.[48]

Alcohol and tobacco companies use similar social media strategies. The marketing of Juul e-cigarettes to young people provides an instructive case study. Its e-cigarette digital advertising emphasized the appealing flavors and the cool, high-tech look of their products. Juul was called the "iPhone of e-cigs" by one enthusiastic reviewer.[49] Digital and other promotion of e-cigs, including the deployment of young brand ambassadors, who used social media to promote Juul, contributed to a surge in their use by adolescents and young adults, a factor that amplified the toll of lung-related injuries and deaths from e-cigarettes first reported in 2019.[50]

Based on a study of Juul's marketing practices between 2015 and 2018, researchers at Stanford University concluded:

> JUUL's advertising imagery in its first 6 months on the market was patently youth oriented. For the next 2 ½ years it was more muted, but the company's advertising was widely distributed on social media channels frequented by youth, was amplified by hashtag extensions, and catalyzed by compensated influencers and affiliates.[51]

When Juul's marketing practices came under attack in Congress, the media, and in court, its executives responded with defensive indignation, insisting that they did not advertise to youth and were determined to offer only a product that would help smokers quit cigarettes, not to addict young people to nicotine.[52] Their defense seemed a little like the Medellín Cartel or Purdue Pharmaceuticals insisting they never intended for anyone to misuse their products. Of interest, few public commentators faulted Facebook and other social media platforms for enabling Juul to market its products so ubiquitously.

The extent to which social media platforms have penetrated the lives of millions of people and the conveniences they provide to consumers make their current power seem inevitable and the goal of limiting exposure appear at best quixotic. In fact, however, no democratic referendum on what people really want from their social media has been carried out. Would parents and communities choose to limit the ability of Big Food, Alcohol, and Tobacco companies to partner with Big Tech to market products associated with preventable ill-nesses, premature deaths, and widening health inequities? If parents and con-sumers were asked whether they wanted to end the now mostly surreptitious monitoring of that marketing for the purpose of better targeting and selling more of these products to children, young people, Blacks, and Latinxs, what would they decide? For now, GAFAM and unhealthy product producers have mostly avoided such public debates, leaving them confident that their current power and political savvy is sufficient to defeat such measures.

POLLUTION AND UNSUSTAINABLE CONSUMPTION

Tech companies and their corporate partners also undermine well-being by contributing to the surge in consumption that fuels human-induced climate change, pollution of oceans and soil by plastics, destruction of rain forests, and an ideology that valorizes consumption as a path to identity and fulfillment.[53]

As Tatiana Schlossberg explains in her book *Inconspicuous Consumption*, the reach of e-commerce magnifies each of these costs.[54] More than two-thirds of Americans have ordered something online, accounting for about 9 percent of all retail in the US, adding about $474 billion to the economy each year.[55] In 2018, retail e-commerce sales worldwide reached almost $3 trillion and since 2011, the percentage of shopping that takes place online has doubled.[56] The quarantines imposed to control COVID-19 further accelerated this shift to e-commerce.

In addition, e-commerce generates waste at every stage. Even though Amazon strives for less polluting packaging, the 608 million packages it ships every year lead to more cut forests, energy use, and waste disposal. As compa-nies compete for quicker delivery, they use more air transport, which is more polluting than ships, rail, or trucks. Every day e-commerce leads 100,000 planes to take off; 20 million parcels to be delivered; and 1.1 million smart-phones to be transported. Although only 1 percent of global cargo by volume travels on planes, it represents 35 percent of the dollar amount of global trade.[57] Boeing estimates that the proportion of commerce that travels by air will double in the next two decades.[58]

In the popular imagination, companies like Amazon, Google, and Facebook live in the cloud—making them poster children for clean twenty-first-century industries. In reality, however, tech companies depend on hardware, software, and an infrastructure that have a physical presence. An investigative team from *The Washington Post* found that the industry relied on polluting supply chains across the world. Cobalt is a metal used in the production of lithium-ion batteries for smartphones, laptops, and electric vehicles. Sixty percent of the world's cobalt supply comes from the Congo, where an estimated one hundred thousand miners, including children, use hand tools to extract cobalt from underground tunnels. Deaths and injuries are common and mining exposes communities to air and water pollution linked to health problems.

In response to *The Post* investigation, Apple said it planned to increase scrutiny of its cobalt suppliers, primarily companies based in China.[59] But as one cobalt industry analyst told *The Post*, concern about cobalt "comes to the fore every now and then. And it's met with much muttering and shaking of the head and tuttering—and goes away again." The deregulatory spirit of modern capitalism, elevated to new heights by the Trump Administration, has made it easier for tech companies to disregard this tuttering.

Graphite is a mineral used to make lithium-ion batteries. In Guangxi, an autonomous region of the People's Republic of China, factories produce graphite that is sold to Samsung, Panasonic, and until recently, Apple. These companies promote their batteries as the clean technology that will reduce global warming but in Guangxi, these factories pollute the air and water, damage crops, and cover homes and belongings in gray ash. Villagers told *The Post* reporter that cleanup efforts have failed because local officials are allied with company executives and value economic growth more highly than health.[60]

Lithium, another metal used to produce batteries, is mined in Argentina and Chile in the Atacama Desert. The indigenous communities worry that the mines will deplete already scarce water. A hand-painted sign in one community reads, "We don't eat batteries. They take the water, life is gone." Panasonic, Tesla, and Apple are some of the companies that buy lithium mined in Atacama. An Apple spokesperson told *The Post*, "Apple is deeply committed to the responsible mining of materials for our products. . . .We will soon launch on-site evaluations of our major lithium producers."[61] Like other health-damaging industries, tech companies have learned that promising investigation and action after public disclosure of harmful practices is less expensive than anticipating and preventing such pollution.

Designing products with short life spans is another strategy to increase consumption. Early in the twentieth century, Alfred Sloan, a longtime leader of General Motors, developed the concept of planned obsolescence, the practice of designing a product with an artificially limited life span, so that it becomes obsolete, unfashionable, or no longer functional after a period of time.[62] In contrast to Henry Ford, who built sturdy, affordable cars to grow a mass market for his Model Ts, Sloan built flashy, status-enhancing cars to encourage consumers to trade up after a short while. The historian Daniel Boorstin explained that Sloan:

> [aimed at] what he called the mass-market class. He saw that the future of the American economy lay not merely in providing machines to do things never done before. For Americans would always be reaching for a slightly better, slightly more appealing, slightly newer machine to do what was already being done. The American economy, then, would have to grow by *displacing objects that*

were still usable. . . . Americans would climb the ladder of consumption by abandoning the new for the newer.[63]

A century later, Zuckerberg, Cook, Bezos, Schmidt, and other tech CEOs are following Sloan's path with gusto. The new features of iPhones 10, 11, and 12 are today's equivalent to the Cadillac's changing fins in the 1950s and 1960s. Following the imperative for capitalist growth, tech companies must be ready to replace each new device they sell with a new, more appealing product before a competitor comes up with something better or cheaper.

In an interview with *The New York Times*, Philip W. Schiller, Apple's head of marketing, explained that after its phenomenal success selling iPods (400 million sold by the end of 2019), "we knew there was a risk that one day a cellphone could play music, that you wouldn't carry two devices, you'd carry one. We wanted to take care of that ourselves and solve that. So we decided we needed to do a phone, a phone that could also replace iPod."[64]

To keep its market share and grow its profits, Apple designed a new product that would make its 400 million iPods obsolete and lead most of them to be discarded. The decision created new jobs and promoted economic growth, but also increased mining for rare metals in environmentally sensitive areas, forced more children to work in these dangerous mines, created mountains of waste, and generated more carbon to transport the new must-have iPhones to their millions of customers and the old iPods to the dump.

Globalization, rapidly changing technologies, more penetrative marketing, and many people's powerful urge to use consumption and brand loyalty to mark status facilitated their task. By 2016, the world generated 44.7 million metric tons of e-waste.[65] Each year, globally, around 1 billion cell phones and 300 million computers are put into production. The EPA estimates that in the United States 152 million mobile phones, 52 million computers, and 36 million monitors are discarded each year, with less than 20 percent of all e-waste being properly recycled.[66]

A recent review of the health hazards of e-waste concluded that exposure contributes to endocrine disruption, reproduction anomalies, brain abnormalities, and disruptions in gene expression, threats that could trigger future global epidemics.[67] Another review reported that e-waste exposure had been linked to changes in thyroid function, changes in cellular expression and function, adverse neonatal outcomes, changes in temperament and behavior, poor educational outcomes, and decreased lung function.[68] Children, especially those working in informal e-waste recycling centers, other e-waste workers, those living close to facilities that contaminated drinking water, and those living in countries with weak regulatory systems were at higher risk than their respective counterparts.

PRIVACY

The tech sector's privacy policies and practices have generated a storm of public debate. Elected officials, journalists, privacy advocates, and even workers at GAFAM companies have raised privacy concerns about how these companies balance their obligations to their shareholders with those to the public.

Over the course of the twentieth century, privacy came to be considered an essential foundation of health as well as a basic human right, with some constitutional protection in the United States. Privacy became the space in which individuals have autonomy to make decisions about their private lives, where they can achieve the dignity that comes with self-sufficiency and independence, and where they can exercise their right to be left alone.[69] In the past, wrote Tim Wu, "privacy was the default, commercial intrusions the exception."[70]

In recent decades, however, two power centers, acting sometimes separately and sometimes together, have challenged the right to privacy. Corporations, especially those of GAFAM, have developed new technologies to invade space that had been private, collecting the most intimate data about personal lives in order to sell to marketers. And, especially after the September 11 attacks, governments have devised new ways to monitor communication and behavior that they perceive as threatening.

A few examples show some of the ways that tech companies intrude on privacy. *The Wall Street Journal* warns that the 5G race could "leave personal privacy in the dust." Fifth generation cellular networks are designed to be faster, smarter, and easier to maintain than their predecessors. But as Randall Stephenson, CEO of AT&T, the multinational telecommunications company, observed, "5G is going to allow sensors all over the place. 4G [the previous version] networks in a square mile can connect thousands of devices. 5G millions of devices."[71] Many people see 5G as a natural and desirable extension of wireless broadband development, but it will bring tech companies faster and more intrusive ways to sell to advertisers and retailers our behavioral data, thus significantly increasing their power to watch and market to users in real time and around the clock.

Drug makers can monitor how many pills their patients are actually swallowing. Retailers can use 5G technology to track shoppers, letting store managers know when a customer is examining a product and using facial recognition software to instantly deliver tailored marketing messages. These new technologies will allow brick-and-mortar retailers to compete with Amazon in predicting and nudging customer behavior.[72]

In a 2013 study, researchers at Cambridge University and Microsoft analyzed the Facebook "Likes" of 58,466 Americans. Using these data, they could accurately "predict a range of highly sensitive personal attributes including sexual orientation, ethnicity, religious and political views, personality traits, intelligence, happiness, use of addiction substances, parental separation, and gender."[73] By selling these insights to marketers, Facebook converts the personal data of its users into a marketable commodity that will be used to target users with tailored advertising messages. Sometimes this leads to macabre results. A man with prostate cancer who used Facebook to look for treatment information, for example, began to get advertisements from funeral homes.[74]

Other privacy concerns arise from big technology companies' efforts to find their way into the country's $3.5 trillion healthcare market. Project Nightingale is a partnership between Google and Ascension, a Catholic healthcare network that is the country's second-largest health system. The project will aggregate data that includes lab results, doctor diagnoses, and hospital records into a database that will provide complete health histories with patient names and dates of both.

At least 150 Google employees have access to the data, although neither patients nor doctors were notified. Privacy experts said it appeared the project did not violate provisions of the Health Insurance Portability and Accountability Act of 1996 (HIPAA), the nation's main medical privacy law, since the law allows medical providers to share data with business partners without telling patients as long as information is used "only to help the covered entity carry out its health care-functions." However, Google is also using the data to design new software that uses artificial intelligence and machine learning to identify suggested changes in that patient's care.[75]

Companies defend their privacy practices vigorously. "If you have something that you don't want anyone to know, maybe you shouldn't be doing it in the first place," suggested Eric Schmidt, then CEO of Google. To which Edward Snowden, the whistleblower who leaked classified intelligence, replied, "Arguing that you don't care about the right to privacy because you have nothing to hide is no different than saying you don't care about free speech because you have nothing to say."[76]

Tech companies claim that customers want the targeted advertising that their surveillance enables so that they can make more informed choices. But in practice, journalist Michael Wolff has observed that "if people can avoid advertising, they do. . . . As soon as they figure out how to circumvent it, they don't go back to it."[77] And tech company executives argue that digital personal assistant like Alexa and Siri use surveillance data to help their customers negotiate the complexities of modern life. But to some users, Tim Wu notes, these services "seem more like a stalker than a valet, following users around the web."[78]

While privacy is a right of individuals, it is also a collective good. The British privacy advocate and academic Simon Davies has written that "society is better off if individuals have higher levels of privacy."[79] And Rikke Frank Jorgensen of the Danish Institute for Human Rights explains, "To me the issue was always political—and always deeply embedded with power. Privacy for me has always been about setting limits to power—be it state or commercial power. . . .It's a fundamental premise for a free and open society—at both individual and societal level."[80]

In Europe, human rights lawyers and activists insisted that the right to privacy included the "right to be forgotten," which meant the right to remove from digital databases information about a person that was untrue, harmful, or obsolete. When Google and a newspaper refused to remove an old story about his business debts, Mario Costeja, a Spanish businessman. filed a court case that eventually went to the European Union's Court of Justice. The court ruled that commercial search firms, such as Google, that gather personal information for profit should remove links to private information when asked, provided the information is no longer relevant. The judges decided that the fundamental right to privacy is greater than the economic interest of the commercial firm and, in some circumstances, the public interest in access to information. "Thanks to this ruling," said Costeja, "there is now the right to be forgotten included in the (European Union's) General Data Protection Regulation, with common rules for 747 million people all over Europe."[81]

Amazon, Google, and other companies regularly announce new privacy initiatives, often after their violations of privacy have attracted attention. But in some basic ways, the business goal of enrolling more users and having them spend more time online is antithetical to the goal of safeguarding privacy. When companies own the data about our personal behavior, beliefs, and preferences, absent regulation, they decide when and how to use that information.

Ultimately, privacy reveals questions of power. Who has the right to draw the line against corporate and governmental intrusions into people's daily lives? In a 2010 interview at the Washington Ideas Forum, Google CEO Eric Schmidt observed that "Google policy is to get right up to the creepy line and not cross it."[82] By allowing Google to define creepy and to draw its own line, our society fails to protect the personal space people need to create healthy, autonomous, and dignified lives. The United States is the only developed nation that lacks comprehensive data-protection rules.

Back in 2011, the Federal Trade Commission negotiated a consent decree that required Facebook to take several steps to make sure it lived up to its promises to give consumers clear and prominent notice and obtain consumers' express consent before their information is shared beyond the privacy settings the company has established.[83] Could regulators have acted more forcefully to protect privacy at that time? In an interview with *The New York Times* in 2019, David Vladeck, the former director of the Bureau of Consumer Protection at the Federal Trade Commission, who imposed the decree, said, "I regret not having done things differently. We struggled with the reporting provisions of both [privacy] consent decrees [with Facebook]. This may have been a failure of our imagination. The idea of privacy audits was floating around, but there were no templates. . . .We did what we could, with biannual privacy assessments. But they turned out to be wholly insufficient."[84]

Democracy

Democracy, a political system in which people have a voice in shaping their lives, is both an end in itself and a means to pursuing life, liberty, happiness, and health. As the philosopher and economist Amartya Sen has shown, democratic governance constrains elites from making harmful decisions and creates institutions and values that protect well-being.[85] Other evidence demonstrates that the psychological consequences of feeling in control of one's life contribute to better health. Various measures of democracy are associated with health outcomes such as life expectancy, child and maternal mortality, suicide, self-rated health, happiness, life satisfaction, and subjective well-being.[86]

A review of the impact of social media on democracy by researchers at the Omidyar Network, a "philanthropic investment firm" created by eBay founder Pierre Omidyar, claims that the rise of social media has eroded democratic processes by:

- exacerbating the polarization of civil society via echo chambers and filter bubbles, the term used to describe the algorithms that ensure that Internet users encounter only information and opinions that conform to and reinforce their own beliefs;
- rapidly spreading mis- and disinformation and amplifying the populist and illiberal wave across the globe;
- creating competing realities that result from users on two sides of an issue being exposed to and interacting only with messages from those who agree with their beliefs;
- enabling malevolent actors to spread disinformation and covertly influence public opinion that can manipulate voters and public opinion;
- capturing unprecedented amounts of data that can be used to manipulate user behavior; and
- facilitating hate speech, public humiliation, and the targeted marginalization of dissenting or minority voices.[87]

These threats to democracy have contributed to the most disruptive political trends of the last few decades: the proliferation of authoritarian and nationalist governments around the world, British voters' decision to exit the European Union, and rising tides of racist and anti-immigrant sentiments. These developments have in turn contributed to higher levels of anxiety, social isolation, anger, and political polarization, key determinants of psychological distress.

Do social media and tech companies *cause* these threats to democracy? The companies themselves emphasize that populist and authoritarian social movements, a proliferation of other small and large media channels, and political polarization are independent perils to democracy—and to their businesses. They claim that their companies are champions of free speech and democracy. In a 2019 speech at Georgetown University, Facebook's Zuckerberg said:

> I've focused on building services to do two things: give people voice and bring people together. These two simple ideas—voice and inclusion—go hand in hand. We've seen this throughout history, even if it doesn't feel that way today. More people being able to share their perspectives has always been necessary to build a more inclusive society.[88]

More pragmatically, GAFAM executives also argue that any efforts to curtail or regulate the industry could cede the field to fast-growing Chinese tech companies[89] or compromise their businesses' democratic rights.

But critics are skeptical of these defenses. In response to Zuckerberg's Georgetown speech, Rashad Robinson, president of Color of Change, a racial justice organization, said:

> Mark Zuckerberg made clear today that he is not only doubling down on a business model that corrupts our democracy, but also fundamentally lacks an understanding of how civil rights, voter suppression, and racism actually function in this country. Under the guise of protecting voice and free expression, Facebook, as in prior elections, is giving Trump and the right-wing a free pass to spread lies, hate and misinformation on the platform.[90]

Tim Wu makes the case that, with power that "rivals or exceeds that of elected government," Big Tech is today the clearest threat to democracy.[91] As Wael Ghonim, a Google executive in Dubai put it, "The system of Facebook is a mobocratic system—if there is a mob of people. . . all organizing around liking content, the content will get massive distribution. The editor became dumb software that just optimizes for whatever sells ads."[92]

Company practices contribute directly and indirectly to threats to democracy. Buzzfeed's study of the impact of Facebook on the 2016 election showed that the twenty highest-performing false election stories from hoax sites and hyper-partisan blogs of the last days of the 2016 campaign did better than the twenty highest- performing real news stories from the *New York Times*, *Washington Post*, Huffington Post, NBC News, and others.[93] This outcome was a result of algorithms optimized for conflict yet ignoring fakeness and targeting individuals most vulnerable to manipulation.

In his 2019 Georgetown speech, Mark Zuckerberg announced that Facebook would not screen its ads for truthfulness. "People having the power to express themselves at scale is a new kind of force in the world—a Fifth Estate alongside the other power structures of society," Zuckerberg proclaimed. Despite the messiness of free speech, he said, "the long journey towards greater progress requires confronting ideas that challenge us. I'm here today because I believe we must continue to stand for free expression."[94]

In an internal Facebook memo published by *The New York Times* in early 2020, Andrew Bosworth, the head of Facebook's virtual and augmented reality division, wrote that even though keeping the current policies in place "very well may lead to" Mr. Trump's re-election, it was the right decision.[95] Whether Facebook's decision not to fact-check its ads was based on a principled commitment to free speech or a more opportunistic desire to help reelect a president averse to regulation or higher taxes, policies that benefited Facebook's bottom line, as the billionaire George Soros charged,[96] is in some sense irrelevant. Either way, one of the largest companies in the nation had the potential to influence, mostly surreptitiously, the outcome of presidential elections in 2016 and 2020.

Tech companies influence the process of democracy in other ways. Tech analyst Kalev Leetaru writing in *Forbes* notes that Twitter can suspend or ban any user from its platform for any reason and users do not possess any legal recourse to appeal their removal from the platform.[97] The company can also delete any post with no legal recourse of appeal. Thus, Twitter controls who can speak to the president of the United States and what they are permitted to say, an important power in times when this medium is the preferred public communication channel of a president.

Authoritarian governments and antidemocratic movements have used the social media platforms created by Facebook, Google, and Twitter to achieve their business goals in ways that leave defenders of democracy with two unpalatable choices. They can leave policing of the platform to the companies themselves, ensuring that profitability will be a primary concern. Or they can turn over regulation to governments often controlled by authoritarian or antidemocratic elites. To date, a third path—public oversight of rules that encourage all players to challenge bad ideas with better ones in order to spark open public deliberation—has proven to be elusive.

GAFAM has also influenced democracy by transforming the environment of mainstream media. By capturing advertising revenues from newspapers and magazines, Facebook and Google have deprived print journalism of a primary source of revenue. Following Google's 2009 purchase for $750 million of AdMob, a digital mobile advertising start-up, Google and Facebook ad revenue soared to almost $135 billion a year. During this same period, ad revenues at newspapers fell from $50 billion in 2005 to $20 billion in 2018. Between 2001 and 2018, the number of reporters working in United States newsrooms dropped from 400,000 in 2001 to 185,000 in 2018.[98] Small newsrooms were hardest hit, depriving residents of many communities of ongoing coverage of the local issues—pollution, education, access to hospital care—that enable more informed citizen participation in shaping policies that influence well-being.

While some media analysts see these changes in media control as the normal working of markets in a capitalist economy, critics like Wu[99] and Siva Vaidhyanathan, a media scholar at the University of Virginia,[100] view the dominance of social media platforms over traditional media as another cost of twenty-first-century capitalism, the consequence of looser antitrust laws, the lack of regulations of the digital economy, and the capture of new technologies by a handful of powerful companies.

Social media platforms have come to play an especially important role in engaging young people in civic and political life. danah boyd, the founder and president of Data & Society, an organization that studies the intersections of technology and society, has written that social media have become the "civil society of teenage culture," a place where young people can freely interact with each other.[101] But Kathryn Montgomery, who studies the role of media in society, has observed that this civil society is curated by corporations who claim the right to design its infrastructure so as to maximize their profits.[102] Thus, Facebook, Instagram, Twitter, and other platforms preferentially promote those opportunities for civic engagement that generate more data to sell to advertisers. These options push out polarizing messages, those that generate many likes and dislikes and not those that encourage deliberation, problem-solving, or critical analysis.

By channeling the routes by which young people engage in civic and political action, tech companies can influence the flow of the river that has often restored and refreshed American democracy—the moral power and passion of mobilized young people. Recent youth activism on police violence against Blacks and systemic racism, immigration policy, gun industry influence, LGBTQ rights, sexual violence, and climate change shows the continuing potential for this force. These movements have effectively used social media to organize and advance their causes. But, as some observers note, social media have also generated new opportunities for political surveillance and repression, corporate co-optation, information overload, and symbolic rather than substantive activism and victories.[103]

Social media and tech companies have a profound influence on equity and fairness, outcomes that are both consequences of and contributors to a sustainable democracy. GAFAM's accumulated capital contributes to income and wealth inequality. Even though most people in this country have some access to digital platforms, the growing stratifications in our society bring different costs and benefits to users. Facebook and Amazon bring distinct messages and market different goods and services to different social classes. When Facebook and PepsiCo. target Black and Latinx youth with sugary beverage marketing, they contribute to inequitable rates of diabetes and other diet-related diseases among people of color compared to whites. By using marketing surveillance data to target and nudge established buying habits with ever-more precision, social media platforms reinforce and exacerbate existing inequalities, widening social and health gaps.

Big tech companies also play an increasingly powerful role in municipal politics, using their money, savvy, and power to seek to overwhelm majority views or traditional views of fair play. In Seattle, for example, the city council approved a tax on local businesses in 2018 in order to expand resources for affordable housing. Amazon and other businesses opposed the measure, threatened to leave the city, and contributed to No Tax On Jobs, a committee created to put a referendum on the ballot to repeal the head tax.[104] The city council soon reversed its decision and repealed the new tax. In Baltimore, Amazon has opened new warehouses, negotiated procurement contracts with local and state governments, and sold data services to medium and large businesses. Although these activities have generated economic growth in the city, they have also led to closures of small businesses, killed union jobs, and exacerbated the gentrification that drives low-income residents out of their neighborhoods or makes them feel unwelcome there.[105] At no time, did Baltimore residents have an opportunity to vote on whether Amazon could transform their city's economy.

As a counterexample, when Amazon and New York City and New York State negotiated a subsidy and tax breaks of $2.6 billion to bring its second headquarters to New York City, an alliance of outraged citizens, activist groups, and elected officials forced New York City and New York State government to negotiate further, leading Amazon to decide to look elsewhere for a better deal.[106] After the COVID-19 pandemic lowered commercial rents in New York City, however, GAFAM companies snapped up new office space, betting that the city would again be a good place to make money.

Resistance and Alternatives

During his efforts to limit J. P. Morgan's domination of financial, railroad, and coal trusts, in 1902 President Teddy Roosevelt declared that "a man of great wealth who does not use that wealth decently is, in a peculiar sense, a menace to the community." He added that the "trusts are the creatures of the State, and the State not only has the right to control them, but it is in duty bound to control them wherever need of such control is shown."[107]

In the next few decades, first Louis Brandeis and then Felix Frankfurter, as Supreme Court Justices and the latter as a presidential adviser, made federal oversight of corporate concentration and regulation of business practices a foundation of US politics and economy.[108] In 1950, Tennessee senator Estes Kefauver, a critic of monopoly business control, argued in support of legislation to strengthen the Sherman Antitrust Act of 1890:

> I think we must decide very quickly what sort of country we want to live in. The present trend of great corporations to increase their economic power is the antithesis of meritorious competitive development. . . . Through monopolistic mergers the people are losing power to direct their own economic welfare. When they lose the power to direct their economic welfare, they also lose the means to direct their political future.[109]

By the 1970s, however, conservative activists and legal scholars, led by Robert Bork, later rejected by the Democrats as a Supreme Court nominee, successfully redefined the goals of antitrust legislation to a narrow focus on the impact of concentration on consumer prices, rather than on the political and economic power of corporations.[110] For the next three decades, the federal government rarely enforced or updated its antitrust laws despite the accelerating concentration of many corporate sectors.

In the run-up to the 2020 presidential elections, however, the monopoly power of corporations again became a political issue, in part due to the political supporters of Senators Bernie Sanders and Elizabeth Warren, and other reformers. At the heart of this debate was the growing power of tech giants such as Google, Amazon, and Facebook to shape the opportunities by which individuals connect to peers, family, commerce, and politics in ways that generate revenue and profit. The 2020 decision by President Trump's Department of Justice to sue Google for unlawfully maintaining monopolies through anticompetitive and exclusionary practices demonstrated the bipartisan appeal of taking on the tech giants.

As resistance to this GAFAM control bubbled up across the country and world and as activists, civil society groups, and public officials worked to create protections from tech domination, new challenges to monopoly consolidation surfaced. To explore the potential, limits, and lessons that can be extracted from these developments, I examine three conflicts about the role and power of tech companies.

PROTECTING CHILDREN

More than three-quarters of eight- to twelve-year-olds use YouTube and many of the 4 billion viewers of a recent YouTube hit video called "Baby Shark," a favorite of two- and three-year-olds, are much younger.[111] Facebook, Instagram, and TikTok are also popular with children. The growing exposure of children to digital media—and therefore digital advertising—has activated parents, psychologists, health professionals, privacy advocates, and some elected officials to set new limits on this form of marketing to children. These advocates assert that since children under thirteen are often unable to distinguish advertising appeals from other types of information, it is wrong to promote products, especially unhealthy products, and to extract behavioral data from children's viewing choices in order to target them for marketing.

As an illustration of the power of digital advertising to influence corporate behavior, in 2019 Kellogg's announced a new cereal for toddlers, Baby Shark, a serving of which contains 150 calories, 190 milligrams of sodium, and 15 grams of sugar.[112] Using the popularity of the song "Baby Shark" generated by YouTube, Kellogg's hoped to reverse its declining cereal sales by convincing toddlers to nag their parents to buy them a brand associated with a song and images they loved—and delivering 40 percent of its calories from sugar.

In September 2019, the Federal Trade Commission, an agency charged with protecting America's consumers, announced a settlement with Google in which the company that owns YouTube agreed to pay a record $170 million fine to settle claims that it had knowingly and illegally harvested personal information from children and used the data to profit from ads targeted at these children.[113] Google also agreed to create a new system that requires video channel owners to identify the children's content they post and bans targeted ads on these child-labeled videos. New York Attorney General Letitia James, whose complaint to the FTC triggered the action, participated in reaching the settlement. She noted that "these companies put children at risk and abused their power, which is why we are imposing major reforms to their practices and making them pay one of the largest settlements for a privacy matter in U.S. history."[114]

The Children's Online Privacy Protection Act (COPPA), passed in 1998, prevents companies from gathering data about children, such as their location or contact information, without first obtaining parental consent. It also bars companies from directing targeted advertising to audiences known to include children. However, limited enforcement and rapidly changing technologies reduced compliance with the law.

The FTC acted against YouTube in part because a coalition of more than twenty advocacy groups—including the Center for Digital Democracy, the Campaign for a Commercial-Free Childhood, and Common Sense Media—had in 2018 sent the FTC a complaint claiming that Google was routinely violating COPPA. Josh Golin, the executive director of the Campaign for a Commercial-Free Childhood, charged that Google had been "actively packaging under-13 content for advertisers" in violation of the law.[115]

Defenders of children's right not to be targeted with ads found the settlement to be inadequate. Senator Edward Markey, a Democrat from Massachusetts and a proponent for stronger protections for children, said that "the FTC let Google off the hook with a drop-in-the-bucket fine and a set of new requirements that fall well short of what is needed to turn YouTube into a safe and healthy place for kids." Jeffrey Chester, the executive director of the Center for a Digital Democracy, observed that "merely requiring Google to follow the law, that's a meaningless sanction. It's the equivalent of a cop pulling somebody over for speeding at 110 miles an hour, and they get off with a warning."[116]

The children's rights, media, and privacy advocates, and elected officials and scholars who have taken up the goal of protecting children's right not to be targeted with personalized digital advertisements have had several successes. They have attracted media and legislator attention, raised public consciousness about the issue, and obliged many elected officials to speak out on protecting children. They have won significant, albeit in their view inadequate, sanctions against Google and Facebook, and persuaded some industry executives to make concessions. They have forced tech executives to endorse children's rights to protection—at least in principle—and to make some modifications in their practices.

At the same time, tech executives have become increasingly concerned about their capacity to continue to set their own rules on behavioral surveillance. In 2019, the FTC announced plans to review COPPA four years earlier than planned, citing new concerns about how the regulations should apply to the education technology sector, voice-enabled connected devices, and platforms that host third-party child-directed messages. One commissioner described the review as "taking care of children and data both," as though, the Center for Commercial-Free Childhood observed, "protecting extracted marketing data is just as important as protecting kids."[117] Some advocates feared that the industry promoted this early review in order to weaken the rules and carve out exceptions.

Google and Facebook reacted to the new limits on surveillance and marketing to children by transferring liability for violations to "content providers," the companies that designed and posted videos for children, even though it was GAFAM who controlled the platforms that distributed the content and extracted the data.

YouTubers, the loose association of individuals and companies that produce videos for children, petitioned the FTC to clarify and reconsider the new COPPA regulations for YouTube creators. Their petition, which attracted more than 870,000 signatures, claimed that calls for "shutting off personalized ads on creators' content will cause more harm than good, especially for children. Quality family-friendly content will shrink, while more mature content will grow—yet kids will still be watching."[118] They urged the FTC to delay any enforcement of COPPA until its review was complete. By shifting the defense of advertising to children to small businesses, a frequent industry tactic, GAFAM was able to step back from its controversial practices.

Mobilizing Tech Workers

A common stereotype portrays tech workers as well-paid engineers, geeky coders, or aspiring billionaires. Across Silicon Valley and other tech industry hotspots, however, a different reality is emerging in which diverse coalitions of tech workers are creating new twenty-first-century variants of labor activism. Consider these examples.

More than four thousand Google workers signed an open letter calling on the company to turn down a contract with the Pentagon that would use artificial intelligence to analyze drone video footage from conflict zones. Such a deal, said the workers, would "irreparably damage Google's brand" and move the company into "the business of war." The signers called on CEO Sundar Pichai to "draft, publicize and enforce a clear policy stating that neither Google nor its contractors will ever build warfare technology."[119] Another petition opposing military work circulated by the Tech Workers Coalition, another labor advocacy group in the Silicon Valley, declared, "Many of us signing this petition are faced with ethical decisions in the design and development of technology on a daily basis. We cannot ignore the moral responsibility of our work."[120] Google subsequently announced it would not renew the Pentagon contract.[121]

More than six hundred workers at an Amazon fulfillment center on Staten Island in New York City signed a petition protesting working conditions at their facility. On Cyber Monday, 2019, the follow-up to Black Friday's shopping frenzy, more than one hundred Amazon workers and their supporters gathered outside the facility to protest working conditions that they say only worsen as they labor to deliver the rush of Christmas and Hanukkah packages. The workers called for more breaks and improved transit benefits to get to work. Prior to the action, a local advocacy organization, Make the Road, had released a report based on leaked company documents and reports filed with the Occupational Safety and Health Agency that showed that injury rates at the Staten Island warehouse were more than three times the industry average.[122] "It has become clear that our safety is a secondary concern in your eyes, lagging far behind line speed," the Staten Island petition said. "There are only weak plans in place to prevent more pain, more injuries, and more deaths as we enter the hardest time of the year."[123]

In 2019, three thousand Amazon workers in Seattle and many tech workers in twenty-five other cities and fourteen countries walked out of work to protect their company's environmental impact, the first walkout of corporate employees in the company's twenty-five-year history (See Figures 7.2a and 7.2b). The workers demanded that Amazon reduce its carbon footprint, acting in support of a larger youth-led international climate strike.[124] A year earlier, sixteen Amazon employees who owned stock in the company had introduced a shareholder resolution asking the company to prepare

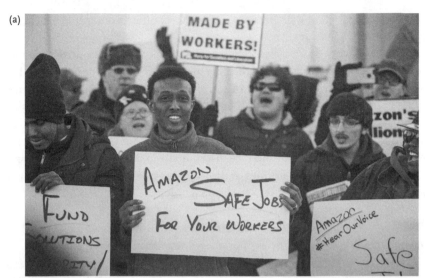

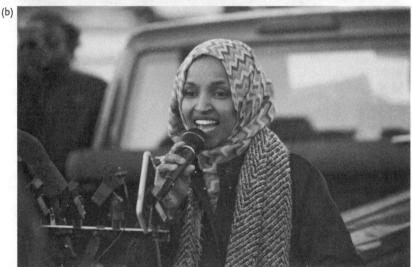

Fig. 7.2 In 2018, East African Amazon workers at a distribution center in Minnesota demanded safer working conditions (left) and US Representative Ilhan Omar spoke to the protesters (right).
Photos: Fibonacci Blue, licensed under CC BY 2.0

a report disclosing the company's carbon reduction strategies.[125] These actions had limited immediate impact but put the company and the media on notice that worker support for harmful corporate policies could not be taken for granted.

Belying the stereotypes, these accounts show that tech workers are developing sophisticated global campaigns to change the company's business practices, improve working conditions, and impose new social responsibilities on the world's wealthiest corporations. Their efforts differ from traditional labor union organizing in several ways.

First, tech workers and their organizations seek to organize across job sectors, employment status, and traditional hierarchies of class, race, and gender. Second, they address a full range of working conditions, including pay, benefits, sex and racial discrimination, sexual harassment, labor rights, and health and safety. Third, they take on the variety of social, political, environmental, and economic issues that confront the tech sector, from climate change to inequality, gentrification, sex and race discrimination, invasions of privacy, and monopoly concentration. Profiles of three groups working in this space clearly illustrate these differences from traditional unions.

Tech Workers Coalition (TWC) started in 2014 via informal meetings hosted by a cafeteria worker turned professional organizer, and an engineer. Their ambitious goal was to bring together tech workers to articulate an alternative to GAFAM's vision of the sector, one centered on workers themselves.[126] As Paige Panter, a TWC organizer, told *Slate*:

> The origin story of Tech Workers Coalition begins with a handful of full-time employees getting in the same room with subcontracted workers, cafeteria workers, security guards, janitors at some of our companies, getting to know each other, sharing about our respective workplace experiences, understanding what they were up against and why they were fighting to unionize, understanding the ways that their fight for economic survival looked different from ours, but at the same time, finding common ground by talking about our struggles at work and how to make a life in the Bay Area, in Silicon Valley.[127]

TWC describes itself as a "democratically structured, all-volunteer, and worker-led organization" that organizes for "activism, civic engagement and education." The group works "in solidarity with existing movements towards social justice, workers' rights, and economic inclusion."[128] TWC campaigns have been strengthened by alliances with scholars, community organizers, immigrant rights activists, and groups like the ACLU. Tech workers have also played an important role in supporting the unionizing efforts of tech's other workers: the service staff on Silicon Valley campuses, who struggle to make ends meet despite working for some of the richest companies in the world.

Panter joined TWC because of her concerns about civic discrimination and the bias that determines who gets hired at what companies for which jobs. In 2014, Google released data on the diversity of their workforce for the first time as the lack of equal representation in tech was finally getting some attention. She became disillusioned by the injustices she was seeing in these workplaces. "I felt like I was getting a front-row seat to the evils of how the VC (venture capital) system works as far as who decides what products get built and deployed in the first place or what problems are valuable to solve. . . . I was starting to see the discrimination in jobs as hard-coded and baked into the system. . . . And so that awareness was growing in me in the sense that top-down interventions seemed like a lost cause."[129]

Among TWC victories were helping hotel workers to win a union at a Hyatt in Santa Clara where tech companies hosted conferences; a protest at Palantir, a data analytics company founded by Peter Thiel, a billionaire friend of President Trump, to highlight the aggressive surveillance programs the firm sold to the Immigration and Customs Enforcement agency; and support for a successful campaign to convince the Orlando, Florida, police department to drop Amazon-produced facial-recognition technology. This last was one of dozens of protests or refusals by tech workers to sell to or accept contracts from the military, police, or immigration authorities.

"Like many workers in many industries before us," TWC wrote, "we too have the skills to self-organize, to refuse to do harm, to make demands, and to fight for the things our communities so desperately need, and to win. . . .We don't have to be complicit, and we don't have to be silent. Talk to your co-workers, look out for one and another and tell the boss Tech Won't Build it!"[130]

Silicon Valley Rising, another tech worker alliance, leads campaigns to create new models for good jobs, responsible employers, and affordable accessible housing in the southern part of the San Francisco Bay area that is the center of the United States technology industry. The group is a coalition of labor, faith, and community organizations that includes subcontracted janitors, shuttle drivers, security officers, and food service workers who serve the tech industry. In recent years, it has partnered with the Teamsters Union to organize an association of gig workers at Uber and elsewhere; helped to organize workers at Apple, eBay, Genentech, PayPal, and Yahoo; supported campaigns to raise the minimum wage in four Silicon Valley cities; and, with allies, won passage of an affordable housing policy for all residents by the regional transit agency.[131]

With a partner, Silicon Valley Rising has launched a responsible contracting initiative to encourage Silicon Valley companies to adopt standards that ensure that all its contractors provide their employees with livable wages and benefits, fair scheduling, safe working conditions, a voice on the job, and opportunities for professional advancement. By launching campaigns that benefited not only tech workers but also homeowners, commuters, and others, Silicon Valley Rising appealed to wider constituencies, building the power to win meaningful improvements.

Athena , a new coalition based in New York City but with a national scope, focuses on one company: Amazon. It seeks to bring together the many organizations resisting Amazon including those opposing monopoly concentration, digital surveillance, and poor working conditions. Athena helped to support the job action at the Amazon warehouse in Staten Island. To guide future action, Athena seeks to analyze Amazon's successes and failures in Seattle, where the company unsuccessfully tried to stack the city council to win more favorable policies; New York City, where a community coalition defeated Amazon's effort to win billions in public concessions in order to build a new headquarters in Queens; and elsewhere. "We're learning from what makes Amazon back down and looking to replicate that as much as possible with as many people as possible," said Dania Rajendra, Athena's director.[132]

After Amazon fired several workers for protesting inadequate protection against COVID-19 infection in its warehouses, Athena organized a letter to CEO Jeff Bezos, demanding that Amazon "listen to workers, reinstate those who have been fired, and start protecting workers' and public health." Almost twelve thousand people signed the letter.[133]

Tech Workers Coalition, Silicon Valley Rising, Athena, and other such alliances face daunting challenges. So far, they have been more successful in launching short-lived campaigns than in creating sustainable organizations. By taking on the array of issues confronting the tech sector, the groups sometimes have trouble setting priorities and using their limited resources effectively. Most of their activities are led by volunteers, making it difficult to win battles in their asymmetrical conflicts with the lobbyists and public relations staff of the world's wealthiest corporations. But what these organizations have shown is that it is possible to win wide public support for an alternative moral vision of the role of the tech industry and that the millions of people whose lives have been changes by the tech industry can come together to demand a voice in those political and economic decisions.

DEFENDING DEMOCRACY

The belief that tech companies have become too big and wield too much economic and political power motivates most of the numerous efforts to resist and seek alternatives to the growing control that these companies exert over people's daily lives. Campaigners, public officials, scholars, civil rights lawyers, and corporate reformers have identified two cross-cutting problems: GAFAM's growing power in the political arena and its threats to the privacy of individual users and to democracy. The underlying cause of these problems, argue these critics, is the monopoly concentration of this sector. As evidence they point to the fact that, as Tim Wu pointed out, in the last several years Facebook purchased 67 unchallenged acquisitions, Amazon bought up 91 companies, and Google acquired 214.[134]

Profiles of a few organizations and individuals who are constructing solutions to these problems illustrate the strategies and tactics they have employed.

Freedom from Facebook, for example, is a coalition that includes the Communication Workers of America, Content Creators Coalition, Democracy for America, Jewish Voice for Peace, MoveOn, Public Citizen, and other groups. Its goals are to "make Facebook safe for our democracy by breaking it up, giving us the freedom to communicate across networks, and protecting our privacy."

On its website, the group succinctly defines the problem in a way that articulates the progressive critique of the company:

> Facebook and Mark Zuckerberg have amassed a scary amount of power. Facebook unilaterally decides the news that billions of people around the world see every day. It buys up or bankrupts potential competitors to protect its monopoly, killing innovation and choice. It tracks us almost everywhere we go on the web and, through our smartphones, even where we go in the real world. It uses this intimate data hoard to figure out how to addict us and our children to its services. And then Facebook serves up everything about us to its true customers—virtually anyone willing to pay for the ability to convince us to buy, do, or believe something. And it is spending millions on corporate lobbyists, academics, and think tanks to ensure no one gets in their way.[135]

In 2018, Freedom from Facebook filed a legal complaint against Facebook with the Federal Trade Commission, calling on the FTC to fully investigate the breach of 5 million users' accounts, seek maximum civil penalties against the company, and require Facebook to spin off WhatsApp, Instagram, and Messenger, three of its subsidiaries.[136]

State attorneys general and other elected officials also joined the debates on protecting privacy and democracy from Big Tech companies. In California, the State Attorney General Xavier Becerra sued Facebook for its failure to respond to dozens of requests for documents, including email correspondence between Mark Zuckerberg, Sheryl Sandberg, and other company leaders. The Massachusetts attorney general is also pressuring Facebook to release more information and the New York attorney general is leading a multistate antitrust inquiry into Facebook. California also recently passed a new privacy law that will give the attorney general a role in regulating digital privacy, a key power in the absence of a comprehensive federal privacy law.[137]

At the federal level, Senator Ron Wyden from Oregon has introduced the Mind Your Own Business Act, which would give the Federal Trade Commission (FTC) the authority to fine companies who mismanage user data, but also to jail and fine company leaders for violating user privacy and lying about their actions. This, he hopes, would be enough to scare Big Tech executives straight and force them to take user privacy seriously. "I hope that this will be the baseline protection for consumer privacy at the largest companies in America," he said. Its fate in Congress is uncertain.[138] And in the 2020 presidential campaign, Mark Zuckerberg and Senator Elizabeth Warren debated the breakup of Facebook. These interchanges forced other presidential candidates to clarify their positions on fighting monopoly concentration.

Human and civil rights groups have also stepped into the fray. In his Georgetown speech, Mark Zuckerberg linked Facebook's efforts to defend free speech and democracy with Frederick Douglass, Martin Luther King Jr., Black Lives Matter, and the civil rights movement. In rebuttal, NAACP Legal Defense Fund president Sherrilyn Ifill wrote that Facebook "has refused to fully recognize the threat of voter suppression and intimidation here at home, especially from users that the company refers to as 'authentic voices'—politicians and candidates for office." After two years of conversations between NAACP, other civil rights groups, and Facebook, and numerous effort to inform Facebook about voter suppression in the real world, Ifill wrote in *The Washington Post* that she is "convinced that Facebook simply is ill-equipped to define what constitutes voter suppression."[139] She went on to observe:

> The civil rights movement was not fought to vindicate free speech rights under the First Amendment. It was a fight to fulfill the promise of full citizenship and human dignity guaranteed to black people by the 14th Amendment. To use the struggle of those extraordinary heroes as a rationale for protecting Facebook users who seek to incite the same kind of division and violence those heroes faced turns that history on its head.

THE COSTS OF BIG TECH

By disrupting previous patterns of social behavior, commerce, and civic engagement to achieve their business goals, the new technology companies have fundamentally changed how our society influences health. More than any other sector, they have transformed how capitalism shapes the daily quest for the pillars of well-being. Enabled by globalization, monopoly concentration, new technologies, and a deregulatory spirit, GAFAM and its fellow tech companies have delivered alluring benefits to billions of people. They have created new ways to connect with family and friends, brought the convenience of having the products consumers want delivered to their front doors with a few clicks, and made the knowledge of the modern world available at one's fingertips.

But the costs have been high. They include:

- a rising burden of depression, anxiety, stress, loneliness, and bullying, especially among children and young people;
- greater access to unhealthy products that worsen the world's most serious health problems and a growing ability for marketers to target vulnerable populations and evade the health regulations forged in the last century;
- increases in personal consumption that will make it more difficult to reduce pollution, slow human-induced climate change, and shrink wide gaps in health among the poor and the better off;
- greater threats to privacy, autonomy, and dignity, generated by tech companies' capacity to extract and sell data about every aspect of our private lives to other companies who use this information to predict and shape consumption, political behavior, and beliefs; and
- a deterioration in democracy precipitated by the growing political power and economic clout of the tech industry and by its development of tools that make it possible to attract users and profits by provoking or aggravating social and political conflicts.

Some might choose the tech benefits despite these problems. But why should a few big companies force hundreds of millions of Americans to accept these companies take-it-or-leave-it options, selected to ensure continued profitability, rather than use our democratic processes to better balance public and private needs?

Clearly, many people are resisting and seeking alternatives. While so far, the opposition to GAFAM is scattered, consisting mostly of time-limited, partially successful campaigns, the cumulative impact has been impressive. The uncritical public celebration of tech companies that characterized its first decade has evolved into a more analytic view, one that seeks to better balance GAFAM's costs and benefits to society. The question of more forceful government anti-trust action and regulatory oversight has returned to the national agenda. The mental health, cognitive, environmental, and political consequences of surveillance capitalism are now the subject of intense interpersonal, familial, and political discussion, the precursor for changes in social norms governing their role.

In the last two decades, a handful of companies have sought to claim for themselves the right to set the rules for what role technology will play in our future and to insist that the world they offer is inevitable and without feasible alternatives. In coming decades, the success of the rising challenges to this assertion will shape health and democracy.

PART III

Conclusion

CHAPTER 8

Transitions from Twenty-first-century Capitalism

She's on the horizon. . . . I go two steps, she moves two steps away. I walk ten steps and the horizon runs ten steps ahead. No matter how much I walk, I'll never reach her. What good is utopia? That's what: it's good for walking.
—*Eduardo Galeano*, Walking Words, *1995*

In modern history, social movements have been a motor force for changing the living conditions that influence well-being, happiness, and social justice. Shaped by shifting global and national economic and political forces and demanding the right to use science, technology, and other innovations to benefit people rather than to generate profits, movements of labor, anti-colonialism, civil rights, women, consumers, LGBTQIA+, disability rights, and environmental activists have won concessions from corporations and wealthy elites that led to better, healthier lives for millions of people and to a more equitable and sustainable planet. In the past and now, successful movements require three ingredients: a shared diagnosis of key problems, a vision for a different world, and strategies for making the transition from current reality to the imagined future.

In previous chapters, I showed how changes in modern capitalism have eroded six key pillars of well-being: food, education, healthcare, work, transport, and social connections. Synthesizing evidence from many sources, I have described how corporations and wealthy elites have modified the rules and operating principles of capitalism that had evolved after World War II. These changes have jeopardized human and environmental health, eroded democracy, and increased inequality. Of course, not everyone agrees with this diagnosis of today's ills but across nations, communities, and social classes, many acknowledge that today's world faces existential threats to survival and that modifying the dynamics and impact of twenty-first-century capitalism is the essential remedy.

The goal of this chapter is to spark a conversation among the many millions of people across the United States and around the world who worry that the costs of twenty-first-century capitalism are too high. These discussions can assist those longing for change to forge a vision and identify strategies to create realistic alternatives that can better promote well-being, a livable planet, more equitable distribution of the necessities of life, and stronger democracies. Such a conversation will also enable the many forces seeking change to reach agreement on their priority goals and to overcome conflicts that have so often weakened recent efforts. It will also provide those ready to work for the change with some common messages and arguments they can use to initiate useful discussions with their peers, families, and communities who are do not yet believe change is possible or even desirable.

IMAGINE

"Imagination is stronger than knowledge," wrote Albert Einstein. "Knowledge is limited, imagination encircles the world." Imagine, if you can, a world where the well-being of people and the planet is the priority.

Imagine a food system that makes healthy food, sustainably grown and produced by decently paid workers, available and affordable to all.

Imagine schools and universities that provide all learners with the knowledge and skills they need to achieve their full potential and contribute to their communities and the world, and use their education to pursue their own and others' well-being and happiness.

Imagine healthcare, accessible to all, that makes prevention of illness and improved quality of life its highest goals and provides care that enables patients to minimize the burden of diseases they encounter and the pain and suffering it imposes.

Imagine work that pays workers what they need for a decent life; ensures that working does not sicken or injure; contributes to a better, more sustainable world; offers pathways to advancement; and allows workers to organize, do their jobs, and enjoy personal and family life outside work.

Imagine transportation that makes it easy for all people to move around their neighborhoods, cities, and beyond; and leaves our streets human-friendly, our air safe to breathe, and our planet fit for life.

Imagine, finally, a way to connect to others—family, friends, peers, businesses, our communities, and the world—that does not require sacrificing mental health, self-confidence, privacy, dignity, civic peace, or commercial access to the most intimate details of our lives.

To many, this vision of another world may seem hopelessly naive, the foolish dreams of idealistic schoolchildren unfamiliar with the realities of today's world, or the fantasies of aging activists and academics who never recovered from the 1960s. It certainly does not seem to be the realistic aspirations of men and women who have to get by in the real world of the third decade of the twenty-first century. Certainly not the achievable goals of the many advocates who have struggled since the 2008 financial crisis to make progress toward a more just and sustainable world.

But consider whether humanity has faced similar grave crises in the past two hundred years—and still found ways to move forward and make progress. Around the world, hundreds of millions of people are dissatisfied with the status quo and already at work seeking to create alternatives. The wealth and scientific knowledge and technology that humanity has created make each of the six visions relatively feasible in the coming decades. Finally, today's generations, especially young people, seem as determined and capable of finding solutions to the deep problems vexing the world today as in the past. These powerful assets for a global movement make optimism an alternative to the deep pessimism that pervades so much of the world today.

Three insights from my many decades as a public health researcher, practitioner, and activist make me optimistic that humans alive today can find the will, skills, and resolve to take up the current challenges. First, improvements in public health, social justice, and democracy have always been driven by social movements and their allies. Why should that be different now?

Second, for at least the last three hundred years, the primary goal of most of these movements has been to make changes in the social and economic arrangements that allocate wealth and power. Many improvements in health, the environment, social justice, and more equitable access to the necessities of life of the past century have come about as a result of the successes of these movements. Many movements active today are already forging our generations' version of such a global mobilization.

Third, health and well-being have consistently proved to be a useful aspiration for bringing together the many constituencies who benefit from changing the status quo. In the Progressive Era, the New Deal, and the movements of the 1960s, improving the well-being of various populations served to motivate, unify, and satisfy many participants in social reforms.

And so to change the future of health in this century, to move away from the gloomy outcomes described in previous chapters, today's activists, concerned citizens, voters, parents, young people, workers, and discriminated against will need to do three things. First, they must bring together the many movements now working for improvements into a more cohesive, unified whole. Second, they must articulate strategies and goals to make changing twenty-first-century capitalism the unifying goal of this emerging movement. Third, those seeking change must find themes and frames that bring together rather than divide. The universal rights to well-being and to living a decent life are examples of such themes highlighted here.

CREATING A COHESIVE MOVEMENT

The many organizations and individuals who constitute the emerging movements for a healthier, more equitable, and sustainable world are the most valuable resources for such a transformation. Analyzing their successes and failures, supporting their efforts to overcome the obstacles they encounter, and synthesizing their practice into guidance that can inform those working on other issues and in different places are urgent tasks for activists and academics.

Why are social movements the medicine of choice prescribed for the ills of capitalism? First, they have a track record of success. In the twentieth century, social movements in the United States worked with reformers in government and civil society to strengthen safety regulations for food and drugs, end child labor, improve worker safety, shorten work hours, end legal segregation, expand voter rights, protect water and air, and reduce discrimination and inequitable access to health resources for Blacks, Latinx, women, and other populations. Each of these reforms contributed to improved well-being, more equitable access to the necessities of life, safer environments, and more opportunities for democratic participation.

Movements also connect constituencies working on different issues or in different places. The civil rights movement started in the South, moved to the North, and focused on education, employment, healthcare, and voters' rights. Leaders like Martin Luther King Jr. and Malcom X linked the effort to end racism in the United States with the global campaign to end US involvement in the war in Vietnam. In a world where media and the demands of daily living separate issues, divide social groups, and isolate individuals, social movements can serve as a cohesive force, assembling the ideas, constituencies, and communications channels that bring people together to achieve common goals.

Compare the potential of social movements for transforming the current economic and political system to three frequently proposed alternatives. For each of the pillars of health, some social actors have suggested that science and technology can solve today's problems. Food and agricultural companies and the scientists they supported claimed that the Green Revolution could end world hunger and reduce diet-related diseases. While some of its discoveries have contributed to these goals, the consolidation of the scientific advances of the Green Revolution in corporate hands facilitated the rise of ultra-processed food and the subsequent rise of diet-related diseases. More than fifty years after the Green Revolution was launched, world hunger and food insecurity remain major global problems.[1]

Similarly, more than fifty years after President Nixon declared war on cancer, cancer deaths have decreased much less than those from other causes and many forms of cancer continue to have dismal survival rates. Science and technology are essential tools for improving life but as long as they are controlled by organizations that seek to use them to benefit their self-interest, their impact will be limited. Social movements can bring the questions of power and control to the forefront.

Another frequently suggested solution to the problems that capitalism imposes is simply to provide more education. Educate consumers to make healthier food and healthcare choices, parents to make better choices of schooling, and workers to choose better jobs and follow safety rules more carefully, claim the proponents of more education, and the problems of those sectors will be significantly diminished. But a growing body of evidence in public health and other disciplines shows that the benefits of education alone are usually modest. Requiring health educators, for example, to inform every smoker, drinker, or unhealthy food eater to resist the multibillion-dollar marketing blitzes designed to persuade people to consume these products is at best a Sisyphean task. Education on its own lacks the capacity to change the structural forces that sustain or encourage unhealthy choices—whereas this is precisely what social movements offer.

A third proposed solution is to use traditional political strategies— legislation, litigation, elections—to achieve change. Advocates of this strategy—most elected officials and many business and civil society groups— claim that these tried and tested means work, albeit sometimes slowly, and are less disruptive than social movements' unconventional or contentious approaches. Of course, traditional politics must play a role and these strategies have contributed to advances in health, the environment, and democracy. But a defining characteristic of twenty-first-century capitalism is the extent to which major corporations and financial institutions have come to dominate politics and modify the formal and informal rules that govern the game in ways that tilt the field to their benefit. For these reasons, politics as usual is less relevant than in the past, another reason why social movements can fill an important gap.

Science, education, and conventional politics will make essential contributions to the efforts to modify modern capitalism but the history of the last several decades shows that by themselves, they lack the capacity to transform a political and economic system that has become increasingly resistant to change. Conventional politics often accept the power-sharing status quo and emphasize incremental rather than transformative changes. In a system characterized by asymmetrical power relationships, following only the rules set by those in power can fail to bring about meaningful reforms.

Despite their potential to create organizational forms that can challenge modern capitalism, contemporary social movements encounter significant obstacles. Reality-based reformers have to acknowledge these weaknesses while also trying to overcome them. Too often, activists and their movements work in silos. Silos describe the boundaries that activists create between their organization, issue, sector, community, and movement and others working for different, albeit connected, goals. On the one hand, such limits are necessary since no one can work on many things at once. On the other hand, this siloing weakens the power of movements, duplicates efforts, and reduces mobilization of additional support. In the food justice movement, for example, those seeking to end hunger and food insecurity, reduce obesity and diet-related diseases, promote sustainable agriculture, or reduce food waste often work separately or even at cross purposes.

Yet each of these goals requires changing the dominant corporate system of food and agriculture. Focusing on the separate goals of each strand rather than the common overarching ones has made the food movement less powerful, less able to win concessions from the highly organized alliance of food and agriculture businesses, and more vulnerable to co-optation by trade groups who offer some factions grants or a seat at the policy table.

And too often the groups working within or across movement sectors frame their choices as binary rather than understanding each choice as a context-specific decision on a continuum of options. Should educational reform movements oppose all charter schools to combat privatization of public services or seek to make those that exist more accountable? Should tech activists work for the breakup of Facebook, Google, and Microsoft or settle for more energetic regulation of their practices? Campaigners frequently squander precious time and energy characterizing those who disagree with their choice as opponents rather than together locating their decisions in the context of a shared strategy. Business leaders will always look to exploit these differences to divide and conquer opposition. By developing principles and forums for such decisions, activists can mitigate the potential damage of these conflicts.

This problem is compounded by the current political climate and resulting lack of safe spaces in which activists who agree on some questions but disagree on others can have open dialogue. The goal is to find common ground where possible and to agree to disagree when not. The excesses of call-out culture, exacerbated by social media and political polarization, often encourage name-calling and shaming rather than critical analysis. As Naomi Klein points out in her book *No Is Not Enough*, when activists do take a step back from daily struggles to analyze lessons and forge strategy across movements and places, they gain powerful new insights and solidarities.[2]

Class, race, and gender hierarchies enable modern capitalists to divide opponents who, united, could pose a much more powerful threat to the status quo. In his book *How to Be an Antiracist*, Ibram X. Kendi describes the intimate relationships between racism and capitalism—he calls them conjoined twins—and the willingness of some activists in both struggles to downplay the costs of the other system of oppression if they believe such concessions give them tactical advantages.[3] Similarly, class, racial, and gender biases within movements impede more powerful alliances against corporate rule. For example, the difficulty the mostly white and middle-class food movement has had in taking up the needs of Black and Latinx farmers and food workers has limited this movement's capacity to win sustainable policy victories.

Some scholars of movements have questioned whether a single cohesive movement is needed or even desirable. Instead they have proposed that contemporary global movements are best considered "a movement of movements," a network or alliance of many social movements that sometimes acts together and sometimes separately.[4] This arrangement, they argue, is more conducive to embedding specific struggles in a particular time and place while still acknowledging global linkages. The World Social Forum, an annual gathering of activists from movements around the world, is a physical representation of the global movement of movements and a concrete opportunity for activists to meet to exchange strategies and plan future actions.[5]

In practice, many social mobilizations that begin with a single issue expand as they grow. In a talk on her lessons from the 1960s movements, the poet Audre Lorde observed, "There is no such thing as a single-issue struggle because we do not live single-issue lives."[6] Current movements such as Black Lives Matter and #Me Too may begin by bringing people together to respond to threats based on race or gender but then confront the ways that these issues are rooted in political economy, history, power, and corporate practices, requiring them to expand their strategic focus and seek new allies.

The decision by Hollywood actors active in #MeToo to use the 2018 Golden Globes Awards to bring media attention to how women domestic, farm, and food service workers experience sexual harassment and discrimination illustrates such expansion. More than three hundred actors raised almost $20 million to help low-wage women workers who had filed sexual harassment and discrimination lawsuits to cover the cost of legal expenses. Ai-jen Poo, the executive director of the National Domestic Workers Alliance, went to the Golden Globes as Meryl Streep's plus-one. She told a reporter, "Domestic workers are coming forward as part of the #MeToo movement to say, not only are we not alone as domestic workers, we are not alone as women working in this economy. Women across the board face this imbalance of power, which makes us susceptible to harassment and abuse, and limits our economic and human potential."[7]

MAKING CAPITALISM THE MOVEMENT'S TARGET

The world's most serious problems—climate change, environmental pollution, racism, sexism, growing inequality, deterioration of health in many populations, threats to democracy—have many causes. And the social movements of the last few decades have had many goals—reversing human-induced climate change, ending police violence and racism, reducing hunger and food insecurity, shrinking the growing gaps in US and global income and wealth, and so on. Why then suggest that an appropriate target for solving the cascade of today's most serious problem would be the social and economic arrangements that characterize modern capitalism? And why should the many social movements striving to rectify the world's wrongs make changing this form of capitalism a priority goal?

As shown in previous chapters, changes in twenty-first-century capitalism have accelerated damage to each of the six pillars of health, the foundations of well-being. The world's response to climate change illustrates the perils of ignoring or covering up growing threats to human and planetary well-being. Decades of inaction and delay have made the challenges of reversing the crises that human-induced climate change has imposed massively more difficult. Evidence suggests that it is imperative to act now to reduce the escalating damage that modern capitalism inflicts on systems to feed, educate, provide medical care to, employ, transport, and connect to others the people of the United States as well as others around the world.

When multiple problems have a common cause, it is more rational and effective to tackle that cause than to separately take on the many disparate roots. Tobacco researchers long understood that other factors contributed to the cancers, heart diseases, circulatory, and other health problems that exposure to tobacco worsened. But in the interest of saving the most lives, preventing disease, and using limited resources wisely, they developed and launched a comprehensive, integrated, global campaign to reduce exposure to tobacco smoke and to shrink the influence of the tobacco industry that had caused the epidemics. It took fifty years to see measurable impact, but we now know that tens of millions of lives have been saved and an unmeasurable burden of human suffering has been averted by forceful action to limit exposure to tobacco smoke and tobacco lobbyists.

A more practical reason further supports a decision to focus on capitalism. Capitalism is a human creation. Since the first corporations were created in the seventeenth century, the capitalist system has evolved continually. Today, while global capitalism shares key essential features, it is not a monolithic or homogeneous system but varies over time and place. Each variant has different arrangements for what is public, what is private, and who decides what, each is forged by the local and national interactions among competing social forces.

Even the most cursory review of history shows that changes in these arrangements are possible, indeed inevitable. In future decades, the Thatcherite dictum that there is no alternative to the current form of capitalism will seem as quaint as the early Christians' assertion that their view of God was the only one possible then and forever.

In my view, while altering the harmful characteristics of modern capitalism is the priority for improving global well-being, other influences on health such as demographic shifts, cultural clashes, urbanization, and migration also require attention. But corporate-controlled globalization, financialization, deregulation, monopoly concentration, and the corporate capture of new technologies, the defining characteristics of twenty-first-century capitalism, are fundamental causes of multiple and growing threats to well-being. This commonality justifies a sharp focus on the system that is the underlying cause.

Does the recommendation to focus efforts on modifying modern capitalism require reformers to agree on a single clear alternative? I think not because what comes next and how to get there will not be decided by the opining of activists, academics. or political leaders. Rather, answers will be found in practice, through intense interactions among the many social groups that always shape these decisions. As the Spanish poet Antonio Machado wrote in 1913, "Traveler, there is no road; the road is made as you go."[8]

Nor does it mean that all reformers need to pledge allegiance to ending capitalism as we know it or to endorse one brand or another of socialism. Identifying clear alternatives to twenty-first-century capitalism, deciding what elements to retain or abandon, and determining what alternatives work best where are critical tasks for the coming decades. Today's priority, however, is to align the many forces harmed by our current system into a more coordinated and effective counter to these threats.

Most important, settling these questions is not a precondition for acting now. Climate change, low-wage jobs, inequitable access to education, and the growing toll from cancer are problems that require action today. By integrating efforts to solve the problems people face in their day-to-day lives with an analysis of changing economic, social, and political realities, those seeking a different world can achieve short-term improvements while setting the stage for more transformative changes in the future. In fact, whether people use or do not use a particular label—reformer, anticapitalist, democratic socialist—is, at least in the short-term, mostly irrelevant. What matters is actual popular support for shared achievable goals.

Even for health professionals and advocates with the more limited goal of improving health, the focus on modern capitalism still makes sense. Two alternative strategies proposed for improving health—clinical medicine and behavioral and lifestyle change—face significant constraints. Clinical medicine seeks to undo the damage that modern life imposes, a task that is both expensive and often of limited efficacy. Addressing lifestyles and eating, smoking, drinking, and other risky behaviors certainly contributes to improving health. But as a growing portion of food available in supermarkets and grocery stores is unhealthy, when many cities have air that is dangerous to breathe, when many public water supplies are contaminated with antibiotics and toxics, when pharmaceutical companies aggressively promote dangerous drugs, and when working conditions are becoming riskier with fewer health and safety protections, asking individuals to take primary responsibility for their health seems both unethical and ineffective.

Growing biomedical and public health evidence highlights the limits of these two strategies, making additional action to address underlying causes of today's major health problem a compelling option. And as I have noted, the public health advances of the last century came not primarily from new drugs or healthy-eating education but from the social movements that improved housing and work conditions, made healthy food more available, and fought to end exclusion and discrimination against women, Blacks, immigrants, and LGBTQIA+s.

USING HEALTH AND WELL-BEING AS A UNIFYING THEME

Modern capitalism contributes to many of the world's most serious problems. Poor health is often the consequence of one group of wealthy, powerful individuals or organizations choosing to act in ways that benefit them at the expense of others, making health a useful lens for identifying opponents, informing strategies, and mobilizing supporters. Why are health and the broader concept of well-being the central focus for this analysis of capitalism? In my view, this emphasis offers clear benefits to those who seek to connect issues, populations, and places. Almost everyone wants to feel better now and in the future. Almost everyone wants to ensure that their families, children, friends, and other people they love have the potential to attain the best health possible. Most people think about health every day, if only in seeking to feel good, avoid pain and unnecessary risks, and protect those they care about.

In these ways, well-being offers a common goal that can bring people together across boundaries that in other circumstances divide them. Well-being also serves to connect the personal and political, two levels of action that feminists of the 1960s and 1970s taught can be effectively linked to nurture sustainable activism.

Throughout human history, people have fought for a better life, improved living conditions, and access to the necessities of life. One useful and appealing framing of this ancient yet modern pursuit is the concept of *buen vivir* (*sumak kawsay* in Quechua), the right to a good life, articulated by indigenous people in Bolivia and Ecuador. Eduardo Gudynas, a leading scholar on the subject, explains, "With buen vivir, the subject of well-being is not [about the] individual, but the individual in the social context of their community and in a unique environmental situation."[9] *Buen vivir*, a concept included in the Bolivian and Ecuadoran constitutions, provides an alternative to the pro-growth, consumerist, and individualistic ideology of health, an alternative that could serve as a rallying call for a movement for sustainable and equitable well-being (See Figure 8.1).[10]

While well-being has the potential to unify across boundaries, the concept also provides a tool for analyzing who is responsible for the living conditions that damage health. Restricted access to higher education, challenges in traveling across urban neighborhoods, or targeted marketing of unhealthy products—each of these experiences connects daily life and feelings of disease with our political and economic system.

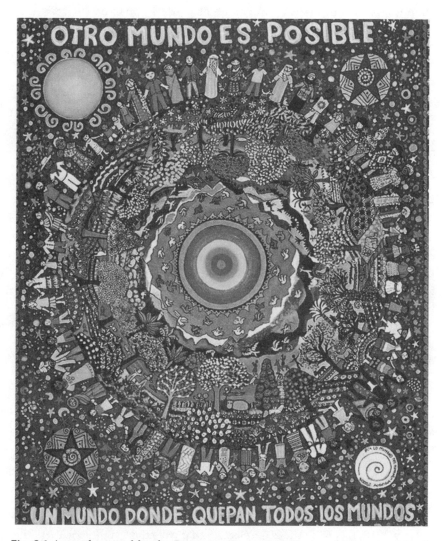

Fig. 8.1 A mural inspired by the Zapatista movement in Mexico which portrays its vision of a world where protecting the planet, growing healthy food, and living well are inseparable goals.

Finally, public health is one of the disciplines that provides evidence that our social, political, and economic arrangements are fundamental influences on patterns of health and disease for both communities and the planet. Scholars and public health professionals have a moral and ethical obligation to use our knowledge to improve the health of populations and to shrink the entrenched inequities in health that characterize today's world.

Practice as the Guide

On one level, taking steps to unify and integrate the goals and strategies of the many movements active today, developing a common focus on changing harmful elements of modern capitalism, and making improved well-being a central movement aim seem straightforward recommendations, difficult of course in practice, but conceptually simple.

On another level, each is a complex task, tried by many with only partial success, and resistant to cookbook recipes. The path forward, I believe, is to ground future efforts to achieve these three goals in the current practices of movements seeking change. Activists around the country and world are developing and testing multiple movements, campaigns, organizational forms, and strategies to modify capitalism in small and big ways, many described in previous chapters. Some of these experiments pass the test of being implementable, others of having an impact, and still others of being replicable and sustainable in other settings. By basing the search for new solutions on this robust body of practice evidence, those seeking alternatives to contemporary capitalism can find the practical, innovative, field-tested, and time-tested ideas that can best advance their goals, as well as failures that suggest avoiding certain paths.

To illustrate this process and to encourage other activists and scholars to join this endeavor, I offer brief profiles of three bodies of practice that I believe offer insights into next steps. In this chapter, I examine the contributions of movements that have made corporations central targets. In the next chapter, I also consider relevant lessons from other powerful recent movements such as Black Lives Matter and #MeToo that targeted the systemic racism and sexism that have worsened the lives of so many Americans—and have been used by modern capitalism to divide potential opponents.

The Green New Deal

In early 2019, following the 2018 election that gave the Democratic Party the majority in the US House of Representatives, Alexandria Ocasio-Cortez, a representative newly elected from New York, and Edward Markey, a veteran senator from Massachusetts, introduced House Resolution 109 and Senate Resolution 59, a package of proposals that came to be known as the Green New Deal.[11]

The idea of an ambitious national plan to reduce climate change while also promoting more equitable economic development and job creation originated in the United Kingdom more than a decade earlier and in subsequent years, the US Green Party promoted its Green New Deal in various state and national elections. But it was the 2019 legislation, which followed several dire warnings from international scientific bodies about the imminent threat of climate change to economic growth, human health, agriculture, and national security[12] that generated intense media, public, policymaker, and corporate interest in the proposal from Ocasio-Cortez and Markey. Four of the candidates in the 2020 Democratic presidential primary endorsed the Green New Deal, ensuring that the topic attracted further attention in national election. By vigorously attacking the Green New Deal, President Trump generated further interest in the idea.

In the words of its proponents, the Green New Deal (GND) was "Green" in the sense that its "aim is to modernize the economy comprehensively so that we no longer have to poison our environment, subsidize decaying infrastructure and sacrifice poor and working-class communities to all manner of pollution and environmental degradation, simply to produce wealth that benefits a tiny fraction of Americans." It was a New Deal "in the sense that it works on a scale not seen in the country since the New Deal and World War II mobilizations."[13]

The legislation itself is broad and ambitious. It calls on the federal government to act to:

- achieve net-zero greenhouse gas emissions through a fair and just transition for all communities and workers;
- create millions of good, high-wage jobs and ensure prosperity and economic security for all people of the United States;
- invest in the infrastructure and industry of the United States to sustainably meet the challenges of the twenty-first century;
- secure for all people of the United States for generations to come clean air and water, climate and community resiliency, healthy food, access to nature, and a sustainable environment; and
- promote justice and equity by stopping current, preventing future, and repairing historic oppression in front-line and vulnerable communities.[14]

Supporters lauded the broad scope and lack of detail, saying this approach invited debate, participation, and improvement by many constituencies. Opponents, however, chided the plan for being vague, confusing, and not including cost estimates. But the proposal successfully triggered robust debate;

local, state, and national activism; and fierce opposition from conservatives and business elites. Thus, the GND plan warrants scrutiny for its capacity to unify movements, highlight the limits of modern capitalism, and enlist new supporters with its broad focus on well-being, sustainable development, and social justice.

The GND offers several characteristics that make it a useful platform for achieving these three goals. First, it brings together what have in the past been mostly separate, often siloed, movements—for slowing climate change, regulating corporations, promoting equitable community development, expanding job training, and pursuing other goals. By putting forth a single plan that includes all these aims, GND encourages supporters (and opponents) to ask: How are these issues connected? What are their common causes? What can we do together to achieve these outcomes?

GND embraces strategic ambiguity—the art of making a claim that can reduce kneejerk opposition—in ways that might be useful for launching other transformative proposals. Is GND a strategy for capitalism to save itself, or one to create an alternative? In support of the former view, proponents cite the benefits to businesses that produce the technology for wind and solar energy, the construction industry that will build the GND infrastructure and improve energy efficiency in existing buildings, and the tech and automobile industries that produce electric cars and other autonomous vehicles.

Advocates of a GND that challenges capitalism note the strong role for government in setting the rules for markets, the public investment needed, and the call for people's participation in making policy decisions that can reduce the disparate impact of climate change on the poor and people of color. Advancing GND in ways that keep both sides of this debate engaged allows wider political support and perhaps less opposition from those on either side.

In the last two decades, changes in capitalism have had different impacts on urban and rural populations and on people living in the North, South, and Midwest. GND proposals that address farming and rural development, infrastructure, food distribution, and job training can benefit each of these groups, perhaps helping to heal the deep urban-rural polarizations and setting the stage for finding other shared goals that benefit the urban and rural poor and middle classes rather than only wealthy elites. Identifying new ways to find common ground among groups now divided by ideology and culture, even when they share long-term interests, is an essential task for a successful movement.

GND also invites participation from other movements not yet fully engaged in climate activism. Anthony Flaccavento, a farmer and political activist in West Virginia, identifies some of the Green New Deal measures that would benefit farmers and eaters: investments in local food and farming infrastructure, support for farmers and land preservation, and increased urban access to locally and regionally grown healthy affordable food. He writes:

A Green New Deal is not the only thing we could do to address emissions and climate change. And it's not the only strategy for creating better jobs, more widely shared prosperity, and a people-centered economy. But it is the only approach I know of that does both. For 40 years, most Americans have been losing ground economically, even as the economy has grown six times faster than our population. During that same period, this same trickle-down economy has . . . launched us on the road to severe changes in the climate and our environment. If a GND offers a roadmap for a better economy and a restored, sustainable ecosystem, what the heck is wrong with that?[15]

In New York City, food justice and health activists, environmentalists, and small farmers have proposed putting food on the Green New Deal menu, both in order to enlist new supporters but also to bring additional benefits. Since the food growing practices that contribute to climate change are those most heavily used by the ultra-processed food industry to produce unhealthy food, changing these practices will have both a climate and health payoff. These activists have successfully persuaded New York City and New York State elected officials to develop their own Green New Deal agendas, a way to spark action at other levels during a time of resistance to climate action at the federal level and also to develop local solutions that can inform national ones in a different political climate.[16]

Second, the GND core goals—reducing climate change, promoting more equitable economic growth, and creating good jobs—can catalyze action at local, regional, national, even global levels. GND thus provides a tool for unifying and integrating activism and pressure within a specific region but also across geographic and political boundaries. It is a practical plan for making the local global and vice versa.

A few examples show the diversity of organizations and causes that have been able to use the GND to make such links. The Sunrise Movement, an organization "building an army of young people to make climate change an urgent priority across America," held sit-ins in Congress to urge quicker action on GND legislation and organized dozens of local action hubs to coordinate advocacy and education in communities across the United States. In September 2019, Sunrise participated in the Global Climate Strike, the largest day of action for climate justice in world history. More than 3 million people chose to #StrikeWithUs at more than 4,000 events in 150 countries.[17]

At Amazon, more than 8,703 workers signed a 2019 open letter to CEO Jeff Bezos, urging him to advocate for "local, federal, and international policies that reduce overall carbon emissions in line with the IPCC report" and to withhold campaign contributions from policymakers who delay action on climate change.[18] It also demanded that Amazon release a company-wide plan to reduce its own carbon emissions and to assist its employees to cope with climate-related crises. By calling media and public attention to the role that big corporations played in supporting or opposing proposals to address climate change, these workers opened another front for GND activism. In 2020, Amazon threatened to fire these critics, further enhancing solidarity and determination of workers who wanted stronger climate action from their employer.[19]

In a third example of GND-inspired activism, Native Americans and other indigenous people have also found ways to use the climate initiative to advance their long struggles to protect their lands and people. Indigenous Environmental Network and Honor the Earth, an indigenous-led environmental nonprofit, helped to prepare the legislation. The resolution requires federal officials to obtain "the free, prior, and informed consent of indigenous peoples for all decisions that affect indigenous peoples and their traditional territories."[20]

New Mexico Representative Debra Haaland, one of the first Native American women in Congress to support the Green New Deal, said, "Communities of color are disproportionately affected by climate change. That's why one of the most important aspects of delivering a Green New Deal for America is making sure that the transition to a renewable economy is equitable and benefits all communities. Making sure provisions in the Green New Deal have language that includes Tribal consultation is part of respecting the status they have as required by law." By recognizing the specific concerns of indigenous people, GND creates a platform for respectful dialogue on the best ways to protect and respect these communities.

A successful movement to modify capitalism will need to make substantive proposals both to change policies that contribute to global warming, wealth inequality, and the rise of low-wage work, for example, and also to strengthen democracy. The GND shows how to combine these strands by including proposals for "peer assemblies," government-constituted bodies to inform implementation of new initiatives;[21] protection of workers' rights to organize; and the previously described mandate for indigenous people to provide "free, prior and informed consent" for new projects.[22]

By putting questions of democracy front and center, GND encourages—and requires—activists to consider simultaneously what to change and how to change it, thus avoiding the tendency of prior movements to focus on one or the other, risking prospects for sustainable growth and increasing political influence.

On another front, GND provides an explicit critique of incrementalism, a mainstream commitment that often reduces success and discourages participation from the disaffected, even as it may help to hold on to more moderate supporters. As Flaccavento, the West Virginia farmer and activist, observes, GND allows activists to:

> put "incrementalism" aside. We can always resurrect it when, if at some point in the future, we've built an economy and a politics that actually works for people, communities, and the land. If we ever get to that point, there will still be need

for tweaking the system. But at this moment, tweaking is not only insufficient, it's utterly counterproductive. It fuels the resentment so many people feel and helps corroborate their belief that we're out of touch.[23]

Another contribution of GND is its capacity to link participants' personal lives and their political activism, an essential task for recruiting new activists and sustaining their engagement. For many climate activists, their fight is intensely personal. Varshini Prakash, the executive director of Sunrise, the climate youth organization, talks about devastation wrought last year by monsoons in South India, where her family originates, and of the threat to her current home in East Boston, "a place where, if we don't take action in the next couple of decades, will cease to exist and will be lost to the seas forever."[24]

Groups like Black Lives Matter underscore that GND proposals must address the disparate racial impact of climate change. "Black, brown, and low-income communities bear the brunt of pollution and environmental degradation, accelerated by climate change," Representative Barbara Lee, one of the ninety co-sponsors of the Green New Deal resolution, observed. "That's why addressing climate change is not just an environmental issue, but also an imperative to achieve racial and economic justice."[25]

For many—young people worried about their future, parents concerned about their children or grandchildren, people living in communities threatened by floods, wildfires, freak storms, drought, or other climate-induced threats—climate change is a recurrent source of anxiety, depression, fear, or stress. By offering these and other people specific actions they can take both to reduce that future threat and to cope with their distress today, GND becomes both a therapeutic and a political intervention. It builds linked communities of support and networks for political action, foundations for successful movements.

While GND offers many benefits to those in search of solutions to the crises of modern capitalism, it also has serious limitations. Its ambiguity, in part a strength, is also a weakness, risking the creation of a movement that lacks the shared intellectual and ideological framework that can unify supporters and help reconcile divergent points of view.

Some critics point out specific gaps. The Green New Deal does not explicitly address land use and protecting farmland. Between 1992 and 2012, according to a report by American Farmland Trust, suburban development devoured nearly 31 million acres of agricultural land, including 11 million acres of prime farmland.[26] Absent a plan to reverse this significant contributor to growing greenhouse gas emissions, it will be more difficult for the nation to meet its climate goals.

No climate plan can address every contributor to carbon emissions but finding ways to identify and fill major gaps in the current policy proposals will be an important priority for GND organizers. Such assessment is necessary both to achieve the broader climate change goals within the time available and to enlist the widest possible political support.

Some critics have lambasted the GND proposal for being politically unrealistic, technologically impossible, and unaffordable. But as *Politico*'s Michael Grunwald has written, these criticisms may be missing the boat:

> The official rollout . . . was met with a barrage of skepticism from well-intentioned fact-checkers, badly intentioned climate trolls, and desperate-to-look savvy pundits, all focusing on the logistical and political impossibilities of transforming the economy as rapidly as the Green New Deal envisions. And they're right: Its goals really do seem impossible to achieve. But they're all missing the point. If anything, they're helping Green New Deal backers to make their point, which is that climate change is an unprecedented emergency that requires unconventional things.[27]

Finally, GND tells a story, the kind of story those seeking alternatives to modern capitalism need to tell and hear. Facts alone will never convince people to abandon one sets of beliefs and lifestyles for another. But the story is compelling: that millions of people can join hands and take action to overcome a handful of greedy, self-serving individuals and organizations who put their own wealth ahead of the well-being and survival of all humanity. And the desired end to this tale is that in taking these actions, we reclaim the world for this and future generations. This powerful narrative, an American tale of collective superheroes, becomes the parable to propel the movement forward.

The COVID-19 pandemic complicated the GND tasks. On the one hand, the pandemic showed the potential for rapid and dramatic declines in the use of fossil fuels. Had world leaders found the will and courage to make a few of the changes over the last two decades that the pandemic triggered in a few weeks, carbon emissions would have grown more slowly, and the world would be farther from a calamitous tipping point. On the other hand, COVID-19–dominated political agendas have pushed climate change off the front burner and made the corporate goal of increased economic growth and consumption at any cost more palatable to some. Moreover, as COVID-19 restrictions relaxed, carbon emissions have risen, confirming the necessity of political commitment to a new way.

GND may or may not survive as a viable policy agenda but it does show the potential to unify issues, movements, and streams of passion by showing comprehensive alternatives to business as usual.

WORKER COOPERATIVES AND THE NEW ECONOMY

A movement to create alternatives to current capitalism needs to develop new organizational forms as well as compelling policy ideas. One such form is the worker cooperative, first introduced more than a century ago, but now attracting renewed interest as a remedy for the deterioration of working conditions unleashed by twenty-first-century capitalism. Worker cooperatives can serve multiple purposes. They provide alternate worksites with better pay, working conditions, and prospects for advancement for low-wage workers than those of traditional companies. They are part of an emerging, more democratic, and equitable economy that can compete with the mainstream for-profit economy. They serve as a visible manifestation of a system that values dignity, community, and well-being. Moreover, worker cooperatives connect to other types of cooperatives—producer, consumer, and housing, for example. This could lay the foundation for a new economy that, over time, can challenge the capitalist status quo. Profiles of two worker cooperatives illustrate the potential and limitations of this organizational form.

Cooperative Home Care Associates (CHCA) was founded in 1985 in the South Bronx in New York City with the mission of providing quality home healthcare by creating quality jobs. It is the largest worker-owned coop in the United States. By 2020, CHCA employed 2,100 home care workers, nearly all African American or Latinx women, of whom about half were also co-op owners. In a community with high unemployment rates, CHCA provided free training and guaranteed high-quality employment for hundreds of women a year, supported by the growing demand for well-trained home health aides. Turnover rates at CHCA are about 20 to 25 percent a year, dramatically lower than the industry average of 66 percent.[28] One way that CHCA maintains its high retention rate is by guaranteeing that workers who stay for three years will be paid for working thirty hours each week as long as they do not refuse any client assignment, a win for an agency seeking stable employees and workers seeking regular dependable work hours.[29]

When Zaida Ramos joined the firm in 1997, she was raising her daughter on public assistance and jumping from one dead-end office job to another. "I earned in a week what my family spent in a day," she told a journalist.[30] After seventeen years as a home health aide at the cooperative, Ramos was able to send her daughter to college, receive full health and dental benefits, earn an annual share in profits, and enjoy flexible hours and a higher than average home care salary. "I'm financially independent. I belong to a union, and I have a chance to make a difference," she said.

Over the years, CHCA found reliable and well-connected partners to help it survive, weather crises, and grow. SEIU Local 1199, the powerful healthcare workers union in New York, organized CHCA's home care workers and then created a joint labor/management committee that offered workers additional opportunities to collaborate with administrators, managers, and union organizers in improving working conditions and operations. CHCA and 1199 also joined forces to lobby the state legislature to adopt fairer reimbursement rates for home care services. In early 2019, when CHCA's largest contractor ceased operations of its health plan, the New York State Department of Health

(DOH) stepped in to find other contractors who could help craft a solution. It helped negotiate an agreement that included new, more stable contractors and new lenders to help CHCA bridge a cash flow problem.

CHCA is still embedded in a capitalist economy and still faces the larger challenges of city and state austerity budgets resulting from tax cuts for the wealthy, a volatile economy, competitive markets, and less political influence than the huge hospital, home care, and insurance industries. But in an industry characterized by isolated workers, low wages, and unstable hours, CHCA has, in the words of Marjorie Kelly and Ted Howard, two scholars of the democratic economy, made its central goal "the creation of good work and good lives, for low-income black women, Latinx women, immigrant women."[31]

More broadly, as Ronnie Galvin, a Black preacher and adviser to the Democracy Collaborative, another organization that supports worker democracy, wrote:

> In the final analysis, if we don't have a movement that is fiercely centered on the reality of Black women who live and endure at this intersection (of class, race and gender), then we will tinker at the margins of a system that is relentless in its pursuit of power, ever-evolving and unafraid to strike back.

However, when this focus on the reality of the most marginalized is maintained, Galvin wrote, "we all win."[32]

The Evergreen Collaborative operates three worker cooperatives in Cleveland, Ohio, located in Cuyahoga County, where the number of manufacturing jobs fell from 241,862 in 1978 to 128,450 in 2000, a 47 percent drop.[33] A city that lost so many jobs appreciates the value of any business that creates jobs and when those jobs are decent paying, sustainable, and contribute to community well-being, they win even greater support. Launched in 2008 by a working group of Cleveland-based foundations, universities, and hospitals, the Evergreen Cooperative works to create living-wage jobs in six low-income neighborhoods in that city.[34]

Evergreen Laundry is the only commercial laundry operator in Cleveland. After working at the worker-owned laundry for a year, new hires are considered for membership in the co-op by their peers. If they are voted in, their pay rises, they contribute a small portion of the increase toward their ownership share, and they become eligible for sharing profits. In 2018, co-op owners received bonuses of up to $4,000. Many of the workers have histories of incarceration and addiction; a failed drug test leads to a probationary period to get cleaned up, a second failure results in termination.

Evergreen also has a homeownership program that combines payroll deductions and property tax abatements to enable workers to buy a city-renovated home in their area, no down payment required. An explicit goal of this program is to lift the Black home ownership rate in Cleveland, now half that of the white rate. Tim Coleman, a driver for the cooperative laundry, told a reporter, "I'm 54 and this is the first house I've owned, and it's right down the street from where I went to high school."[35]

The hospitals and other institutions that contract with the laundry also get benefits. Neither these institutions nor the cooperative is likely to move to another state or nation seeking to pay lower wages, taxes, or other costs, thus both can depend on each other over time. Working with the co-ops also builds goodwill. The chief administrator for the University Hospitals of Cleveland reported, "I can tell you at our annual meetings, it is the one thing people talked about most. People want to know how the cooperatives are doing and what they can do to help."[36] Now Evergreen is helping other cities—including New Haven, Milwaukee, and Buffalo—to establish cooperative laundry services.

Green City Growers, the second Evergreen cooperative business, grows lettuce and herbs in a hydroponic greenhouse, the largest food-production greenhouse in a core urban area in the United States. Produce is sold to grocers, restaurants, institutional food programs, and food service establishments throughout northeast Ohio. The greenhouse allows the co-op to grow year-round and deliver produce to customers within forty-eight hours of harvest.

Green City Growers provides local customers healthier choices for fresh, locally produced wholesome food.[37] In 2018, the greenhouse replaced the high-energy sodium lights with twelve hundred low-energy LED lights, saving money and energy.[38] The lettuces and herbs are grown without use of genetically engineered products or pesticides and since they replace those grown in California or Arizona, they cut down on the food miles traveled to Cleveland, all part of Evergreen's commitment to sustainability.

The third business, Evergreen Energy Solutions, produces next-generation LED lighting systems, solar power, and other energy-efficient solutions for Cleveland-area businesses, institutions, and residential properties. Showing that worker cooperatives can thrive in a number of sectors, Evergreen Energy Solutions helps manufacturers, large institutions, residential developers, and others save energy—from installing solar panels to outfitting offices or parking lots with energy-efficient LED lighting.[39] The company also weatherizes properties and offers support to lead-abatement projects.

By building on the "green jobs" sector that emerged a few decades ago,[40] Evergreen provides pathways and training into the alternative energy, construction, and remediation sectors, all of which provide current and future prospects for decent jobs. Like workers at the other Evergreen co-ops, the workers at Energy Solutions also share profits, are eligible for other benefits, and contribute to a family of businesses that support one another while strengthening the local economy.

In all three businesses, the Evergreen model is to first create jobs, then find and train people to fill them, a different approach than the many business and government workforce development programs that often train unemployed or underemployed people, then leave them to find their own jobs, an often frustrating task.

In sum, worker cooperatives offer powerful benefits to a movement dedicated to modifying modern capitalism. Cooperatives provide multiple entry points and paths out to other varieties of social activism. They attract workers frustrated by the gig economy, community activists seeking to establish new, more humane work opportunities, and "anchor institutions" such as universities and hospitals wanting to contribute more economic benefits to their communities by establishing businesses that will allow them to procure the goods and services they need more locally.

Worker cooperatives also seek partnerships with consumer, credit, energy, or housing cooperatives to begin to create alternative local economies; alliances with labor unions, as in the one between CHCA and 1199, that can open new opportunities for the labor movement; and partnerships with city governments as in New York City, Milwaukee, and Oakland, where public funding helps to support the infrastructure that can grow cooperatives.

Cooperativism can start at the local, national, or even global level, then link or scale up or down as needed. Together these linkages create a "solidarity economy," defined by the political economist Jessica Gordon Nembhard, as "a non-hierarchal, non-exploitative, equitable set of economic relationships and activities geared towards the grassroots."[41] For example, in 2012, Mondragon International, one of the largest cooperatives in the world, with many international projects, based in the Basque region of Spain, joined with the United Steelworkers and the Ohio Center for Employee Ownership to create a template for a union–co-op model and now sponsors several cooperative businesses in Cincinnati and supports other co-ops around the world.[42]

Worker cooperatives have the potential to confront directly and collaboratively the racism and sexism that characterize most mainstream workplaces. By ensuring that all workers have voices in making workplace decisions, Black, Latinx, and women workers can contribute to developing policies and practices that target discrimination, offer equal opportunities for promotions and raises, and create supportive workplaces.

Although worker and consumer cooperativism have evolved on separate paths, they share goals and social critiques. No person is either completely a worker or a consumer and in everyday life, most people switch roles regularly. What some scholars have called multi-stakeholder co-cooperativism can help people bridge this separation. Worker-consumer cooperatives, for example, demonstrate the potential for linking production and consumption into a single people-oriented economy.[43]

Worker and other forms of cooperatives also enable effective responses to market disruptions or failures, offering a clear alternative to the options capitalism offers. CHCA emerged in part in response to the failure of for-profit home care agencies to meet labor needs as more older people required care and healthcare reimbursement rates fluctuated. Similarly, the opening for Evergreen Laundry was the collapse of the largest for-profit laundry service in Cleveland, making hospitals and other customers willing, even eager, to finance alternatives including worker-owned laundries.

In a different way, the failure of companies like Uber, Lyft, and We Work to provide decent pay and benefits for its workers encourages some gig workers to explore creating their own cooperatives to take up this work under more livable terms.

Another advantage is that cooperativism can be a wellspring for values and ideologies that offer practical alternatives to the capitalist ideology that privileges individualism, profit, and markets. Cooperatives offer communities to their workers, expect their input in work decisions, support their lives outside work, invest surplus in community projects rather than return it to investors, and value local sustainable development over higher returns on investment. In these ways, cooperatives demonstrate a different way of organizing lives, economies, and politics—alternatives that ordinary people can experience, assess, and use to guide their future personal and political choices.

Finally, cooperativism enables and requires its participants to connect economic and political democracy, opening the door to new ideas and practices that link the two. Cooperatives, writes Maurie Cohen, a sustainability researcher, "inculcate democratic values and solidaristic social relations that will be essential for easing the process of innovating a new system of social organization over the next few decades."[44]

Cooperatives are of course not a panacea for the ills of society. Like traditional businesses, they too can be victims of the vagaries of the market. Their heterogeneity challenges any unified effect on the economy or movement-building; and their current modest scale make any meaningful impact on overall working conditions at best distant. Nembhard suggests, "Realistically, we need twenty to thirty years to slowly develop more cooperatives, through conversions and bottom-up development, and to strengthen and widen the solidarity economy,"[45] a long wait for those who insist that climate change requires transformative action within the decade.

But what cooperativism, workers co-ops, and the solidarity economy do offer is a coherent social and economic vision, a powerful presence on the ground, and a capacity to engage people from all walks of life in daily activities that can make life better today as well as offer hope for the future.

RESPONSES TO THE COVID-19 PANDEMIC

The COVID-19 pandemic harshly spotlighted the limits of twenty-first-century capitalism to solve human problems. High levels of inequality, the incapacities of deregulated and privatized governments, and the refusal of corporations to value human need over profit contributed to the rapid spread of COVID-19. These trends also worsened the pandemic's inequitable distribution of illness, death, and economic distress.

But the spotlight's glare also lit up the pandemic's silver lining. It showed that communities and nations can mobilize quickly to change deep-seated habits to confront an imminent threat. It showed that ordinary people can claim agency to meet their own and others' needs and challenge government and corporate failures. The pandemic sparked new cross-cutting alliances of those harmed by capitalism and enabled some public officials to propose more transformative reforms of economic and political structures.

Three stories—of mutual aid organizations, policy proposals to revitalize safety nets and challenge monopolization, and the valorization of essential workers—illustrate just a few of the pathways to resistance and creation of alternatives that the pandemic opened.

Mutual aid. Mutual aid describes the voluntary reciprocal exchanges of resources and services for the joint benefit of participating individuals and organizations. It is neither charity nor government-controlled services. Dean Spade, a scholar and practitioner of mutual aid, writes that "expanding mutual aid strategies will be the most effective way to support vulnerable populations to survive, mobilize significant resistance and build the infrastructure we need for coming disasters."[46]

The mutual aid efforts inspired by the pandemic show the potential for this strategy to build a movement that can confront the recurrent crises and disasters that characterize modern capitalism. In its first weeks, the pandemic overwhelmed existing safety net and social protection programs. Food assistance programs closed down or limited services as a result of missing volunteers, inadequate food supplies, or a surge in demand. In two months, more than 20 million American workers lost their jobs and even newly funded unemployment programs were unable to support all those eligible, much less the many low-wage, gig, and undocumented workers excluded from most publicly funded programs. As a result, millions of workers lost their health insurance, feared missing rent payments or being evicted, or were unable to keep up debt repayments.

Across the nation, thousands of groups formed to meet these overwhelming needs. In Colorado, librarians assembled and distributed food packages for older people and for children who no longer received meals at school. In Seattle, a collective provided material and informational help to "undocumented, LGBTQI, Black, Indigenous, People of Color, Elderly and Disabled, folks who are bearing the brunt of this crisis."[47] In New York City, dozens of groups provided child care, delivered food and medicine, and performed other services for healthcare, food service, and other essential workers, and for those who were ill. Unlike charity programs, mutual aid groups had no eligibility requirements, no forms to fill out, and no moralistic lectures delivered with the help. If people asked for support, they were assisted.

In some places, mutual aid groups organized or supported rent strikes (See Figure 8.2). On May 1, 2020, tens of thousands of people across the country participated in a rent strike with the slogan "Can't Pay, Won't Pay." A national poll that week had shown that nearly a quarter of Americans were unsure whether they would be able to afford their May 1 rent or mortgage payments.[48] In Los Angeles, a landlord evicted a tenant who had just been diagnosed with COVID-19. The landlord changed the tenant's locks, turned off her power, and threw her belongings into the street. A rapid mobilization by members of the Los Angeles Tenant Union ensured that she could return to her apartment and quarantine in peace. For years, the LA union had been organizing tenants to roll back rent increases and push their landlord to guarantee needed repairs. As one organizer put it, these actions alchemized "shared vulnerability into shared power,"[49] a good description of the potential of mutual aid.

Integrating grass-roots activism with legislative action. Social movements in the United States often have trouble coordinating grass-roots activism, mass mobilizations that include confrontations or civil disobedience, and legislative advocacy for new laws or budget allocations. Often these are seen as conflicting or contradictory strategies and activists believe they have to endorse

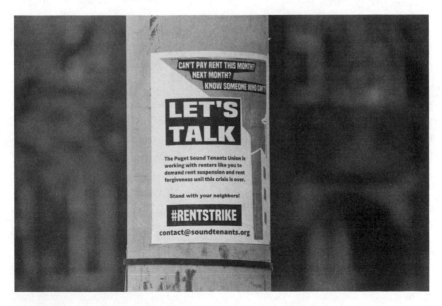

Fig. 8.2 The Puget Sound Tenants Union organized tenants from the northwest coast of Washington State to demand the suspension of rent collection during the COVID-19 pandemic.
Photo: © JohannMG / Shutterstock

one or the other. The responses to the pandemic showed once again the benefits of working in all three domains, a lesson further reinforced by the activism triggered by the police killing of George Floyd and other manifestations of systemic racism.

In response to tenant and citizen activism on rent strikes, for example, US Representative Ilhan Omar, a Democrat from Minnesota, introduced the Rent and Mortgage Cancellation Act, which would provide rent and mortgage forgiveness. "In 2008 we had the ability to bail out Wall Street. This time we need to bail out the American people who are suffering," said Representative Omar.[50]

The pandemic also focused attention on the costs of the monopoly concentration of the last two decades. As cases spread, all levels of government had trouble finding suppliers of masks, ventilators, and essential medicines. Price gouging and price fixing also made it harder for hospitals to get the supplies they needed. The continued growth of online retailers such as Amazon and the acquisition sprees of Big Tech companies who had capital to spare further endangered competition. As a result, Senator Elizabeth Warren and Representative Alexandria Ocasio-Cortez introduced the Pandemic Anti-Monopoly Act to "impose a moratorium on risky mergers and acquisitions—and stop large corporations from exploiting the pandemic to engage in harmful mergers." "As we fight to save livelihoods and lives during the coronavirus pandemic," said Warren, "giant corporations and private equity vultures are just waiting for a chance to gobble up struggling small businesses and increase their power through predatory mergers. We're introducing legislation to protect workers, entrepreneurs, small businesses, and families from being squeezed even more by harmful mergers during this crisis and any future national emergency."[51]

While these bills had little chance of approval by the Republican Senate or president, they put new issues on the national agenda, introduced ideas that could be discussed in the 2020 election and beyond, forged new alliances, and reinforced the idea that activism and progressive legislation could together in time lead to meaningful changes in the lives of disenfranchised populations.

Redefining essential work. The September 11 attacks brought new recognition to the bravery and dedication of the first responders and emergency workers who went into burning buildings and rescued trapped victims. But proponents of the subsequent war in Iraq soon sought to convert that public respect into militaristic and patriotic support for the war.

The reconsideration of work precipitated by COVID-19 seems different. In cities and towns across the country, people turned out every evening to applaud and thank the healthcare workers who cared for COVID-19 patients. Soon the people who fed healthcare workers and those who delivered food to them and others and those who helped to keep communities functioning—food store workers, bus and subway workers, teachers, home care attendants, postal deliverers, and truck drivers were also recognized as workers essential to collective survival. Suddenly the hedge fund guys, the media celebrities, and the billionaires who has been celebrated by popular media seemed less important. As Rev. William Barber, the co-chair of the Poor People's Movement, and Joe Kennedy III, the congressman from Massachusetts, wrote, transforming service workers into essential workers reminds everyone that we cannot survive without them.[52]

The pandemic also created new opportunities for worker organizing. When large clusters of COVID-19 infections occurred in an Amazon warehouse in Pennsylvania, among apple pickers in Washington, and at a Tyson Foods pork processing plant in Indiana, it was clear employers needed to do more to protect their workers. Labor unions and worker organizations brought these issues to the media and Congress.

The epidemic thus created new policy imperatives. Many essential workers risk sickness or death due to their service or travel to the job, so there is a need to keep the workers and their families healthy, protect their families' financial future, compensate workers for their exposure to COVID-19, and incentivize their continued work within essential industries.[53] On this last point, some labor activists argued that the pandemic offered an opportunity to move beyond "hazard pay"—higher wages for risky work—by ensuring that no workers should be required to work in unnecessarily dangerous conditions.

Other labor groups highlighted the near dismantlement of the federal occupational health and safety apparatus under President Trump and initiated by Labor Secretary Alexander Acosta and continued by Secretary Eugene Scalia. In testimony before the Senate Judiciary Committee, Rebecca Dixon, the executive director of the National Employment Law Project, told senators how employers in the food manufacturing, home care, and other sectors had ignored CDC recommendations for personal protective equipment and social distancing to prevent infection and how the Occupational Safety and Health Administration had failed to take action to protect workers. Instead, industry was asking Congress and the president to eliminate their liability for workplace infections.

"To truly honor frontline workers," testified Dixon, "Congress must help ensure workers are safe from needless risk of infection, rather than giving irresponsible employers a pass to put workers in harm's way. . . . If we focus on helping the most vulnerable in our country weather these dangerous times, we will lift the conditions of everyone, and create the most vibrant nation and economy possible."[54]

One Fair Wage, an organization dedicated to ending the practice of allowing lower minimum wages for tipped food service workers, also advanced its case during the pandemic. Building on prior victories that had established a single $15 per hour minimum wage in seven states—California, Montana,

Alaska, Washington, Nevada, Oregon, and Minnesota—the group insisted that federal and state unemployment packages created in response to the pandemic be based on a single $15 per hour minimum wage rather than with a lower tipped-workers rate. They also organized online town hall meetings of unemployed food service workers, registered them to vote, and created a relief fund that provided direct assistance to more than one hundred thousand unemployed food workers.

In the advocacy for adequate unemployment compensation, Saru Jayaraman, president of One Fair Wage, also insisted on advancing their broader agenda—paid sick and family leave, safe working conditions, and fair work hours. "After COVID," said Jayaraman, "nothing is going to be the same. We can't go back. We don't want to go back." She insisted that COVID-19 presented the food worker movement with the opportunity and necessity to reimagine how food work should be organized and compensated in the future.[55]

The refusal to go back also provides an opportunity to underline the racist and sexist features of low-wage and service work. Not only has COVID-19 hit people of color much harder, the economic collapse it triggered has had a disproportionate financial and social impact on the Black, Latinx, and women workers concentrated in low-wage jobs. By making these inequities a target for change, labor groups like One Fair Wage set the stage for collaboration with Black Lives Matter, #MeToo, and other organizations dedicated to ending systemic oppression based on race, gender, and their intersection.

Modern capitalism manufactures precarious workers, precarious economies, and precarious living conditions. When natural and unnatural disasters push people living in these circumstances further into poverty and instability, their well-being suffers. By mobilizing and strengthening the ties among the many communities harmed by the virus, communicating the specific ways that corporate elites worsened and profited from the pandemic, and providing direct support to those most harmed, movements for a healthier world can show that it is possible to respond to crises without sacrificing the most vulnerable.

Green New Deal, workers cooperatives, and the responses to COVID-19 offer three foundations for building a movement that has the mission, vision, and capacity, over time, to transform twenty-first-century capitalism. They are not of course the only practices worthy of exploration. I have also described more sectorally focused or place-based initiatives in each chapter, organizations such as Via Campesina, a global group that organizes small farmers on a variety of issues; the broad coalition of teachers, parents, young people, and civil rights groups launched by the Caucus of Rank and File Educators to resist corporations and take back schools in Chicago; and Silicon Valley Rising, an alliance that leads campaigns to create new models for good jobs, responsible employers, and affordable accessible housing in the Silicon Valley.

Each of these and many other examples provide living proof that there are two, three, many alternatives to modern capitalism unfolding in front of our eyes. More than any academic text or party doctrine, these examples illuminate the path toward other worlds, with activists, residents, and leaders together working out the details and future steps. These field-tested, cross-cutting models illustrate ways to stitch together the many now-siloed, single-issue, single-place patches of activism into a single quilt. Such a quilt communicates the potential for a more unified vision of a different world that offers all it covers and all who stitched it together shared goals, strategies, and tactics.

By presenting these practical tools to all those dissatisfied with the ways that modern capitalism has worsened their daily lives, confronted their search for dignity with disrespect, jeopardized individual and collective well-being and privacy, or eroded their democratic rights, the creators of this quilt offer the movement of movements a starting point for identifying the next steps towards another, better world.

CHAPTER 9

From Now to Next

How to Build a Movement for Another World

Vision without action is just a dream, action without vision just passes the time, and vision with action can change the world.

—Nelson Mandela

For those who believe that the solution to major problems confronting humanity today is more activism and stronger movements, many promising signs provide hope. In the last few years, activism motivated by roiling political, economic, and cultural changes has bubbled up, creating new opportunities to build a more coherent, integrated, and powerful movement. The stories of resistance and building alternatives described in chapter 8 provide additional inspiration.

Recent national elections launched millions of young people, women, working people, LGBTQIA+ people; those concerned about the environment; Blacks, Latinxes, and immigrants fighting voter suppression; and others into electoral politics, movement building, and community organizing. These mobilizations bring political discussions and debates into households, communities, workplaces, and schools across the country. The growing threats of climate change, police shootings of Blacks and other people of color, resurgent discrimination against sexual minorities and immigrants, gun violence and mass shootings, and sexual violence against women also sparked mass demonstrations, street protests, and other forms of activism. In 2018, the largest number of workers walked off their jobs or participated in strikes since the 1980s, with five hundred thousand walking off their jobs in 2018, up from about twenty-five thousand in 2017, according to the Bureau of Labor Statistics.[1]

In 2020, the failure of government and businesses to protect people against the COVID-19 pandemic; the police killings of George Floyd, Breonna Taylor, Rayshard Brooks, and others; and the deeper systemic racism these killings manifested pushed many millions more into activism. The continued expansion and growing sophistication of #MeToo also brought more women and some men into activism. Across the conflicts that pushed people into activism was a growing current of anger and outrage, a feeling of enough is enough. The combined impact of these shattering events was a growing determination not to go back, but to seek a truly different world.

Of course, not all of this activism was effective, not all of the political debates changed minds, no consensus emerged that defined a clear path forward, and certainly the future of capitalism was not the headline in most of these conflicts. But only an ostrich with its head in the sand could deny that millions of people were dissatisfied with the status quo and willing to take action to make things better for themselves and their communities. And only the most ardent market fundamentalists could fail to notice that underlying much of the dissatisfaction were the practices of twenty-first-century capitalism and its roots in inequity, racism, and planetary destruction.

In this chapter, I ask what ordinary citizens, activists of all stripes, health professionals, and others can do tomorrow and over the next decades to build a social movement that can create alternatives to the world created by twenty-first-century capitalism. My starting points are the premises presented in chapter 8: that modern capitalism is the fundamental cause of the world's most serious problems, that only a massive social movement will have the capacity to bring about feasible and meaningful reforms, that existing movements and campaigns are the basic ingredients for any recipe for change, and that human and planetary well-being constitute a powerful mobilizing idea for this movement.

My goal is to spark strategic conversations among those seeking to advance the transition from the current form of capitalism to a less damaging, healthier, happier, and more sustainable world. I discuss first what such a movement could do, then how it could achieve these goals.

A note of caution: readers hoping for a detailed blueprint for building a successful movement will not find those architectural specifications here. Over the last century, many movements and organizations have proposed such plans; some have served to bring together new alliances or clarify shared policy and political agendas. Too often, however, these prescriptions divide rather than unify diverse constituencies, become out of date quickly, or miss opportunities for wider framing of the problems or solutions. For these reasons and because I believe that strategic directions for a movement to create alternatives to modern capitalism must be forged in practice, I propose not a plan but broad goals and approaches for a stronger, more effective movement.

Six specific goals can anchor the development of a more cohesive, integrated movement to modify twenty-first-century capitalism. Each is based on practice described in this book and tested in the field around the United States and the world. The six suggested here are both substantive proposals for a starting shared agenda but also illustrations designed to inspire others to add to or modify these suggestions. This list suggests goals that a movement can promote for government, business, and civil society action.

1. Grow the Public Sector

For each pillar of well-being, a public sector offers alternatives to and competes with commercial markets. In public education and healthcare, for example, a robust public sector provides affordable, accessible, and sometimes good-quality services to millions of Americans. Strengthening and protecting these services and resisting corporate incursions can slow modern capitalism's penetration of daily lives and compete with privatized services degraded by profit extraction. Broad public support for improved and more equitable access to healthy food, high-quality education, and effective and affordable healthcare gives campaigns for these reforms the potential to mobilize people across communities, classes, and race/ethnicities.

In food, governments spend billions of dollars a year on public benefits such as the Supplemental Nutrition Assistance Program (SNAP, formerly known as Food Stamps) and WIC, a program for pregnant and new mothers and their young children. Billions more are spent on school and other public institutional food programs. Other public dollars are used for agricultural subsidies, usually to the biggest industrial growers of the least healthy crops: corn, sugar, and soy. By insisting that public expenditures on food have to meet public goals such as reducing hunger, diet-related disease, and carbon and greenhouse gas emissions, governments and food activists can insist that tax dollars spent on food be used to improve food choices for taxpayers rather than to benefit giant food companies.

In healthcare, in 2018 seven for-profit and not-for-profit US hospital systems and three private foundations announced an ambitious project to create a nonprofit generic drug company that could combat high drug prices and shortages regularly faced by American patients. Called Civica Rx, the new enterprise sought to guarantee a built-in market for the drugs that the nonprofit company would supply.[2] It purchased drugs often in short supply in US hospitals from European drug makers and promised that all hospitals would pay the same prices for its drugs with no discounts or special process for big users. It also partnered with European for-profit pharmaceutical companies to purchase drugs often in short supply. Whether the hybrid approach tested by Civica Rx can provide a meaningful alternative to Big Pharma and whether it is scalable remains to be seen, but such models may be feasible in other sectors as well.

In transportation, the public sector should defend mass public transit against incursions from Uber and Lyft and insist that tax-funded spending on transportation or on autonomous vehicle research and development must produce benefits to the public. Environmental, health, and social justice activists can bring sunlight onto the many public handouts now going to private transportation providers, welfare for the rich that often fails to benefit the public.

In employment, the public sector has become a substantial part of the national economy and provides an accessible entry point for public policies that improve working conditions and pay. The leading role that state and local governments have played in advancing a higher minimum wage, paid parental leave, and paid sick time illustrates this. The public sector can become a forceful advocate, showing by example how wage, tax, and job policies can lead to higher wages, better benefits, safe working conditions, opportunities for advancement, rights to organize, and sustainable economic development. The public sector can set an example for improving pay and working conditions for workers often harmed by twenty-first-century capitalism: women, people of color, recent immigrants, young people, and those with disabilities. Especially in tight labor markets, these policies would force private companies to match the public sector and would also help to stimulate the economy in productive ways.

Free or highly subsidized public higher education will ensure that every American has the education needed to succeed, as well as health and social benefits that a college degree confers across one's lifetime. The pension funds of public sector workers can be used to leverage private businesses to pursue more responsible labor, environmental, investment, and other practices.

Finally, in the tech industries, the public sector can protect public access to digital technologies, create public alternatives to privatized and profit-seeking communications channels, and find new ways to use new digital technologies to promote democracy, protect privacy, and hold governments accountable.

In these and other areas, only the public sector has the mandate and resources to make human and planetary well-being a priority. Only public sector initiatives have the potential to overcome the rising and imminent threats that climate change and the growing burden of chronic disease pose to the nation and the world. Only the public sector can make reducing inequity an explicit goal. Only a robust public sector can force corporations to make the needs of "stakeholders" other than shareholders a priority rather than an empty promise.

On the one hand, shrinking the public sector and characterizing it as a failure in solving human problems have long been key tenets both of neoliberal capitalism and the current conservative movement. But as the failures of contemporary capitalism to meet human needs become more apparent, an equally central tenet of American beliefs is that taxpayer money should benefit the public, not private interests, setting the stage for what must become a central debate of the next decade. By promoting the idea that a strong public sector helps almost everyone, a movement can unify now mostly categorical struggles, build support for an alternative to market solutions, and offer meaningful assistance to those most harmed by current capitalism.

To complicate this seemingly simple goal, efforts to expand the public sector must also forcefully resist the corporate capture of this space and the corruption that private interests can bring to government. Walking this tightrope confronts a movement with many opportunities to crash to the ground but as always, the proper balance will emerge from a concrete analysis of how best to support the public sector in specific circumstances.

2. Strengthen Democracy

The most problematic developments of twenty-first-century capitalism have largely depended on the success of corporations and wealthy elites in changing the rules of democracy to enable them to better advance their interests. Specific examples include the Citizens United Supreme Court decision, reduced protection of labor rights, a more inequitable tax system, and the growing role of lobbying and campaign contributions in shaping state and federal policies. The successes of the alliance between corporations, the wealthy, and conservative movements—funded in large part by a handful of billionaires—in suppressing voter registration and participation, defeating campaign finance reform, capturing the federal courts, and supporting deregulation and privatization of education, healthcare, and transportation have further eroded democracy.

Strong democracies make it easier for majorities to win changes in policy and allocations of wealth and power. More democratic communities better engage citizens in civic activities and better support the human quest for dignity, meaning, and autonomy. A movement to transform capitalism can succeed only if it can begin to reverse recent declines in democracy. Too often, groups working on public health, the environment, education, or related issues have seen protecting democracy as someone else's fight. Democracy activists have had trouble connecting the reforms they advocate to well-being, safer environments, or better schools.

How can these two branches of activism find better alignment? Activists have demonstrated a few possible starting points. They have, for example, sponsored educational campaigns to show some of the specific ways that corporate spending on elections and campaign contributions leads to laws or policies that weaken public health protections, undermine successful public schools, produce more pollution, or lead to declines in health.[3] Others have advocated new laws that require corporations to disclose money used to influence public opinion in their required filings with the Securities and Exchange Commission. They have proposed laws to require corporate CEOs, foundations, and other "dark money" operations that underwrite political commercials to have their names listed as sponsors. They have supported the activities and election campaigns of progressive state attorneys general who use the law to monitor corporate interference with democracy, through tax-exempt and corporate foundations' involvement in politics.[4]

Some activists have proposed a 28th Amendment to the US Constitution or other legislative strategies to establish that corporations are not persons and do not have the political or legal rights of human beings. Others have suggested resurrecting and expanding the now-defunct Fairness Doctrine to require all media—radio, TV, and digital media—to give equal time to that purchased by corporations and their allies to civil society and advocacy groups to inform and educate the public on major public policy issues.[5]

When every health and social justice activist asks, "How can I strengthen democracy to better achieve the reforms I seek?" and every democracy advocate asks, "How can I better connect our democracy goals to the campaigns to improve the lives of ordinary people?" then these two essential streams of support for transforming the current political and economic system will begin to form a more powerful force for change than either can muster on its own.

Today, most of these democratic reforms seem aspirational, a heavy lift from current practice. But not so long ago segregation was legal in the United States and gay marriage illegal. Not so long ago women could not vote and not so long ago, few people challenged mass incarceration as a viable strategy to prevent crime or questioned giving the police more rather than less funding to make communities safer. These political realities changed over decades because movements mobilized, communities protested, and courageous political leaders demanded change. By creating a public rationale for strengthening democracy in order to make people's lives better, activists can set the stage for the next democratic reforms, whether they take a year, a decade, or a century.

3. Confront the Roles that Systemic Racism and Sexism Play in Inequitably Distributing Health and Disease

Through law, culture, economics, and social norms, African Americans, and other people of color in the United States experience higher rates of premature death and preventable illnesses, worse diets, more polluted environments, poorer housing, more police violence, and riskier working conditions. While systemic racism has many roots, throughout history, US corporations have benefited from the racism that allows them to pay people of color lower wages, make them work in riskier jobs, sell them more unhealthy products, and distract white workers from demanding more from employers by encouraging them to fight Blacks instead. Some big corporations have changed their hiring, philanthropic, and public relations strategies to address racism but too often these modifications have served to modernize or sanitize but not end racism.

Corporations have also benefited from paying women less, assigning them to less desirable jobs, failing to provide adequate support for parenting, targeting them with predatory marketing, and distracting male workers from making more demands on their employers by encouraging them to discriminate against women instead.

These racist and sexist practices—and their intersection—are essential foundations for both early and modern capitalism, powerful props for the perpetuation and evolution of oppression, and daunting obstacles to creating alternative social and economic systems.

Black Lives Matter and #MeToo and their organizational cousins have shown that millions of people have been moved into political action by the outrage and anger that racist and sexist structures evoke. Any movement that hopes to change the world has to listen to, connect with, and embrace these movements. Racism and sexism contribute to shorter and less healthy lives and undermine dignity and self-sufficiency; thus aligning those seeking to end these systems of oppression and those seeking alternatives to modern capitalism promises more success for each. (See Figure 9.1). The history of racism and sexism in undermining and weakening social movements in the United States requires an unyielding focus on this goal.

4. Transform the National Discussion on Taxes and Regulation

As a result of their recent successes in modifying democracy and governance, corporations and wealthy elites have dramatically changed the rules on taxes and regulation in ways that have harmed the public good. Corporations and the wealthy are now paying a lower portion of their income in taxes than at any time in recent history. With the rushed confirmation of Supreme Court Justice Amy Coney Barrett in 2020, this business-friendly alliance ensured its continued control of the nation's highest court.

Similarly, since the early 1980s, deregulation, defunding, and lack of strict enforcement of the health, environmental, and consumer protections that had been passed in the 1960s and 1970s enabled corporations to endanger well-being, the environment, safe working conditions, and equity in both new

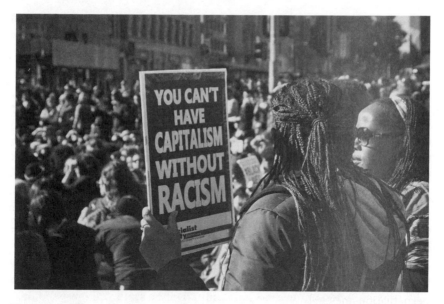

Fig. 9.1 A poster at a Black Lives Matters demonstration calls out the links between racism and capitalism.
Photo:

and old ways.[6] The Trump presidency has made deregulation a top priority. The administration appointed industry officials to lead the dismantling of regulatory agencies, cut funding for enforcement, and turned over responsibility for writing new regulation to industry insiders.[7]

Public opinion polls show that substantial majorities of Americans support fair taxation, oppose polices that allow the wealthy and corporations to avoid paying their fair share, and support regulations that protect the public. According to a Gallup Poll, for the last fifteen years about 70 percent of the public believed that corporations were paying too little in taxes, yet recent policies have further lowered corporate taxes, another example of elected officials ignoring public opinion in favor of the interests of the wealthy.[8]

Similarly, a 2019 Pew Center Poll on regulation showed that 63 percent of US adults say stricter environmental regulations are "worth the cost," while only 30 percent say such regulations "cost too many jobs and hurt the economy," according to the Pew Research Center. Two years earlier, 59 percent had said stricter environmental regulations were worth the cost. Thus, despite the increase in public support for stronger regulation, the Trump administration significantly weakened these rules.

How can a movement capitalize on these discrepancies between majority public opinion and governmental enthusiasm to enact policies that favor big business? Public Health Awakened, an activist public health group, has suggested some ways to change the national discussion on taxes.

They call on activists to clearly reveal and challenge the elite narrative on taxes. This narrative claims that Americans live "in a world of scarcity, where we don't have enough resources to achieve what we want, where the government is considered corrupt or inefficient, and where 'middle class' is used as a code to protect resources for white communities."[9]

Public Health Awakened proposes that social justice campaigns advance a counter-narrative that says that tax policy should be moral statements of what our society stands for: fairness, equal opportunity, and a better future for all. Corporate taxes and taxes on the wealthy, they note, are much lower than in the recent past, suggesting that fairer taxes would restore American values. The group also calls on activists to promote the view that taxes fight fires, improve public education, protect food and water—in short allow Americans to enjoy the standard of living they have achieved and to continue to better their lives.

Various activist groups have proposed a variety of specific campaigns to advance these ideas on taxes. These include calls to repeal the 2017 Trump tax bill;[10] sponsor referendums and ballot initiatives on state caps on spending;[11] and enact wealth taxes, inheritance taxes, stock and property transfer taxes, and capital gains taxes that seek to rebalance the share of taxes paid by the ultrawealthy.[12] Requiring polluters, rather than taxpayers, to contribute to a fund for cleanups, as the Environmental Protection Agency's Superfund program originally did, until funding was switched to general revenues, provides an incentive for preventing problems.[13] Others have suggested linking revenue streams from specific taxes targeted at the ultrawealthy to popular programs such as expanded child care, free college, or improved access to prescription drugs. Taxes that enhance equity such as the Earned Income Tax Credit could be expanded to counteract other taxes and policies that exacerbate inequity.[14]

By linking these disparate efforts into a coordinated campaign to create a fairer tax system, one that enables people in this country to live better lives and better respects majority views on taxes, a movement can win new supporters and unify now mostly separate struggles.

Social justice, environmental, and public health campaigns have also promoted approaches to regulation that challenge neoliberal deregulatory initiatives.[15] For example, some have opposed preemption, a practice used by businesses to pass laws that prevent one level of government, usually state or local governments, from passing stronger laws than those of another level, usually the federal level. The food and agriculture, firearms, pharmaceutical, and automobile industries, for example, have sought to preempt lower levels of government from filling gaps in the relatively weak federal regulations these industries have achieved, a strategy that undermines democracy and exposes many Americans to higher health risks.[16] The successes of the California Air Resources Board in strengthening regulation of air pollution from automobiles, described in chapter 6, illustrate a successful alliance between a state government and local activists to overcome the opposition of the automobile industry and, in some cases, the federal government.

The environmental justice movement has used environmental law, civil rights law, and human rights law in international settings to insist that health and environmental regulations must reduce the disparate burden of environmental and occupational exposures on low-income people and communities of color, making equity a desired outcome of regulation.[17]

Each of these tax and regulatory initiatives, some already successful and others still aspirational, has important specific goals but also contribute to a national conversation that is greater than the sum of its parts. Since the 1980 election of Ronald Reagan, conservatives and corporations have led a vigorous and well-funded campaign both to cut taxes and roll back regulations but also to make these actions appear to be in the public interest as well as their own financial interest. Challenging these myths and presenting evidence of the harm that austerity budgets inspired by tax cuts and worsening public health triggered by deregulation can help to create the climate in which the public support for fair taxation and effective regulation can be translated into government practice.

5. Focus on Cities

Any movement to transform modern capitalism must represent the interests of both rural and urban areas and acknowledge the similar and differing threats to well-being, economic development, and sustainability in these different regions. For the next period, however, cities make an especially promising setting for growing a movement to challenge modern capitalism.

First, in both the United States and around the world, most people live in cities. According to the United Nations, about 55 percent of the world's population lives in urban areas, expected to rise to 68 percent over the coming decades.[18] In the United States, about 80 percent of the population lives in urban areas.

Second, corporations and other businesses are most active in cities, the homes of their headquarters, their investors, their biggest markets, and their most aggressive marketing. This urban footprint and the visible impact of corporations on city living makes corporations readily accessible to urban activists. The rapid and successful mobilization of a broad cross section of New Yorkers to oppose Amazon's 2018 demand for more than $2 billion in tax cuts and subsidies to build its headquarters in the city is one visible manifestation of this.[19]

After Amazon pulled out, Alexandria Ocasio-Cortez, the congresswoman from the Queens district where Amazon had planned to build its new headquarters, explained the local opposition, "This is going to displace us, and we want a seat at the table. . . . And when we got a seat at the table, Amazon just said, 'We're not going to budge one bit.' We shouldn't be inviting bullies to our neighborhood."[20]

Third, in both the United States and around the world, city governments have demonstrated they can join together to confront, for example, the fossil fuel, firearms, pharmaceutical, and food industries, initiating tougher regulations, stronger public policies, and more emphasis on promoting equity than other levels of government.[21] Recent battles for affordable housing,[22] "sanctuary cities,"[23] alternative food outlets,[24] and public education[25] show the potential for bottom-up as well as top-down urban resistance.

Finally, cities have dense social networks and a history of resistance to corporate intrusions, making them fertile grounds for growing stronger, deeper social movements to challenge the harms from capitalism. Many of the most successful movements of the twentieth century had their roots in cities and many cities have generations of activists who can provide lessons, leadership, and inspiration to emerging movements. For these reasons, cities are also good testing grounds for finding common ground and shared actions among, for example, movements for food justice, educational equity, healthcare for all, and public transit. Population density, overlapping networks, and histories of resistance facilitate such integration within urban areas.

Cities need rural and less developed areas for food, water, and trees, and nonurban areas need cities for markets, entertainment, employment, and culture. Modern capitalism has often divided these populations and pitted them against each other. A successful movement can find opportunities to create common ground.

Another model for urban activism and partnerships with city governments is the Milano Urban Food Policy Pact, an agreement signed by 209 cities with more than 450 million inhabitants from around the world.[26] Mayors, community organizations, and activists in cities around the nation are also working together to end gun violence and build safer communities, showing ways to influence gun industry practices, even in the absence of federal support.[27] Finding ways to connect these now mostly separate urban activist alliances into a more cohesive network that can challenge corporate control locally, nationally, and globally will be an important goal for the future.

In the past, cities have often served as sites for creating alternatives to unfettered capitalism. The three case profiles—Green New Deal, worker cooperatives, and the political responses to COVID-19—each thrive in cities but also show the potential of bringing urban, suburban, and rural communities and activists together. By nurturing grass-roots activism in fertile urban spaces, a movement can contribute new forms of support to activism in other spaces.

6. Make Science and Technology Public Property

New developments in science, technology, and engineering—some created both in the public and private sectors—have contributed to important advances in health, nutrition, environmental protection, as well as to more convenient and labor-saving products. But in many cases, corporations and other private-sector organization have won control of these new discoveries and used them to benefit their own economic interests at the expense of public well-being.

For this reason, a successful movement to improve human lives must win back public control of scientific and technical knowledge. It must also set firm restrictions on the potential to use new knowledge to harm others or to benefit one small group at the expense of humanity or the planet.

Activists and scientists have initiated a variety of campaigns to make science more accountable and accessible to the public. Some groups have sought greater protection of public intellectual property and criticized protection for private intellectual property that leads to withholding life-enhancing goods or services from those unable to pay market prices.

For example, with members in the United States and other countries, groups like the Union for Affordable Cancer Treatment, Médicin Sans Frontières, Medicines Patent Pool, and Knowledge Ecology International have challenged pharmaceutical companies' intellectual property rights by fighting for open licenses,[28] compulsory licensing, or price negotiations, all strategies to make essential medicines more available to those now denied access.[29]

In universities and research institutes, independent scholars have proposed and, in some cases, won new rules to reduce conflicts of interest between corporate funders and academics to make funding more transparent. As universities increasingly turn to corporations for new funding, these sometimes uphill battles will require academics and administrators to clarify whether their core allegiance is to the corporations that fund them or to the intellectual community that expects full reporting of results, disclosure of conflicts, and the primacy of public over private interests.[30]

Proponents of drawing a sharper line between research seeking primarily to increase profits and investigations designed mainly to improve the world have proposed a variety of policies to distinguish these two approaches. They suggest that corporations (and those they support) and scientific journals disclose their funding of research; report all results, negative or positive; and sanction individuals and institutions who violate these rules or make false or misleading scientific claims.[31]

Another approach is to provide public support from state or federal sources to conduct applied research on salient threats to health, on the presumption that public funding reduces the likelihood that commercial forces will sponsor self-serving studies.[32] State-funded studies on air pollution, regional food systems, and transportation have sometimes informed public sector approaches to these problems.

Some have also proposed that if corporations want to fund research on social issues, they give the money to a wholly independent third party to administer and oversee the research.[33] Finally, on the policy side, all parties involved in setting public policy or lobbying—elected officials, advocacy groups, lobbyists, professional organizations, and scientists should be required to disclose any corporate contributions, fees, or paid lectures they accept.

The capacity of activists and reformers to win greater public support for policies that protect public interests depends heavily on their success in presenting credible scientific evidence to support such proposals. Industry groups and scientific consultants hired by industry often seek to discredit any evidence that interferes with their business aims, making the protection of scientific integrity an important goal. By establishing principles that reduce conflicts of interest and monitoring their implementation, academics and advocates working on different issues in different sectors can help to create a culture of accountability and integrity that discourages the misuse of science.

Not every campaign or movement organization will be able to include each of these goals in all their work. But many will be able to weave these ideas into their ongoing organizing and education and thus create wider opportunities for public discussion and debate. As they succeed, these and other ideas about a healthier, more sustainable political and economic system will become a fuller part of the national discourse and make it the norm for universities and researchers to value human need over corporate profit. By creating viable alternatives to the ideology espoused by twenty-first-century capitalism, this emerging movement can plant the seeds for a different world.

HOW TO DO IT

Creating a movement that has the vision, skills, and power to catalyze changes to twenty-first-century capitalism that jeopardizes humanity's well-being and survival seems both impossible and inevitable. Impossible because how can fragmented, imperfect, and contradictory strands of activism become a force that can successfully challenge the dominant institutions on earth? Inevitable because throughout history, people have never abandoned for long their efforts to create better lives and overcome threats to survival.

The success of any movement, however, will depend as much on the daily success of engaging more people, building stronger organizations, and bringing material and emotional benefits to participants as on the intellectual analyses or policy agendas of these movements. Thus, any popular mobilization for change must ask not only what it should do but also how it engages participants, makes decisions, and communicates with others.

What lessons can be extracted from a review of these "how" practices of the activists, organizations, and movements that have been working to modify our current capitalist system? And what other insights come from analyses of other recent social movements, such as those for women's, LGBTQIA+, Black, and immigrant rights? Finally, what lessons can those seeking to change capitalism learn from the sometimes successful conservative movements for gun rights, restricting voting, shrinking government, and opposing abortion and reproductive rights?

To inform practice and to encourage others to propose additional recommendations, I suggest a few.

1. Present Problem, Vision, and Strategies in Ways that Unify across Sectors and Issues

One of the greatest obstacles to effective movements for social change is the continued siloing by issue, sector, and population. Both lumpers and splitters have their roles in activism but defining ground rules for smart lumping may help to build a stronger, more cohesive movement. The Green New Deal (GND) and workers cooperatives each demonstrate some concrete ways to broaden their appeal. They create multiple entry points—by issue, location, population, and strategy—into their activism. They frame the issue expansively to invite others in. They pay attention to the personal as well as to the political lives of their members. The starting point for most GND activists is the urgent sense that the world needs to act to reduce global warming, but they understand that by devising solutions that create jobs, make cities more livable, expand access to healthy food, reduce the effects of systemic racism, and widen democracy they can attract many additional supporters.

Some movement strategists emphasize framing as a task that requires choosing the right words to engage rather than offend potential supporters. But the question goes much deeper: how can activists align and reconcile their world views with those of others who may agree with their diagnosis, but not their prescription, or approve some but not all of their goals? The needed skills involve listening better, searching for common ground more skillfully, and finding new ways to compromise while sticking to core values.

On every campaign, organizers can ask, "How can we describe the problem in ways that connect to the widest cross-section of people?" "How can we best engage the widest range of participants in developing solutions to the identified problem?" and "How can we achieve results that bring real and tangible benefits to a wide range of participants?"

In practice, of course, not all constituencies will identify shared interests. In some cases, potentially valuable partners may have conflicting interests. Construction workers, for example, may support some climate-harming infrastructure development projects because they need jobs and the wages to support their families. Their concerns must be addressed. For example, some Green New Deal projects explicitly emphasize the need to create alternative jobs and provide training for displaced workers. Another approach is to appeal to deeply held higher values: the need to protect the well-being of one's children and grandchildren.

And a more pessimistic option is to acknowledge that some groups may not be ready to join alliances for reform. Some coal miners, for example, still hope that their jobs can be saved, despite the growing evidence this will not happen, and the persistent risks that mining poses to their own, their families', their communities', and the planet's health. In these cases, searching for other partners may be the most viable option. Of note, however, those coal miners who do see the necessity of alternatives make the most persuasive organizers.

2. Make It Easy to Connect Personal and Social Activism

In an understandable reaction to the individualism celebrated in capitalist ideology, many on the political left in the United States discount individual resistance to capitalist intrusions in favor of more collective action. They argue that such personal responses—recycling, eating vegan, practicing yoga, limiting screen time, riding a bike instead of driving a car—are symbolic acts that fail to address the underlying political and economic structures. They also worry that these individual responses can become a substitute for acting for more fundamental changes.

This binary view has two major flaws. First, people's most intensive and dissatisfying interactions with capitalism come in their intimate personal daily lives. It's too hard to find affordable healthy food for their families, too hard to pay back their college debts and still get ahead, or too hard to get treatment for their own or their family member's diabetes or cancer and manage the other tasks of daily life. If more people in the United States are going to join a movement to create alternatives to twenty-first-century capitalism, it will be their personal experiences that will motivate them to do so. To declare that irrelevant is to sacrifice our most promising asset. Mutual aid responses to COVID-19, climate change, and economic crises offer the potential to link meeting immediate needs with confronting systemic flaws.

Second, and closely related, the most successful movements of the past century—the labor, civil rights, women's, and LGBTQIA+ movements, as well as the conservative gun rights, anti-abortion, and white nationalist movements—have understood that the personal is political and the political personal. Yes, these movements had ideas and values that attracted members, but their strength and success came from providing ways for participants to connect their daily experiences to the vision of a different world. Any successful movement to change the most powerful system on the planet must match and exceed this capacity of earlier movements.

How can activists and organizers do this? Successful movements have identified a few approaches that appear to be effective in engaging new supporters.

Protect children. Enlisting parents and families in defending their children against predatory marketing of unhealthy foods and beverages, social media companies that enable cyberbullying, or media that use violence and sexuality to generate profit has helped some groups to expand parents' goals from protecting their own children to protecting all children in their community or nation. Few organizations or individuals are willing to publicly defend putting children at risk, making the protection of children a unifying theme for public campaigns.

Support those who resist defining identity by consumption. After the September 11 attacks, President George W. Bush famously urged Americans to "go shopping for their families" and he encouraged Americans to "go to Disneyworld," as part of his effort to renew confidence in the safety of air travel. To be fair, Bush was appealing for resilience to external attack, but the normality he promoted was to buy more, travel more, and consume more, the very habits that endangered the world's environment and widened national and global inequalities.

For many Americans, reducing their personal consumption has been a way to demonstrate their commitment to a more sustainable and equitable world. Riding a bike, walking, or taking mass transit instead of driving; repairing rather than discarding dated or broken digital devices; limiting screen time for oneself or one's children; recycling, foraging, or repurposing food, clothes, or furniture that many send to the dump—all these are paths to rethinking how people relate to the world. Resisting the branded identities corporations seek to impose helps people reclaim their self-definition. Creating ways to connect to people, relax, and have fun that do not depend on corporations, marketing, and branding opens the door for thinking about living differently.

By themselves, of course, these gestures will not change the world. But these acts of defiance and autonomy serve as starting points for more collective action, as examples, as triggers to conversations and debate, and thus open paths to transformation. By supporting and encouraging people to make changes in their personal lives, activist organizations help to create a culture of autonomy and independent thinking, a critical challenge to capitalist ideology.

Create spaces free of corporate influence. While corporations have claimed an ever-larger role in people's daily lives and inner consciousness, it is also true that most Americans still have ongoing and meaningful interactions with organizations that are relatively autonomous from corporate influence. These places can become sites for resisting capitalist encroachment. A few examples:

- Many schools have removed soda from their vending machines and cafeterias, and some have asked parents and teachers not to drink soda inside the school. Their goal is not to encourage prohibition of Coke and Pepsi but to make a statement that schools should be about health, not about the creation of new markets, and that parents and teachers can say no and mean it, thus rejecting soda companies' efforts to get their children to nag them into acquiescence.
- Libraries, schools, and youth organizations have organized classes and workshops on media literacy and teach children to analyze and resist corporate marketing.
- Health clinics and doctors' offices have refused entry to pharmaceutical company sales agents, the detail men and women who seek to persuade doctors to prescribe their products and patients to ask for them.[34] Some have also banned infant formula makers from distributing free products and their "educational" materials with misleading or false claims about the health benefits of infant or toddler formula.
- Mutual aid organizations have worked with local community organizations to create food programs and food-growing cooperatives, funds that make emergency grants or loans, and child care cooperatives—all noncommercial enterprises that help people to deal with COVID-19 or other emergencies.

These and similar acts open spaces where parents, children, teachers, health professionals, and others can discuss corporate influences on well-being, denormalize predatory marketing, act to reclaim public space, and regain some measure of autonomy (See Figure 9.2). These can lead to public policies that support more public noncommercial spaces—bans of advertising of unhealthy products on public transit, a measure London took in 2018;[35] limits on social media advertising to children under thirteen or eighteen;[36] or mandates that public radio and television stations must offer free equal time to opponents of unhealthy products, a measure that helped reduce cigarette smoking in the United States in the late 1960s and early 1970s.[37] By connecting efforts to change community institutions with those designed to enact new local or national policies, each of these campaigns becomes stronger than either one on its own.

3. Take the Long View

By temperament, many activists are impatient; they want results—to end misery or confront wrongdoing, both admirable characteristics. But as Moms

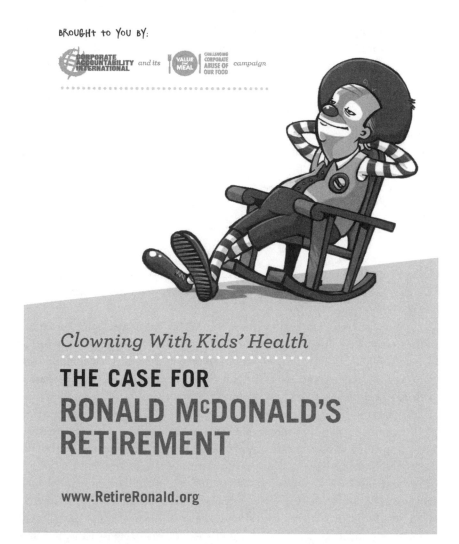

Clowning With Kids' Health

THE CASE FOR
RONALD McDONALD'S RETIREMENT

www.RetireRonald.org

Fig. 9.2 Corporate Accountability International, a national advocacy organization, led a campaign to urge McDonald's to retire Ronald from its public advertising which targeted children. By 2020, McDonald's had stopped using the clown in its advertising.
Photo: Courtesy of Corporate Accountability International

Demand Action, a group seeking to end gun violence and reduce the role of gunmakers in gun policy, has observed, activism to change the most powerful economic and political system on earth today should be seen as a marathon, not a sprint.[38] Unrealistic expectations for quick victories can end up dampening participation and slowing achievements. What practical strategies have movements and leaders used to nurture a longer view?

Some groups have created multigenerational leadership teams so that boomers who have experienced victories after twenty or thirty years of uphill activism can engage with Gen Xers and millennials who sometimes unrealistically hope for quicker victories. Organizations have created action plans that identify short- as well as long-term markers of progress to enable participants to periodically assess if they are moving in the right direction. Others have studied similar struggles or campaigns in other times and places to develop realistic timelines needed to achieve different levels of change.

Another approach encourages activists to maintain other aspects of personal life. COVID-19 mutual aid organizations organized online concerts, art shows, and dances to help people cope with quarantine and loss. Long-time activists can underscore the necessity of this by telling stories of their own burnout or that of others; nothing is more inefficient than losing the energy and wisdom of an experienced movement participant.

4. Find Ways to Talk about Race, Class, and Gender That Recognize How These Stratification Systems Have Weakened Movements

As I observed earlier in this chapter, capitalism has long depended on its ability to use race, class, gender, and other social characteristics to keep opponents divided. Successful movements overcome this obstacle by directly confronting systemic racism and sexism but also by developing internal processes to challenge these divisions.

One starting point is simply to talk about race, class, and gender within activist campaigns and movements. Problems not discussed cannot be overcome, so finding relatively safe ways to begin these discussions is an obvious starting point. Another path is to reach out to organizations working on related issues but rooted in communities of different race, class, or gender. Such conversations can be painful—or joyous—but they are necessary to identify common ground, differences, and shared goals.

Many organizations hire consultants to lead dismantling racism and other stratification systems workshops and training sessions, and others establish internal working groups to guide organizational efforts to dismantle the practices that oppress or divide people. Organizations rooted in indigenous communities or communities of color will need to decide if and how they can best work with organizations that are mostly white and what principles and values can guide their search for common ground.

Exploring the historical intersections between capitalism, racism, sexism, and other forms of oppression and the pathways by which these systems of power interact to undermine well-being and social justice can be useful conversations. These may help activists of differing backgrounds to identify similar and dissimilar experiences and needs, an important step in developing common strategies. When organizations and movements commit to acting together to dismantle the systems of oppression that harm one another's communities, they forge a unity in practice that can transcend the histories of division.

It is challenging to define the line that separates useful if painful exploration of differences from those interactions that only weaken constituencies that have the potential to work together. The parallel rises of movements to confront sexism and racism in all their manifestations and of "cancel culture," the practice of severing from those perceived to have offended some deeply held value, have made it difficult for some progressive movements to find the right balance. Some organizations have borrowed from the restorative justice movement, and developed guidelines for independent assessment of the claims and counterclaims and for conversations between accusers and accused that consider just resolutions.

In some cases, the shared goal of improved well-being for all people might be a starting point for reconciling different perspectives. On the population level, the harms of capitalism are disproportionately allocated to people of color, women, and low-income communities. At the individual level, however, people of all backgrounds can be adversely affected by inequality, climate change, pollution, and inadequate healthcare and educational systems. Even the grandchildren of billionaires will struggle to survive in a world with cataclysmic weather, even the children of the wealthy now struggle to get into the right college, and even global jet-setters have to worry about COVID-19 or its successors. Emphasizing the shared experience of living on this planet together may help some to see others as allies in confronting the dangers that contemporary capitalism erects.

5. Make Leadership Development a Priority

A movement to modify capitalism will require two, three, many generations of leaders. New leaders are needed from the populations most harmed by the status quo, most experienced in fighting for their survival, and most knowledgeable about the specific structures and policies that damage their lives and their communities. This includes leaders from indigenous, Black, Latinx, immigrant, and other low-income communities. It also includes children and young people, the motor force of many social movements of the last several decades, who bring energy and passion to their struggles. It includes women, the population that holds up half the sky, but often experience more than half the burden of suffering that modern capitalism imposes.

Women have proved to be effective movement leaders, finding in their gendered upbringing the patience, fierceness, and communication skills needed to build movements. These and other groups will also need to replace current leaders who age out or burn out, suggesting that movement organizations need the type of succession plans that every corporation develops. Current leaders need to make developing new leaders a priority, and also need to learn how to step out of the way. Some emerging leaders do not need "development" but rather the space to try new ideas and practices.

How can organizations ensure succeeding generations of leadership? One way is to create safe and non-hierarchical spaces and platforms where old, new, and emerging leaders can exchange ideas, analyze practices, and share skills. Larger organizations, progressive philanthropies, and universities can create fellowship programs for new and emerging leaders, places where they can develop the skills and social networks they will need to be effective leaders. Leaders as well as participants will also need deeper understanding of the changing dynamics of modern capitalism and the skills to identify opportunities for successful campaigns and reforms. Movement organizations, sometimes in equitable partnerships with universities, can create workshops, reading groups, formal and informal academic programs, and other forums that can provide these skills.

6. Challenge Capitalist Ideas

While the political power of corporations and their allies is formidable, their domination of the public's ideas, consciousness, and feelings may be an even bigger obstacle to creating alternatives to twenty-first-century capitalism. Thus, a movement that seeks to open paths to such alternatives must find ways to replace key tenets of capitalist ideology. These problematic tenets include the beliefs that individual solutions are always better than collective ones, that problems in capitalism are the result of a few "bad apples" rather than the rules of the system, that market solutions to social problems are always preferable to government ones, and that there is no realistic alternative to the current status quo. Weakening the hold of these ideas is an essential task for a movement that aspires to a healthier, more sustainable world.

Another strategy is to denormalize the acceptability of capitalist practices that endanger health and the environment. The tobacco control movement, for example, sought to "denormalize"—to make socially and morally unacceptable—tobacco industry practices of advertising to children and lying about the evidence on the harmful health effects of cigarettes.[39] Many of this movement's policy and cultural successes resulted from these changes in norms.

Denormalizing, for example, predatory marketing of unhealthy food to children; misrepresenting the findings of scientific research on the harms of alcohol, medicine, or defective cars; or profiteering during a pandemic could build policy maker and public support for more effective laws and policies to end these common corporate practices.

In the case of tobacco, the lawsuits against the tobacco industry forced the release of documents that showed the tobacco industry covered up and withheld evidence on the harmful effects of their products, actions that further diminished their credibility as participants in setting public policies. Shaming the victims of misleading advertising or the individuals with whom activists disagree is inappropriate, but bringing shame on organizations that profit by hurting others in order to encourage them to stop seems the height of civic responsibility.

7. Use Multiple Strategies

A consistent theme of studies of social movement activism and personal accounts of activists is that multiple strategies work better than single ones. In the campaigns to reduce the harmful health impact of the tobacco industry, research has shown that the combination of cigarette taxes, smoking bans in public places, access to treatment, and media and counter-marketing campaigns together reduce smoking more effectively than any single approach.

So if the question for activists is whether to favor social media or face-to-face communications, the answer is "both." Adversarial or collaborative strategies? Both. Incremental or transformative demands? Again, both. In these and other questions of strategy, avoiding binary choices and exploring a continuum of options increases the likelihood of success. No group can do everything but developing a portfolio of strategies and deploying them over time increases pressure on opponents. Distributing some activities and strategies to appropriate partners increases the scope of activism without burdening a single group.

In the civil rights movement, unlikely partners sometimes worked together to capitalize on different strengths and appeals. Martin Luther King Jr. could tell presidents and politicians, "If you don't deal with me, you'll have to deal with the radicals. You choose." Climate activists appealing to banks and other financial institutions to disinvest from fossil fuel companies can say, "Take steps now to address public concerns about your record on climate change or face the wrath of the children and the politicians they will elect in coming years and the investors whose wealth you may lose." These multipronged strategies do not require one reform faction to disparage another, simply to capitalize on their respective strengths and appeal.

8. Find Effective Ways to Interact with Corporations

Movements seeking to change the way corporations do business must inevitably interact with these organizations and their leaders. In the last few decades, thousands of coalitions and alliances have led campaigns to modify harmful corporate practices, some described in previous chapters. What have we learned from the successes and failures of these confrontations that can guide future efforts to convince corporations to make concessions or bring about health-enhancing changes?

Three different strategies warrant consideration: partnerships with corporations to achieve shared goals (public-private partnerships), campaigns designed to pressure corporations to reduce harmful practices (corporate social responsibility or corporate accountability), and efforts to convince government to limit damaging corporate practices (regulation). While many activist organizations use all three strategies, each has distinct advantages and disadvantages.

Public private partnerships. Mainstream politicians and civil society organizations often encourage activists to work with corporations. Their arguments can be compelling: corporations have the technical knowledge, the resources, and the self-interest to solve even those problems they have created. Corporations are not as constrained by democracy and can act more quickly, an advantage for rapidly emerging problems. The default rationale for corporate partnerships is often "there-is-no-alternative." In this view, corporations and their allies are the most powerful entities on earth and will be so for the foreseeable future, so it would be hopelessly naive to imagine solutions that are not endorsed by these interests. This view posits such partnerships as the path of least resistance, an attractive option for overburdened and fearful public officials and public health professionals.

Two considerations make me question these arguments. First, there is almost no empirical evidence from independent researchers that corporate partnerships lead to meaningful reforms. Recent academic reviews summarizing what is known conclude that the evidence presented on their benefits is often misleading, scant, or would have occurred even in the absence of partnerships.[40] Many scholars endorsing partnerships reported conflicts of interest such as financial support from one of the corporate partners.[41] Other reviews identify unintended consequences such as the co-optation of more meaningful reforms, the exaggerated or undeserved burnishing of corporate credibility, and the successful use of these partnerships to divert the conversation away from stronger corporate regulation.[42]

Moreover, for understandable reasons, as Buse and Waxman point out, partnerships sometimes focus on relatively affluent countries that offer a reasonable chance of success, rather than on those that are poor[43]. In this way, they may exacerbate inequalities.[44]

So the case for corporate partnerships appears to be a faith-based one. Its proponents believe that corporations (and by extension modern capitalism) should be able to help solve the problems they create so they urge public health and corporate representatives to work together to make that happen. They suspend the demand for evidence made in other circumstances and ignore the literature that suggests that highly asymmetrical partnerships have trouble achieving real consensus.

As Jeffrey Marks, a philosopher and public health ethicist who studies public private partnerships, has observed, "We imperil public health, as well as the integrity of public health agencies, when we confound the common good and common ground. It is time to explore new paradigms in public health and perhaps revisit and revise some old ones."[45] In the final analysis, Marks warns, collaboration with industry actors "can imperil the core functions of governments and intergovernmental bodies; hamper their ability to promote the public good; undermine their integrity; and erode public trust."[46]

A second, more nuanced concern is that considering partnerships with corporations as a yes/no choice simplifies more complex questions. Under what circumstances should corporations, health and environmental officials, and civil society advocates sit down to negotiate? What should be the ground rules for such talks? Who should decide who talks to whom about what?

A few examples illustrate the expansion of possibilities when these questions are asked. In the Framework Convention on Tobacco Control, the international treaty to limit the harm from tobacco and the tobacco industry, Section 5.3 forbids the involvement of tobacco industry representative in government deliberations on tobacco policy.[47] Implementation has been variable, and the tobacco industry still uses national litigation and other strategies to challenge tobacco control policies.[48] But Section 5.3 provides a clear line that governments, public health professionals, and advocates can use to draw attention to industry interference in public policy.

Boyd Swinburn, an Australian researcher who studies the role of the food industry in child obesity, uses the term "public private interactions" rather than partnerships, as he believes the latter creates inevitable conflicts of interest.[49] He suggests public health researchers and advocates spell out the ground rules for these interactions in advance of meeting. Several organizations have suggested guidelines for such encounters.[50]

In the United States, the Sunshine Act, a law that was passed as part of the Affordable Care Act of 2010, requires public disclosure of payments from pharmaceutical, medical device, biologic, and medical supply manufacturers to physicians and hospitals to promote their products. A study of the impact of the Sunshine Act on Medicare prescriptions before and after its implementation found that industry payments to physicians dramatically declined after implementation and that such payments had been significantly associated with increased prescription costs, branded prescribing, and prescribing for high-risk medications.[51]

These experiences suggest that interactions between advocates for corporate reforms and corporations can lead to reductions in harmful practices.

However, the many misleading claims that corporate leaders make about such partnerships, the fact that there is asymmetrical access to resources and political influence between advocates and corporations, and the potential for co-optation require those entering such agreements to spell out their goals clearly. These agreements also need to set explicit ground rules and establish independent monitoring of impact. Some advocates have proposed a quid pro quo for agreeing to talk to corporations in which businesses commit in advance to end any funding of lobbying and campaign contributions designed to undermine public health protections.

Corporate campaigns. A second strategy, corporate campaigns, has been developed by civil society, health, environmental, and labor groups to pressure corporations to end practices that activists consider to be harmful.[52] The campaigns to force Nestlé to end misleading promotion of its infant formula products, encourage banks and financial institutions to disinvest from fossil fuel companies, and force McDonald's to "retire" Ronald McDonald and its business strategy of marketing unhealthy fast food directly to young children are examples of such strategies. Organizations such as Save Our Walmart, Silicon Valley Rising, and the Tech Workers Coalition, described in previous chapters, show how worker organizations can bring together a variety of constituencies who are harmed by a company to develop common strategies to compel change.

Other corporate campaigns target investors. The logic of using investors to drive change in corporate practices is that investors have what most companies want most—capital that can be invested to generate additional profits. This gives investors the power to make demands on corporate executives as a condition for investing new resources or maintaining current investments. Moreover, persuading investors to put their money here rather than there does not explicitly challenge conservative views on the role of government, regulation, and individual responsibility. This approach may therefore generate less business opposition than other tactics.

Some campaigns to persuade investors to disinvest from harmful industries have been quite successful. Fossil Free describes itself as "a global movement to end the age of fossil fuels and build a world of community-led renewable energy for all." In the last few years, it has supported campaigns that have helped to convince 381 universities to divest all funds from fossil fuel companies. In late 2019, it claimed that these efforts had led investors responsible for $11 trillion to divest from oil, coal, and gas companies fueling the climate crisis.[53]

Finally, some campaigns are launched by corporations themselves to demonstrate their responsibility and concern for the public. Some blend public relations and marketing. Mixify, a marketing campaign by the American Beverage Association (ABA), the beverage industry trade association, launched in 2015, promotes balance in what you "eat, drink and do." "Balance" is defined as "crossing cats with dragons"; finding it will keep you "feeling snazzier than the emoji of the dancing lady in red."[54] As food activist Anna Lappe notes, "Mixify is just one tactic [ABA] is deploying to try to fix a core image problem" and to present a responsible face in the low-income communities it targets for marketing sugary beverages.

Legislation and litigation. A third strategy is to choose governmental institutions and processes—legislation, elections, or litigation—to bring about changes in corporate practices. The successful campaigns to require more employers to pay minimum wage, offer paid sick leave and parental leave, or to drop new acquisition efforts because of their impact on monopoly, are examples of this approach, described in previous chapters.

By mastering a variety of strategies for interacting with corporations and by analyzing which strategies work best under what circumstances, activist campaigns can avoid the Johnny-one-note tendency to repeatedly deploy the same strategies, especially when they are not the most appropriate.

9. Identify Vulnerabilities of Corporations

In their efforts to defeat labor organizing campaigns or regulations or taxes, corporations and their allies have learned that a careful assessment of their opponents' vulnerability can help them to achieve their objectives more effectively and efficiently. Savvy investors have organized law firms, public relations and lobbying companies, communications specialists, and social media influencers to help corporations advance their agendas. Social movements need to identify similar allies who can study their opponents and present strategic guidance for successful campaigns.

Can movement activists learn from this approach? A review of the evidence on social change campaigns designed to change corporate practices suggests a few strategies that organizations have used to build on their own strengths while exploiting the vulnerabilities of corporations.

Many successful campaigns have found that a corporation's brand identity is often its corporate Achilles Heel, as the brand is often its most cherished asset. The 2010 campaign by Corporate Accountability International (CAI) to retire Ronald McDonald made the case that McDonald's core strategy of predatory marketing of unhealthy food to children, symbolized by the clown Ronald, was inherently unethical and antisocial. The group called on McDonald's to abandon this strategy and its symbol. The campaign organized parents and teachers to end McDonald's events at schools, organized doctors to speak out against fast-food marketing to children, and sent children to confront McDonald's CEO at a shareholder meeting.

As a result of these and other activities, CAI reports, half of the hospitals with a McDonald's on-site have shuttered the outlet in their facility; and tens of thousands of people, the second-largest school district in the country, and the largest US teachers' union have called on McDonald's to stop McTeacher's Nights. In addition, the company slashed spending on Happy Meals marketing and rolled out several other expensive but largely ineffective efforts to increase sales and improve its image.[55] In 2020, McDonald's did in fact retire Ronald.

In an interview, Naomi Klein, the author of *No Logo*, her 2000 book that challenged the ways consumer companies like Starbucks and Nike used branding, highlighted the potential for activists to use this branding against companies. "The flip side of relationship marketing is that it makes companies vulnerable," Klein said. "Just as people are becoming more like brands, brands are becoming more like people. Nike is a celebrity, and that's not just because of Michael Jordan. Nike used Michael Jordan to get there, but now it's a celebrity in its own right. That means that when Nike gets caught using sweatshop labor, it's celebrity news. Everybody wants to talk about it."[56]

Another lesson from the campaigns against Nestlé, McDonald's, Purdue Pharma, and Nike is the power of using moral arguments. Profiting from promoting infant formula to mothers whose infants' future health and survival would be better served by breast milk, encouraging young children to nag their parents to buy them food that will put them at risk of obesity and diabetes, paying doctors to prescribe Oxycontin and other painkillers that contribute to tens of thousands of preventable overdoses, and selling Nike sneakers and other gear made by sweatshop workers is plain wrong.

Sometimes activists believe they will win their case by assembling the most compelling scientific evidence, whose power will overwhelm opponents of the action they propose. But moral and ethical arguments plus evidence are almost always more persuasive than evidence alone and can sometimes win over allies unmoved by data.

Tobacco control activists use the term "denormalization" to describe their goals in making the promotion of tobacco, especially to children and young people, morally unacceptable as well as illegal.[57]

How campaigns choose their specific targets provides another opportunity to plan more effective campaigns. McDonald's was not the only food company aggressively marketing unhealthy food to young children but its visibility, its position as an industry leader, and its brand vulnerability led Corporate Accountability International to focus its campaign on this industry leader. This probably increased media coverage, enabled CAI to reach more people, and allowed them to enlist new partners who might have been less attracted to a lesser, unknown target.

A variant of this approach is to select "high road" companies as partners in order to pressure less responsible sectors of the industry. The Restaurant

Workers Opportunity Center, an organization that supports low-wage restaurant workers, found a few restaurants willing to follow "high-road" practices on wages, benefits, and shifts. These high-road restaurants demonstrated to others in the sector that it was possible both to make a profit and to treat workers with respect. At least some restaurant owners found they could attract customers with their commitment to high-road practices.[58]

Some corporations and business sectors prefer a single standard for regulation, rather than the chaos of multiple standards or regulations across jurisdictions and markets. Part of the success of the California Air Resources Board (CARB) in getting some cooperation from the national and even global auto industries for their tough state automobile emissions standards is that automakers believed it was less cumbersome to produce vehicles that met California's more stringent and expensive standards than to produce different products for every state or nation. CARB knew how big the California market was, enabling them to press their advantage.[59]

A final strategy activist can use to take advantage of corporate vulnerabilities is to look for waves they can surf to success. By the time supporters of tougher policies to limit promotion of sugary beverages were ready to implement policies such as sugary beverage taxes, portion size limitations, and changes in sugar labeling on packages, the amount of sugary beverages sold each year had already begun to decline. It may be that early failed efforts to adopt new beverage policies contributed to the changes in norms and attitudes but reinforcing an existing trend is almost always an easier lift than reversing a rising one. By looking for such waves to ride, activists can get their campaigns higher on the beach. They can also use successes to build support for additional policy measures to sustain and expand these changes.

Movements operate in a symbolic realm as well as in the rough and tumble of daily politics. Since the United States has a long history of successful struggles to improve living conditions and rein in corporate excesses, using these symbols in contemporary activism can borrow some of their glitter. The Flint autoworkers' sit-down strike in 1936, Rosa Parks's refusal to move to the back of the bus in 1955 and the subsequent Montgomery Bus Boycott, and the Seattle street demonstrations against the World Trade Organization meeting in 1999 each illustrate part of the history and diverse tactical repertoire of US activism. Borrowing some of these symbols helps movements to connect to these previous struggles, illustrates their deep roots in US history, and connects this generation of activists to previous ones.

CAN WE CREATE ANOTHER WORLD?

Those of us living on the planet today did not choose to be born in the time when the world has to decide what follows modern capitalism. But here we are, needing to ask what tools, what skills, and what values are needed to protect the world today. At worst, this generation will witness further declines that could precipitate the extinction of a survivable planet. At best, it will bequeath to our children, grandchildren, and their progeny a world where they can be happier, healthier, and freer than we are today.

By acknowledging that change takes time and progress is not linear, movement activists and their peers can set realistic goals, weather the inevitable setbacks, and learn to analyze defeats to inform future success.

Humility and patience can also help with sorting out what can be decided by whom and when. While it would certainly be helpful to reach consensus on the exact framework of a social and economic system that would bring us a healthier world, these are not decisions that can be made by leaders, activists, or academics on behalf of others. Social movements succeed when they engage many people to act over time to improve their lives. Short-term wins lead to longer-term successes when those who have created the changes together chart the actions that will amplify and accelerate change. This practice-grounded approach increases the likelihood for sustainable transformations.

A people too afraid, depressed, or apathetic to resist or change the organizations that are worsening their lives cannot protect the well-being of their children and their grandchildren or the planet that sustains them. Leaders too timid, unwilling, or incapable of assessing the costs, benefits, and alternatives to a system that benefits the wealthy at the expense of the many cannot successfully confront the challenges of the twenty-first century. But every generation has faced similar challenges. And always some individuals, organizations, and movements have found ways to bring together their fellow residents of this planet to organize for improved well-being, more decent lives, and a safer future for humanity.

Like those who came before us, those of us living today have a choice. We can accept the dogma that only the current form of capitalism can solve the world's problems and that any costs this system imposes are bearable because they are inevitable. Or we can together create another future.

NOTES

Note to readers: Following contemporary referencing practices, these notes include hyperlinks only for references not readily accessible on common search engines.

CHAPTER 1
1. Marc Benioff , "What Is Required from Corporate Leadership?" World Economic Forum 2020, Davos, Switzerland, January 21, 2020, https://www. weforum.org/events/world-economic-forum-annual-meeting-2020/sessions/ stakeholder-capitalism-what-is-required-from-corporate-leadership.
2. Feike Sybesma , "What Is Required from Corporate Leadership?" panel discussion at World Economic Forum 2020, Davos, Switzerland, January 21, 2020, https://www.weforum.org/events/world-economic-forum-annual-meeting-2020/sessions/stakeholder-capitalism-what-is-required-from-corporate-leadership.
3. K. Schwab, "Davos Manifesto 2020: The Universal Purpose of a Company in the Fourth Industrial Revolution, 2020," World Economic Forum, December 4, 2019, https://www.weforum.org/agenda/2019/12/davos-manifesto-2020-the-universal-purpose-of-a-company-in-the-fourth-industrial-revolution.
4. T. Wu, "The Revolution Comes to Davos," *New York Times*, January 26, 2020.
5. Klaus Schwab, quoted in D. Zak, Will Davos Save the World, or Put It Out of Its Misery? Washington Post, January 24, 2020.
6. Zak, "Will Davos Save the World?"
7. PwC, "Navigating the Rising Tide of Uncertainty: Key Findings from PwC's Twenty-third Annual CEO Survey, 2020."
8. K. Schwab, "5 Trends in the Global Economy—and Their Implications for Economic Policymakers," World Economic Forum, October 9, 2019, https://www.weforum.org/agenda/2019/10/global-competitiveness-report-2019-economic-trends-for-policymakers/.
9. S. Meredith, "BlackRock CEO Says the Climate Crisis Is about to Trigger 'a Fundamental Reshaping of Finance.'" CNBC, January 14, 2020.
10. IPCC, "2019: Summary for Policymakers." In *Climate Change and Land: An IPCC Special Report on Climate Change, Desertification, Land Degradation, Sustainable Land Management, Food Security, and Greenhouse Gas Fluxes in Terrestrial Ecosystems*, ed. P.R. Shukla et al., (Geneva: Intergovernmental Panel on Climate Change, 2019); IPCC, "2019: Summary for Policymakers." In *IPCC Special Report*

on the Ocean and Cryosphere in a Changing Climate, ed. H. O. Pörtner et al., (Geneva: Intergovernmental Panel on Climate Change, 2019).

11. Greenpeace International, "Davos Financial Players Pump US$1.4 Trillion into Fossil Fuels," January 21, 2020.

12. D. Gelles and S. Sengupta, "Big Business Vows to Fight Climate Change," *New York Times*, January 25, 2020.

13. C. Coffey, P. E. Revollo, R. Harvey, M. Lawson, A. Parvez Butt, K. Piaget, D. Sarosi, J. Thekkudan, "Time to Care Unpaid and Underpaid Care Work and the Global Inequality Crisis," Oxfam International, January 2020.

14. Zak, "Will Davos Save the World, or Put It Out of Its Misery?"

15. "Edelman Trust Barometer 2020," January 19, 2020.

16. "Edelman Trust Barometer 2020."

17. Harvard University Institute of Politics, "Survey of Young Americans' Attitudes toward Politics and Public Service," March 18–April 3, 2016.

18. Pew Research Center, "Public Trust in Government: 1958–2019," April 11, 2019.

19. "2018 Edelman Trust Barometer Global Report, 2018," January 21, 2018.

20. J. Ray, "Americans' Stress, Worry and Anger Intensified in 2018," Gallup Poll, April 25, 2019, https://news.gallup.com/poll/249098/americans-stress-worry-anger-intensified-2018.aspx.

21. Blue Cross Blue Shield, "Major Depression: The Impact on Overall Health," May 2018.

22. N. Goldman, D. A. Glei, M. Weinstein, "Declining Mental Health among Disadvantaged Americans," Proceedings of the National Academy of Sciences, 2018:201722023.

23. T. Yilmazer, P. Babiarz, F. Liu, "The Impact of Diminished Housing Wealth on Health in the United States: Evidence from the Great Recession," *Social Science and Medicine* 130 (2015): 234–41.

24. A. Arenge, S. Perry, A. Tallevi, "Poll: Majority of Millennials Are in Debt, Hitting Pause on Major Life Events," NBC News, April 4, 2018.

25. T. Andres, "Divided Decade: How the Financial Crisis Changed Housing," *Marketplace*, December 17, 2018.

26. G. Holland, "L.A.'s Homelessness Surged 75 Percent in Six Years: Here Is Why the Crisis Has Been Decades in the Making," *Los Angeles Times*, February 1, 2018.

27. R. Grant, D. Gracy, G. Goldsmith, A. Shapiro, I. E. Redlener, "Twenty-five Years of Child and Family Homelessness: Where Are We Now?" *American Journal of Public Health* 103, no. S2 (2013): e1–0.

28. See A. Case and A. Deaton, "Mortality and Morbidity in the Twenty-first Century," Brookings Papers on Economic Activity 2017 (2017): 397–476; and A. Case and A. Deaton, *Deaths of Despair and the Future of American Capitalism* (Princeton, NJ: Princeton University Press, 2020).

29. U. E. Bauer, P. A. Briss, R. A. Goodman, and B. A. Bowman, "Prevention of Chronic Disease in the Twenty-first Century: Elimination of the Leading Preventable Causes of Premature Death and Disability in the USA," *The Lancet* 384 no. 9937 (2014): 45–52.

30. A. Alwan, "Global Status Report on Noncommunicable Diseases 2010," World Health Organization, 2011.

31. R. Micha, J. L. Peñalvo, F. Cudhea et al., "Association between Dietary Factors and Mortality from Heart Disease, Stroke, and Type 2 Diabetes in the United States," *JAMA* 317, no. 9 (2017): 912–24.

32. Gallup Poll, "Nutrition and Food," October 14–31, 2019.

33. C. Funk, B. Kennedy, and M. Hefferon, "Public Perspectives on Food Risks," Pew Research Center, November 19, 2018.
34. L. Sanders, "2017 Food and Health Survey: Food Confusion," International Food Information Council Foundation, September 13, 2017, https://foodinsight.org/2017-food-health-survey-food-confusion/.
35. Gallup Poll, "Healthcare System, 2019," https://news.gallup.com/poll/4708/healthcare-system.aspx.
36. A. Maccagnan, S. Wren-Lewis, H. Brown, and T. Taylor, "Wellbeing and Society: Towards Quantification of the Co-benefits of Wellbeing," *Social Indicators Research* (2018): 1–27.
37. New Economics Foundation, "Happy Planet Index 2016 Methods Paper," https://static1.squarespace.com/static/5735c421e321402778ee0ce9/t/578dec7837c58157b929b3d6/1468918904805/.
38. E. M. Lawrence, R. G. Rogers, and T. Wadsworth, "Happiness and Longevity in the United States," *Social Science and Medicine* 145 (2015): 115–19.
39. R. Costanza, I. Kubiszewski, and E. Giovannini et al., "Time to Leave GDP Behind," *Nature* 505, no. 7483 (2014): pg #.
40. S. Zuboff, *The Age of Surveillance Capitalism: The Fight for a Human Future at the New Frontier of Power* (London: Profile Books, 2019); H. Heller, *The Birth of Capitalism: A Twenty-first-century Perspective* (London: Pluto Press; 2011); E. O. Wright, *How to Be an Anticapitalist in the Twenty-First Century* (Brooklyn, N.Y.: Verso Books, 2019).
41. G. Rose, "The Future of Capitalism," *Foreign Affairs*, January–February 2020, 8.
42. F. L. Block, *Capitalism: The Future of an Illusion* (Berkeley: University of California Press, 2018).
43. Planetary health has been defined as "the health of human civilization and the state of the natural systems on which it depends." ("The Bigger Picture of Planetary Health," *The Lancet Planetary Health* 3, no. 1 [2019]: e1).
44. W. Gossett, quoted in *Planning, Regulation, and Competition: Automobile Industry—1968, Hearings by United States Congress*, 90ᵗʰ Cong., 7 (1968),https://play.google.com/books/reader?id=Q9YVAAAAIAAJ&hl=en&pg=GBS.PA7.
45. D. Eisenhower, "Eisenhower's Farewell Address (audio transcript)," January 17, 1961. https://www.youtube.com/watch?v=CWiIYW_fBfY
46. J. K. Galbraith, *The Age of Uncertainty* (London: Trafalgar Square, 1977), pg 257.
47. A. Murphy, "America's Largest Private Companies 2019," *Forbes*, December 17, 2019. https://www.forbes.com/sites/andreamurphy/2019/12/17/americas-largest-private-companies-2019/#31818ce75261
48. See "Fortune 2018 Annual Global 2000 List" and "Fortune 2003 Annual Global 2000 List." Total assets in 2018 equaled $189 trillion and in unadjusted dollars; the total was $65 trillion in 2003.
49. A. Lundeen and K. Pomerleau, "Corporations Make Up 5 Percent of Businesses but Earn 62 Percent of Revenues," *Tax Foundation*, November 25, 2014, https://taxfoundation.org/corporations-make-5-percent-businesses-earn-62-percent-revenues/.
50. "69 of the Richest 100 Entities on the Planet Are Corporations, Not Governments, Figures Show," Global Justice Now, October, 17, 2018, https://www.globaljustice.org.uk/news/2018/oct/17/69-richest-100-entities-planet-are-corporations-not-governments-figures-show.
51. "Tupperware! The Rise of American Consumerism," *American Experience*, February 4, 2004.

52. US Bureau of Economic Analysis, "Shares of Gross Domestic Product: Personal Consumption Expenditures (DPCERE1Q156NBEA)," retrieved from FRED, Federal Reserve Bank of St. Louis, August 13, 2020, https://fred.stlouisfed.org/series/DPCERE1Q156NBEA.

53. US Bureau of Economic Analysis, Personal consumption expenditures per capita [A794RC0A052NBEA], FRED, Federal Reserve Bank of St. Louis, n.d., https://fred.stlouisfed.org/series/A794RC0A052NBEA.

54. "US Business Cycle Expansions and Contractions," National Bureau of Economic Research, September 20, 2010.

55. R. J. Gordon, *The Rise and Fall of American Growth* (Princeton, NJ: Princeton University Press, 2016), 13–18.

56. Peterson Institute for International Economics, "What Is Globalization? And How Has the Global Economy Shaped the United States?" February 4, 2019.

57. R. Dobbs, T. Koller, S. Ramaswamy et al., "Playing to Win: The New Global Competition for Corporate Profits," McKinsey Global Institute, September 2015.

58. United Nations Conference on Trade and Development, *Key Statistics and Trends in International Trade* (Geneva, Switzerland: United Nations, 2019).

59. T. R. Tørsløv, L. S. Wier, and G. Zucman, "The Missing Profits of Nations" (working paper 2470, National Bureau of Economic Research, June 2018; revised April 2020).

60. United Nations Department of Economic and Social Affairs, "The Number of International Migrants Reaches 272 Million, Continuing an Upward Trend in All World Regions, Says UN," September 17, 2019.

61. R. Moodie, D. Stuckler, C. Monteiro, Lancet NCD Action Group et al., "Profits and Pandemics: Prevention of Harmful Effects of Tobacco, Alcohol, and Ultra-processed Food and Drink Industries, *The Lancet* 381, no. 9867 (February 23, 2013): 670–79; D. Stuckler, M. McKee, S. Ebrahim, and S. Basu, "Manufacturing Epidemics: The Role of Global Producers in Increased Consumption of Unhealthy Commodities Including Processed Foods, Alcohol, and Tobacco," *PLoS Medicine*, June 26, 2012, doi 2012;9(6):e1001235.

62. "Latin America: The Fastest Growing Latin American Industries for 2013–2015," Global Intelligence Alliance, April 26, 2012.

63. R. Labonté, A. Ruckert, A. Schram, "Trade, Investment and the Global Economy: Are We Entering a New Era for Health?" *Global Social Policy* 18, no. 1 (2018): 28–44; D. McNeill, P. Barlow, C. D. Birkbeck et al., "Trade and Investment Agreements: Implications for Health Protection," *Journal of World Trade* 51, no. 1 (2017): 159–82; S. Friel, L. Hattersley, and R. Townsend, "Trade Policy and Public Health," *Annual Review of Public Health* 36 (2015): 325–44.

64. Campaign for Tobacco Free Kids, "Philip Morris v Uruguay: Findings from the International Arbitration Tribunal," July 2016.

65. E. Crosbie and S. Glantz, "Philip Morris Gets Its Ash Kicked in Uruguay, Where Will It Next Blow Smoke?" AP News, July 31, 2016.

66. C. Drake, "Disparate Treatment for Property and Labor Rights in US Trade Agreements," *UCLA Journal of International Law and Foreign Affairs* 22 (2018): 70.

67. D. Bacon, "The New NAFTA Won't Protect Workers' Rights," *The Nation*, November 8, 2019.

68. C. Hawkes, "The Role of Foreign Direct Investment in the Nutrition Transition," *Public Health Nutrition* 8, no. 4 (2005): 357–65.

69. D. McNeill, P. Barlow, C. D. Birkbeck et al., "Trade and Investment Agreements: Implications for Health Protection," *Journal of World Trade* 51, no. 1 (2017): 159–82.

70. S. E. Clark, C. Hawkes, S. M. Murphy, K. A. Hansen-Kuhn, and D. Wallinga, "Exporting Obesity: US Farm and Trade Policy and the Transformation of the Mexican Consumer Food Environment," *International Journal of Occupational and Environmental Health* 18, no. 1 (2012): 53–64.

71. J. Page and B. McKay, "The World Health Organization Draws Flak for Coronavirus Response," *Wall Street Journal*, February 12, 2020.

72. R. M. Orrange, *The Corporate State: Technopoly, Privatization and Corporate Predation* (Abingdon, Oxfordshire: Routledge, 2020).

73. J. Brecher, T. Costello, and B. Smith, *Globalization from Below the Power of Solidarity* (Boston: South End Press, 2000).

74. G. R. Krippner, "The Financialization of the American Economy," *Socio-Economic Review* 3 (2005): 174.

75. Krippner, "The Financialization of the American Economy," 173–208.

76. S. Donnan, "Financial Sector in Advanced Economies Is Too Big, Says IMF," *Financial Times*, May 12, 2015.

77. R. Foroohar, *Makers and Takers: The Rise of Finance and the Fall of American Business* (New York: Crown Books, 2016).

78. S. Brill, *Tailspin: The People and Forces Behind America's Fifty-year Fall—and Those Fighting to Reverse It* (New York: Vintage, 2019), 71–72.

79. Brill, Tailspin, 92.

80. E. Stewart, "What the Republican Tax Bill Did—and Didn't—Do, One Year Later," Vox, December 22, 2018.

81. "Financialization" is defined as a "pattern of accumulation in which profit making occurs increasingly through financial channels rather than through trade and commodity production" (Krippner, "The Financialization of the American Economy," 173–208).

82. N. Pace, A. Seal, A. Costello, "Food Commodity Derivatives: A New Cause of Malnutrition?" *The Lancet* 371, no. 9625 (2008): 1648–50.

83. P. Whoriskey and D. Keating, "Overdoses, Bedsores, Broken Bones: What Happened When a Private-equity Firm Sought to Care for Society's Most Vulnerable?" *Washington Post*, November 25, 2018.

84. Business Roundtable, "Statement on Corporate Governance," September 1997, http://www.ralphgomory.com/wp-content/uploads/2018/05/Business-Roundtable-1997.pdf.

85. The Business Roundtable, "Statement on the Purpose of a Corporation," August 19, 2019, https://opportunity.businessroundtable.org/wp-content/uploads/2019/12/BRT-Statement-on-the-Purpose-of-a-Corporation-with-Signatures.pdf.

86. P. Goodman, "Big Business Pledged Gentler Capitalism: It's Not Happening in a Pandemic," *New York Times*, April 14, 2020.

87. P. Nolan, D. Sutherland, and J. Zhang, "The Challenge of the Global Business Revolution," *Contributions to Political Economy* 21 (2002): 91–110.

88. Ibid.

89. H. Hveem, "Global Market Power," in *The Palgrave Handbook of Contemporary International Political Economy* (London: Palgrave Macmillan, 2019), 43–58.

90. S. Teles and B. Lindsey, *The Captured Economy: How the Powerful Enrich Themselves, Slow Down Growth, and Increase Inequality* (New York: Oxford University Press, 2017), 8.

91. T. Wu, *The Curse of Bigness: Antitrust in the New Gilded Age* (New York: Columbia Global Reports, 2018), 71.

92. Nolan, Sutherland, and Zhang, "The Challenge of the Global Business Revolution," 91–110.

93. P. M. Danzon, A. Epstein, and S. Nicholson, "Mergers and Acquisitions in the Pharmaceutical and Biotechnology Industries" (working paper no. 10536, National Bureau of Economic Research, June 2004).

94. M. Boldrin and M. K. Levine, *Against Intellectual Monopoly* (New York: Cambridge University Press, 2008).

95. B. Fulton, "Health Care Market Concentration Trends in the United States from 2010 to 2016," *Health Affairs* 36, no. 9 (2017): 1530–38.

96. S. Teles and B. Lindsey, *The Captured Economy*, 20.

97. B. Jessop, "Fordism and Post-Fordism: A Critical Reformulation," in *Pathways to Industrialization and Regional Development* (Abingdon, Oxfordshire: Routledge, 2005), 54–74.

98. J. M. Keynes, The General Theory of Employment, Interest and Money. (Basingstoke, Hampshire: Palgrave Macmillan. 2007 [1936]).

99. N. Chorev, "On the Origins of Neoliberalism: Political Shifts and Analytical Challenges," in Handbook of Politics: *State and Society in Global Perspective*, ed. Kevin T. Leicht and Craig Jenkins (New York: Springer, 2010, 127–44.

100. Chorev, *On the Origins of Neoliberalism*, 127.

101. D. Harvey, *A Brief History of Neoliberalism* (New York: Oxford University Press, 2007).

102. A. Saad-Filho, "Coronavirus, Crisis, and the End of Neoliberalism," MR Online, April 18, 2020.

103. E. S. Savas, *Privatization and Public-private Partnerships* (New York: CQ Press, 2000).

104. R. Reagan, The President's News Conference, August 12, 1986," https://www.reaganfoundation.org/media/128648/newsconference2.pdf.

105. C. Hartney and C. Glesmann, "Prison Bed Profiteers: How Corporations Are Reshaping Criminal Justice in the US," National Council on Crime and Delinquency, May 2012.

106. G. Hodge, *Privatization: An International Review of Performance* (Abingdon, Oxfordshire: Routledge, 2018).

107. Andrew Calabrese, "Privatization of the Media," In *The International Encyclopedia of Communication*, ed. W. Donsbach (Oxford: Blackwell Publishing, 2008).

108. J. D. Michaels, *Constitutional Coup: Privatization's Threat to the American Republic* (Cambridge, MA: Harvard University Press, 2017), 1–10.

109. S. E. Gollust and P. D. Jacobson, "Privatization of Public Services: Organizational Reform Efforts in Public Education and Public Health," *American Journal of Public Health* 96, no. 10 (2006): 1733–39.

110. P. J. Cooper, *The War against Regulation: From Jimmy Carter to George W. Bush* (Lawrence: University Press of Kansas, 2009).

111. Cooper, *The War against Regulation from Jimmy Carter to George W. Bush*.

112. D. Jacobs, "Rising Income Inequality in the U.S. Was Fueled by Ronald Reagan's Attacks on Union Strength and Continued by Bill Clinton's Financial Deregulation," *LSE American Politics and Policy*, August 12, 2014.

113. G. Otero, *The Neoliberal Diet: Unhealthy Profits, Unhealthy People* (Austin: University of Texas Press, 2018), 39–43.

114. N. Popovich, L. Albeck-Ripka, and K. Pierre-Louis, "The Trump Administration Is Reversing 100 Environmental Rules," *New York Times*, May 20, 2020.

115. "Tracking Deregulation in the Trump Era," The Brookings Institution, August 6, 2020, https://www.brookings.edu/interactives/tracking-deregulation-in-the-trump-era/.

116. Grover Norquist, "Conservative Advocate," interview by Mara Liasson, *Morning Edition*, NPR, May 25, 2001.

117. M. Prasad, *Starving the Beast: Ronald Reagan and the Tax Cut Revolution* (New York: Russell Sage Foundation, 2018).

118. M. Gardner, L. Roque, and S. Wamhoff, *Corporate Tax Avoidance in the First Year of the Trump Tax Law*, Institute on Taxation and Economic Policy, December 2019.

119. Ibid.

120. R. Phillips, S. Wamhoff, and D. Smith, "U.S Offshore Shell Games 2014: The Use of Offshore Tax Havens by Fortune 500 Companies," US PIRG Education Fund and Citizens for Tax Justice, 2014, https://www.ctj.org/pdf/offshoreshell2014.pdf.

121. D. Mccoy, S. Chigudu, and T. Tillmann, "Framing the Tax and Health Nexus: A Neglected Aspect of Public Health Concern," *Health Economics, Policy and Law* 12, no. 2 (2017): 179–94.

122. W. H. Wiist, "Public Health and Corporate Avoidance of US Federal Income Tax," *World Medical and Health Policy* 10, no. 3 (2018): 272–300.

123. N. Klein, *The Shock Doctrine: The Rise of Disaster Capitalism* (New York: Allen Lane, 2007).

124. W. K. Tabb, *The Long Default: New York City and the Urban Fiscal Crisis* (New York: NYU Press, 1982).

125. N. Freudenberg, M. Fahs, S. Galea, and A. Greenberg, "The Impact of New York City's 1975 Fiscal Crisis on the Tuberculosis, HIV, and Homicide Syndemic," *American Journal of Public Health* 96, no. 3 (2006): 424–34.

126. M. Karanikolos, P. Mladovsky, J. Cylus et al., "Financial Crisis, Austerity, and Health in Europe," *The Lancet* 381, no. 9874 (2013): 1323–31; R. McGahey, "The Political Economy of Austerity in the United States," *Social Research* 80, no. 3 (2013): 717–48.

127. D. Stuckler and S. Basu, *The Body Economic: Why Austerity Kills* (New York: Basic Books, 2013).

128. G. Morley, J. Ives, and C. Bradbury-Jones, "Moral Distress and Austerity: An Avoidable Ethical Challenge in Healthcare," *Health Care Analysis* 27, no. 3 (2019): 185–201.

129. R. Hohle, *Racism in the Neoliberal Era: A Meta History of Elite White Power* (Abingdon, Oxfordshire: Routledge, 2017).

130. G. Dutfield, *Intellectual Property Rights and the Life Science Industries: A Twentieth Century History* (Abingdon, Oxfordshire: Routledge, 2017).

131. D. Cantor, ed., *Cancer in the Twentieth Century* (Baltimore: Johns Hopkins University Press, 2008).

132. J. Anderson, *Devices and Designs: Medical Technologies in Historical Perspective* (London: Palgrave Macmillan, 2006).

133. P. Basu and B. A. Scholten, "Technological and Social Dimensions of the Green Revolution: Connecting Pasts and Futures," *International Journal of Agricultural Sustainability* 10 (2012): 109–16.

134. D. MacAray, "The Man Who Saved a Billion Lives," *The Huffington Post*, October 15, 2013.

135. P. Hazell, "Green Revolution: Curse or Blessing?" *International Food Policy Research Institute*, 2002, https://oregonstate.edu/instruct/css/330/three/Green.pdf.

136. D. Noble, *Forces of Production: A Social History of Industrial Automation* (Abingdon, Oxfordshire: Routledge, 2017).

137. D. F. Noble, *America by Design: Science, Technology, and the Rise of Corporate Capitalism* (New York: Oxford University Press, 1979).

138. V. Bush, *Science the Endless Frontier* (Washington, DC: United States Government Printing Office, 1945).
139. S. Krimsky, *Conflicts of Interest in Science: How Corporate-funded Academic Research Can Threaten Public Health* (New York: Simon & Schuster, 2019).
140. J. Brathwaite and P. Drahos, *Global Business Regulation* (Cambridge: Cambridge University Press, 2000), 69.
141. Brathwaite and Drahos, *Global Business Regulation*, 62–63.
142. Access Campaign, "Spotlight on: TRIPS, TRIPS Plus, and Doha," Médecins sans Frontieres, 2017, https://msfaccess.org/spotlight-trips-trips-plus-and-doha.
143. Access Campaign, "Spotlight on: TRIPS, TRIPS Plus, and Doha."
144. World Trade Organization, World Intellectual Property Organization, World Health Organization *Promoting Access to Medical Technologies and Innovation: Intersections between Public Health, Intellectual Property and Trade* (Geneva: World Health Organization, World Intellectual Property Organization, World Trade Organization, 2012).
145. M. Boldrin, D. K. Levine, *Against Intellectual Monopoly* (New York: Cambridge University Press, 2010).
146. United Nations General Assembly, "International Covenant on Economic, Social and Cultural Rights, Article 15.1. (b) and (c)," adopted December 16, 1966, 993 U.N.T.S. 3 (entered into force January 3, 1976), G.A. Res. 2200 (XXI), 21 U.N. GAOR Supp. (no. 16), 49, U.N. Doc. A/6316 (1966).
147. A. Brandt, *The Cigarette Century: The Rise, Fall, and Deadly Persistence of the Product that Defined America* (New York: Basic Books, 2009).
148. B. Penders, J. M. Verbakel, A. Nelis, "The Social Study of Corporate Science: A Research Manifesto," *Bulletin of Science, Technology and Society* 29, no. 6 (2009): 439–46.
149. D. Michaels , *Doubt Is Their Product: How Industry's Assault on Science Threatens Your Health* (New York: Oxford University Press, 2008).
150. N. Oreskes and E. Conway, *Merchants of Doubt: How a Handful of Scientists Obscured the Truth on Issues from Tobacco Smoke to Global Warming* (London: Bloomsbury Press, 2011).
151. M. Kakutani, *The Death of Truth: Notes on Falsehood in the Age of Trump* (New York: Tim Duggan Books, 2018), 171.
152. S. Lukes, *Power: A Radical View* (London: Palgrave Macmillan, 2005), 64.
153. E. S. Herman and N. Chomsky, *Manufacturing Consent* (New York: Pantheon Books, 1988); B. Penders and A. P. Nelis, "Credibility Engineering in the Food Industry: Linking Science, Regulation, and Marketing in a Corporate Context," *Science in Context* 24, no. 4 (2011): 487–515.
154. E. L. Bernays, "The Engineering of Consent," *The Annals of the American Academy of Political and Social Science* 250, no. 1 (1947): 113–20.
155. L. F. Powell Jr. "Confidential Memo: Attack on American Free Enterprise System," August 23, 1971, http://reclaimdemocracy.org/corporate_accountability/powell_memo_lewis.html.
156. B. Moyers, "How Wall Street Occupied America," *The Nation*, November 21, 2011.
157. Federal Election Commission, "Statistical Summary of 18-Month Campaign Activity of the 2017–2018 Election Cycle," August 30, 2018, https://www.fec.gov/updates/statistical-summary-18-month-campaign-activity-2017-2018-election-cycle/.

158. J. Mayer, *Dark Money: The Hidden History of the Billionaires behind the Rise of the Radical Right* (New York: Doubleday, 2016).

159. A. Lutz, These 6 Corporations Control 90 Percent of the Media in America," *Business Insider*, June 14, 2012.

160. J. Temple, "The Worst Thing that Could Happen to Local News," *The Atlantic*, August 15, 2019.

161. C. Kang, "Antitrust Bill May Help Newspapers," *New York Times*, January 13, 2020.

162. K. Phillips-Fein, *Invisible Hands: The Making of the Conservative Movement from the New Deal to Reagan* (Jakarta: Yayasan Obor, 2009).

163. Mayer, *Dark Money* .

164. D. Callahan, *The Givers: Wealth, Power, and Philanthropy in a New Gilded Age* (New York: Vintage, 2017).

165. D. Matthews, "The Case against Billionaire Philanthropy," Vox, December 17, 2018; I. Kapoor I. "Billionaire Philanthropy: 'Decaf Capitalism,'" in *Handbook on Wealth and the Super-rich* (Cheltenham, Gloucestershire, UK: Edward Elgar Publishing, 2016), 113–31.

CHAPTER 2

1. S. J. Vermeulen, B. M. Campbell, J. S. Ingram, "Climate Change and Food Systems," *Annual Review of Environment and Resources* 37 (2012): 195–222.

2. W. Willett, J. Rockström, B. Loken, "Food in the Anthropocene: The EAT–Lancet Commission on Healthy Diets from Sustainable Food Systems," *The Lancet* 393, no. 10170 (2019): 447–92.

3. UNICEF, "Malnutrition Prevalence Remains Alarming: Stunting Is Declining Too Slowly While Wasting Still Impacts the Lives of Far Too Many Young Children," March 2020.

4. American Heart Association, "Heart Disease and Stroke Statistics-2019 At-a-Glance," 2019.

5. S. M. Krebs-Smith, J. Reedy, C. Bosire, "Healthfulness of the US Food Supply: Little Improvement Despite Decades of Dietary Guidance," *American Journal of Preventive Medicine* 38, no. 5 (2010): 472–77.

6. CDC, "Prevalence of Overweight and Obesity among Adults: United States, 2003–2004."

7. G. Sacks, B. Swinburne, E. Ravussin, "Combining Biological, Epidemiological, and Food Supply Data to Demonstrate That Increased Energy Intake Alone Virtually Explains the Obesity Epidemic," US International Conference on Diet and Activity Methods, Washington, DC, June 2009, http://www.icdam.org/.

8. B. Wilson, *The Way We Eat Now: How the Food Revolution Has Transformed Our Lives, Our Bodies, and Our World* (London: Hachette UK, 2019).

9. C. A. Monteiro, G. Cannon, R. B. Levy et al., "Ultra-processed Foods: What They Are and How to Identify Them," *Public Health Nutrition* 22, no. 5 (April 2019): 936–41.

10. Ibid.

11. C. A. Monteiro, J. C. Moubarac, G. Cannon, S. W. Ng, B. Popkin, "Ultra-processed Products Are Becoming Dominant in the Global Food System," *Obesity Reviews* 14 (2013): 21–28; E. H. Zobel, T. W. Hansen, P. Rossing, B. J. von Scholten, "Global Changes in Food Supply and the Obesity Epidemic," *Current Obesity Reports* 5, no. 4 (2016): 449–55; B. M. Popkin, "Nutrition, Agriculture and the Global Food System in Low and Middle Income Countries," *Food Policy* 47 (2014): 91–96.

12. A. Gearhardt, C. Davis, R. Kushner, and K. Brownell, :The Addiction Potential of Hyperpalatable Foods," *Current Drug Abuse Reviews* 4 (2011): 140–45.

13. E. M. Steele, D. Raubenheimer, S. J. Simpson, L. G. Baraldi, C. A. Monteiro, "Ultra-processed Foods, Protein Leverage and Energy Intake in the USA," *Public Health Nutrition* 21, no. 1 (2018): 114–24.

14. S. Vandevijvere, L. M. Jaacks, C. A. Monteiro et al., "Global Trends in Food and Drink Product Sales and Their Association with Adult Body Mass Index Trajectories," *Obesity Reviews* supplement, *Future Directions in Obesity Prevention* 20, no. 2 (2019): S10–19.

15. L. G. Baraldi, E. M. Steele, D. S. Canella, C. A. Monteiro, "Consumption of Ultraprocessed Foods and Associated Sociodemographic Factors in the USA between 2007 and 2012: Evidence from a Nationally Representative Cross-sectional Study," *BMJ Open* 8, no. 3 (2018): e020574.

16. J. M. Poti, M. A. Mendez, S. W. Ng, and B. M. Popkin, "Is the Degree of Food Processing and Convenience Linked with the Nutritional Quality of Foods Purchased by US Households?" *American Journal of Clinical Nutrition* 101, no. 6 (2015): 1251–62.

17. Monteiro, Cannon, Levy et al., "Ultraprocessed Foods," 936–41.

18. A. Fardet, "Minimally Processed Foods Are More Satiating and Less Hyperglycemic than Ultraprocessed Foods: A Preliminary Study with 98 Ready-to-eat Foods," Food and Function 7, no. 5 (2016): 2338–46.

19. M. Zinöcker and I. Lindseth, "The Western Diet–Microbiome-host Interaction and Its Role in Metabolic Disease," *Nutrients* 10, no. 3 (2018): 365.

20. Ibid.

21. F. Juul, E. M. Steele, N. Parekh et al., "Ultraprocessed Food Consumption and Excess Weight among US Adults," British Journal of Nutrition 120 (2018): 90–100; B. Srour, L. Fezeu, E. Kesse-Guyot et al., "Consommation d'aliments ultra-transformés et risque de maladies cardiovasculaires dans la cohorte NutriNet-Santé," *Livre des abstracts, Journée Francophone de Nutrition*, Nice, France, November 28–30, 2018, 61; M. Lavigne-Robichaud, J.-C. Moubarac, S. Lantagne-Lopez et al., "Diet Quality Indices in Relation to Metabolic Syndrome in an Indigenous Cree (Eeyouch) Population in Northern Québec, Canada," *Public Health Nutrition* 21 (2018) 172–80; ibid.; L. Schnabel, C. Buscail, J. M. Sabate et al., "Association between Ultra-processed Food Consumption and Functional Gastrointestinal Disorders: Results from the French NutriNet-Santé Cohort," *American Journal of Gastroenterology* 113, no. (2018): 1217–28; T. Fiolet, B. Srour, L. Sellem et al., "Consumption of Ultraprocessed Foods and Cancer Risk: Results from NutriNet-Santé Prospective Cohort," *The BMJ* 360 (2018): k322; M. Askari, J. Heshmati , H. Shahinfar, et al. Ultra-processed food and the risk of overweight and obesity: a systematic review and meta-analysis of observational studies. *International Journal of Obesity.* 44(2020):2080–2091.

22. A. Afshin, P. J. Sur, K. A. Fay et al., "Health Effects of Dietary Risks in 195 Countries, 1990–2017: A Systematic Analysis for the Global Burden of Disease Study 2017" 393, no. 10184 (2019): 1958–72.

23. J. Breda, J. Jewell, A. Keller, "The Importance of the World Health Organization Sugar Guidelines for Dental Health and Obesity Prevention," *Caries Research* 53, no. 2 (2019): 149–52.

24. Institute of Medicine and National Research Council, *U.S. Health in International Perspective: Shorter Lives, Poorer Health* (Washington, D.C., National Academies Press, 2013), 145.

25. R. A. Ferdman, "Where People around the World Eat the Most Sugar and Fat," *Washington Post*, February 5, 2015.

26. B. M. Popkin and C. Hawkes, "Sweetening of the Global Diet, Particularly Beverages: Patterns, Trends, and Policy Responses," *The Lancet Diabetes & Endocrinology* 4, no. 2 (2016): 174–86.

27. S. Bhat, M. Marklund, M. E. Henry et al., "A Systematic Review of the Sources of Dietary Salt around the World," *Advances in Nutrition* 11, no. 2020: 677–86.

28. L. J. Harnack, M. E. Cogswell, J. M. Shikany et al., "Sources of Sodium in US Adults from Three Geographic Regions," *Circulation* 135, no. 19 (2017): 1775–83.

29. S. Greer, L. Schieb, G. Schwartz, S. Onufrak, and S. Park, "Association of the Neighborhood Retail Food Environment with Sodium and Potassium Intake among US Adults," *Preventing Chronic Disease* 11, no. 130340 (2014).

30. V. Bouvard, D. Loomis, K. Z. Guyton et al., "Carcinogenicity of Consumption of Red and Processed Meat," *The Lancet Oncology* 16, no. 16 (2015): 1599–600.

31. P. Wilde, J. L. Pomeranz, L. J. Lizewski et al., "Legal Feasibility of US Government Policies to Reduce Cancer Risk by Reducing Intake of Processed Meat," *The Milbank Quarterly* 97, no. 2 (2019): 420–48.

32. L. Zeng, M. Ruan, J. Liu et al., "Trends in Processed Meat, Unprocessed Red Meat, Poultry, and Fish Consumption in the United States, 1999–2016," *Journal of the Academy of Nutrition and Dietetics* 119, no. 7 (2019): 1085–98.

33. A. Clonan, K. E. Roberts, and M. Holdsworth, "Socioeconomic and Demographic Drivers of Red and Processed Meat Consumption: Implications for Health and Environmental Sustainability" *Proceedings of the Nutrition Society* 75, no. (2016): 367–73.

34. R. Micha, J. L. Peñalvo, F. Cudhea et al., "Association between Dietary Factors and Mortality from Heart Disease, Stroke, and Type 2 Diabetes in the United States," *JAMA* 317, no. 9 (2017): 912–24.

35. K. D. Hall, A. Ayuketah, R. Brychta et al., "Ultra-processed Diets Cause Excess Calorie Intake and Weight Gain: An Inpatient Randomized Controlled Trial of Ad Libitum Food Intake," *Cell Metabolism* 30, no. 1 (2019): 67–77.

36. G. Otero, G. Pechlaner, G. Liberman, E. Gürcan, "The Neoliberal Diet and Inequality in the United States," *Social Science & Medicine* 142 (2015): 47–55.

37. A. M. Reese, *Black Food Geographies: Race, Self-reliance, and Food Access in Washington* (Chapel Hill: University of North Carolina Press, 2019).

38. Otero, *The Neoliberal Diet*, 93–98.

39. Ibid., 99.

40. A. Brones, "Food Apartheid: The Root of the Problem with America's Groceries," *Guardian*, May 15, 2018.

41. E. A. Beverly, M. D. Ritholz, L. A. Wray, C. J. Chiu, E. Suhl, "Understanding the Meaning of Food in People with Type 2 Diabetes Living in Northern Appalachia," *Diabetes Spectrum* 31, no. 1 (2018): 14–24.

42. M. Mialon, P. Sêrodio, F. B. Scagliusi, "Criticism of the NOVA Classification: Who Are the Protagonists?" *World Nutrition* 9, no. 3 (2018): 176–240.

43. S. J. Vermeulen, B. M. Campbell, J. S. Ingram, "Climate Change and Food Systems," *Annual Review of Environment and Resources* (2012): 37.

44. K. Hamerschlag, "Meat Eaters Guide to Climate Change + Health," Environmental Working Group, 2011.

45. H. C. Godfray, P. Aveyard, T. Garnett et al., "Meat Consumption, Health, and the Environment," *Science* 361, no. 6399 (2018): eaam5324.

46. A. Drewnowski and C. Rehm, "Energy Intakes of US Children and Adults by Food Purchase Location and by Specific Food Source," *Nutrition Journal* 12 (2013): 59.
47. "What to Do When There Are Too Many Product Choices on the Store Shelves," *Consumer Reports*, March 2014.
48. A. Malito, "Grocery Stores Carry 40,000 More Items than They Did in the 1990s," Market Watch, June 17, 2017.
49. T. Mathisen, "Supermarkets Wage War for Your Dollars," NBC Today, January 27, 2011.
50. M. Morris, "40 Ways Grocery Stores Are Scamming You!" August 6, 2018.
51. N. Bose, "Walmart CEO Points to New Company Culture, Cuts Profit Forecast," Reuters, October 16, 2018.
52. B. Ladd, "Playing to Its Strengths: Why Walmart Must Focus on Its Stores and Logistics," *Forbes*, September 9, 2018.
53. T. Hsu, "Walmart Is Finding Success in the Aisle," *New York Times*, August 17, 2018, B3.
54. M. Horst, S. Raj, C. Brinkley, "Getting Outside the Supermarket Box: Alternatives to 'Food Deserts,'" *Progressive Planning* 207 (2016): 9–12.
55. R. Patel, *Stuffed and Starved: The Hidden Battle for the World Food System* (New York: HarperCollins, 2007), 239.
56. "How Many Products Does Walmart Grocery Sell—July 2018?" ScrapeHero, 2018.
57. B. Morgan, "7 Ways Amazon and Walmart Compete—a Look at the Numbers," *Forbes*, August 21, 2019.
58. S. Schmidt, "Walmart's Competitive Advantage: 3 Key Success Factors," Marketresearch.com, August 13, 2018.
59. Hsu, "Walmart Is Finding Success in the Aisle."
60. "Wal-Mart Consumer Reviews," Consumer Affairs, March 19, 2019, https://www.consumeraffairs.com/retail/walmart.htm?page=3#sort=recent&filter=none.
61. Schmidt, "Walmart's Competitive Advantage."
62. "Walmart," Statista Profile, 2018.
63. M. Corkery, "How Walmart, the Big Seller, Is shopping for a Fight with Amazon," *New York Times*, May 9, 2018.
64. "Share of Walmart and Walmart Supercenter Customers in the United States as of 2016, by Income," Statista, 2018.
65. B. C. Lynn, "Breaking the Chain: The Antitrust Case against Walmart," *Harper's Magazine*, July 31, 2006, 1.
66. A. Bonanno and S. J. Goetz, "Food Store Density, Nutrition Education, Eating Habits and Obesity," *International Food and Agribusiness Management Review* 15, no. 4 (2012): 1–26.
67. R. Volpe, A. Okrent, and E. Leibtag, "The Effect of Supercenter-format Stores on the Healthfulness of Consumers' Grocery Purchases," *American Journal of Agricultural Economics* 95, no. 3 (2013): 568–89.
68. J. Hausman and E. Leibtag, "Consumer Benefits from IncreasedCompetition in Shopping Outlets: Measuring the Effect of Wal-Mart," *Journal of Applied Economics* 22, no. 7 (2007): 1157–77.
69. D. R. Bell and J. M. Lattin, "Shopping Behavior and Consumer Preference for Store Price Format: Why "Large Basket" Shoppers Prefer EDLP," *Marketing Science* 17, no. 1 (1998): 66–88.

70. Walmart, "Walmart and HumanaVitality Partner for First-of-its-kind Healthier Food Program Designed to Incentivize Wellness in America, September 19, 2012, . https://corporate.walmart.com/newsroom/2012/09/19/walmart-and-humanavitality-partner-for-first-of-its-kind-healthier-food-program-designed-to-incentivize-wellness-in-america

71. Hsu, "Walmart Is Finding Success in the Aisle."

72. Walmart, store pick up, baby department, https://www.walmart.com/search/?cat_id=5427_133283_1001699&grid=true&ps=40&query=toddler+formula#searchProductResult.

73. Partnership for a Healthier America, "About PHA," n.d., https://www.ahealthieramerica.org/partnership-for-a-healthier-america-pha-2.

74. Partnership for a Healthier America, "Walmart Commitment," January 20, 2012, https://www.ahealthieramerica.org/articles/walmart-commitment-311.

75. Partnership for a Healthier America, "In It for Good: 2015 Annual Progress Report, Executive Brief," https://www.ahealthieramerica.org/documents/23.

76. L. S. Taillie, S. W. Ng, B. M. Popkin, "Packaged Food Purchases at Walmart and Other Food Retail Chains Changes in Nutritional Profile from 2000 to 2013," *American Journal of Preventive Medicine* 50, no. 2 (2016): 171.

77. L. Smith, S. W. Ng, B. M. Popkin, "Can a Food Retailer-Based Healthier Foods Initiative Improve the Nutrient Profile of US Packaged Food Purchases? A Case Study of Walmart, 2000–2013," Health Affairs (Project Hope)" 34, no. 11 (2015): 1869.

78. A. Bhattarai, "Americans Are Buying More Food at Walmart," *Washington Post*, August 17, 2017.

79. I. Ken, "Profit in the Food Desert: Walmart Stakes Its Claim," *Theory in Action* 7, no. 4 (2014): 13.

80. B. Huber, "Walmart's Fresh Food Makeover: Can the Retailer Known for Its Poverty Wages Solve the Problem of Urban 'Food Deserts'?" *The Nation*, September 14, 2011.

81. A. Drewnowski, C. D. Rehm, "Energy Intakes of US Children and Adults by Food Purchase Location and by Specific Food Source," *Nutrition Journal* 12, no. 1 (2013): 59.

82. Statista, "Number of Establishments in the United States Fast Food Industry from 2004 to 2018, May 15, 2013, https://www.statista.com/statistics/196619/total-number-of-fast-food-restaurants-in-the-us-since-2002/.

83. C. D. Fryar, J. P. Hughes, K. A. Herrick, N. Ahluwalia, "Fast Food Consumption among Adults in the United States, 2013–2016," NCHS Data Brief, no. 322, October 2018, 1–8.

84. M. Hartman, "Does McDonald's Have Too Many Items on the Menu?" *Marketplace*, May 23, 2013.

85. E. Brelsford, "McDonald's 10 Most Popular Menu Items May Surprise You," *One Country*, January 10, 2017, https://www.onecountry.com/lifestyle/mcdonalds-most-popular-menu-items/.

86. R. Gebeloff and R. Abrams, "Thanks to Wall St., There May Be Too Many Restaurants," *New York Times*, October 31, 2017.

87. E. Teixeira, "Franchise Fast-Food Industry Continues Consolidation as Sonic Drive-In Chain Is Acquired," *Forbes*, September 26, 2018.

88. P. H. Howard, *Concentration and Power in the Food System: Who Controls What We Eat?* (New Delhi: Bloomsbury Publishing), Kindle.

89. A. Chapin, "McDonald's Seeks 'Nocturnivores' for Midnight Breakfast," *MacLeans*, August 22, 2012.

90. M. A. McCrory, A. G. Harbaugh, A. Appeadu, S. B. Roberts, "Fast-food Offerings in the United States in 1986, 1991, and 2016 Show Large Increases in Food Variety, Portion Size, Dietary Energy, and Selected Micronutrients," *Journal of the Academy of Nutrition and Dietetics* 119, no. 6 (2019): 923–33.

91. J. Maze, "Among QSRS, the Big Get Bigger," *Restaurant Business*, May 2, 2019, https://www.restaurantbusinessonline.com/financing/among-qsrs-big-get-bigger.

92. C. Roberts, R. Ilieva, C. Willingham, N. Freudenberg, "Reducing Predatory Marketing of Unhealthy Foods and Beverages in New York City: Policy Options for Governments and Communities," CUNY Urban Food Policy Institute, 2019.

93. J. L. Harris, W. Frazier, S. Kumanyika, A. G. Ramirez, "Increasing Disparities in Unhealthy Food Advertising Targeted to Hispanic and Black Youth," *Rudd Report*, 2019.

94. J. Littman, "Global Fast Food Market to Surpass $690B by 2022," *Restaurant Dive*, July 15, 2019.

95. H. Timmons, "Breastfeeding Is Winning! So Companies Are Pushing 'Toddler Milk' to Neurotic Parents," *Quartz*, February 9, 2014.

96. UNICEF, Breastfeeding, July 29, 2015, https://www.unicef.org/nutrition/index_24824.html.

97. D. B. Jelliffe and E. P. Jelliffe, "The Infant Food Industry and International Child Health," *International Journal of Health Services* 7, no. 2 (1977): 249–54.

98. World Health Organization, "International Code of Marketing of Breast-milk Substitutes," 1981.

99. UNICEF, "International Code of Marketing of Breast-milk Substitutes Update," January 12, 2005.

100. "Baby Food in the US—Analysis," Euromonitor International, September 2018.

101. K. Browne, "Do Toddlers Need Their Own Milk?" *Choice*, July 7, 2014.

102. UConn Rudd Center for Food Policy & Obesity, "Nutrition and Marketing of Baby and Toddler Food and Drinks," January 2017.

103. K. McKeever, "Perfecting Infant Formula with BabyNes," City Dads Group, March 9, 2016.

104. "Best Performance Coming from Toddler Milk Formula," Euromonitor International, 2018.

105. "Toddler Milk Formula Performs Well in Saturated Developed Markets," Euromonitor International, 2018.

106. See, for example, S. I. Granheim, K. Engelhardt, P. Rundall et al., "Interference in Public Health Policy: Examples of How the Baby Food Industry Uses Tobacco Industry Tactics," *World Nutrition* 2, no. 2 (2017): 288–310; B. Jasani, K. Simmer, S. K. Patole, S. C. Rao, "Long Chain Polyunsaturated Fatty Acid Supplementation in Infants Born at Term," Cochrane Database of Systematic Reviews, issue 3, art. no: CD000376; R. J. Boyle, D. Ierodiakonou et al. "Hydrolysed Formula and Risk of Allergic or Autoimmune Disease: Systematic Review and Meta-Analysis," *The BMJ* 352 (2016): i974.

107. C. White, "Ranjit Chandra: How Reputation Bamboozled the Scientific Community," *The BMJ* 351 (2015): h5683.

108. J. L. Pomeranz, M. J. Palafox, J. L. Harris, "Toddler Drinks, Formulas, and Milks: Labeling Practices and Policy Implications," *Preventive Medicine* 109 (2018): 11–16.

109. S. I. Granheim, K. Engelhardt, P. Randall P, "Interference in Public Health Policy: Examples of How the Baby Food Industry Uses Tobacco Industry Tactics," *World Nutrition* 8, no. 2 (2017): 288–310.

110. J. Maalouf, M. E. Cogswell, M. Bates et al., "Sodium, Sugar, and Fat Content of Complementary Infant and Toddler Foods Sold in the United States, 2015," *The American Journal of Clinical Nutrition* 105, no. 6 (June 2017): 1443–52.

111. K. Singer, C. N. Lumeng, "The Initiation of Metabolic Inflammation in Childhood Obesity," Journal of Clinical Investigation 127, no. 1 (2017): 65–73.

112. M. B. Vos, S. H. Abrams, S. E. Barlow et al., "NASPGHAN Clinical Practice Guideline for the Diagnosis and Treatment of Nonalcoholic Fatty Liver Disease in Children: Recommendations from the Expert Committee on NAFLD (ECON) and the North American Society of Pediatric Gastroenterology, Hepatology and Nutrition (NASPGHAN)," *Journal of Pediatric Gastroenterology and Nutrition* 64, no. 2 (2017): 319.

113. Bayer, "Products for the Health of Humans, Animals and Plants," nd, https://www.bayer.com/en/product-portfolio-of-bayer.aspx.

114. D. Meyer, "As Bayer's Roundup Cancer Costs Accumulate, Questions Linger about the Wisdom of Its Monsanto Merger," *Fortune*, March 30, 2019.

115. R. Bender, "How Bayer-Monsanto Became One of the Worst Corporate Deals— in 12 Charts," *Wall Street Journal*, August 28, 2019.

116. BASF, "Precision Agriculture in the Digital Era," n.d., https://www.basf.com/cn/en/media/BASF-Information/Food-nutrition/Precision-agriculture-in-the-digital-era.html.

117. "What Is Palm Oil?" PalmOil Investigations, n.d., https://www.palmoilinvestigations.org/about-palm-oil.html.

118. P. Tullis, "How the World Got Hooked on Palm Oil," *Guardian*, February 19, 2019.

119. Grand View Research, "Palm Oil Market Is Anticipated to Grow to $88 Billion by 2022: New Report by Grand View Research, Inc., July 27, 2015, https://www.globenewswire.com/news-release/2015/07/27/755234/10143225/en/Palm-Oil-Market-Is-Anticipated-To-Grow-To-88-Billion-By-2022-New-Report-By-Grand-View-Research-Inc.html.

120. US FDA, "Final Determination Regarding Partially Hydrogenated Oils (Removing Trans Fat), https://www.fda.gov/Food/IngredientsPackagingLabeling/FoodAdditivesIngredients/ucm449162.htm.

121. E. J. Brandt, R. Myerson, M. C. Perraillon, T. S. Polonsky, "Hospital Admissions for Myocardial Infarction and Stroke before and after the Trans-Fatty Acid Restrictions in New York," *JAMA Cardiology* 2, no. 6 (2017): 627–34.

122. A. Mancini, E. Imperlini, E. Nigro, C. Montagnese, A. Daniele, S. Orrù, P. Buono, "Biological and Nutritional Properties of Palm Oil and Palmitic Acid: Effects on Health," *Molecules* 20, no. 9 (2015): 17339–61.

123. N. A. Muhamad, N. Mustapha, M. F. Baharin et al., "Impact of Palm Oil versus Other Oils on Weight Changes: A Systematic Review," *Food and Nutrition Sciences* 9, no. 7 (2018): 915.

124. Q. Wang, A. Afshin, M. Y. Yakoob et al., "Impact of Nonoptimal Intakes of Saturated, Polyunsaturated, and Trans Fat on Global Burdens of Coronary Heart Disease," *JAMA* 5 (2016): e002891.

125. G. Scrinis, C. A. Monteiro, "Ultraprocessed Foods and the Limits of Product Reformulation," *Public Health Nutrition* 21, no. 1 (2018): 247–52.

126. P. Tullis, "How the World Got Hooked on Palm Oil," *Guardian*, February 19, 2019.

127. O. Milman, "US Investors Ploughing Billions into Palm Oil, Claims Report," *Guardian*, July 26, 2016.

128. European Commission, "Energy for the Future: Renewable Sources of Energ" (white paper, Community Strategy and Action Plan, November 26, 1997).

129. A. Lustgarten, "Palm Oil Was Supposed to Help Save the Plant. Instead It Unleashed a Catastrophe," *The New York Times Sunday Magazine*, November 25, 2018, 42.

130. Tullis, "How the World Got Hooked on Palm Oil."

131. Ibid.

132. Lustgarten, "Palm Oil Was Supposed to Help Save the Plant," 42.

132 Tullis, "How the World Got Hooked on Palm Oil."

133. Lustgarten, "Palm Oil Was Supposed to Help Save the Plant," 42.

134. S. N. Koplitz, L. J. Mickley, M. E. Marlier et al., "Public Health Impacts of the Severe Haze in Equatorial Asia in September–October 2015: Demonstration of a New Framework for Informing Fire Management Strategies to Reduce Downwind Smoke Exposure," *Environmental Research Letters* 11, no. 9 (2016): 094023.

135. S. Balaton-Chrimes, "Sustainable Palm Oil Must Consider People Too," *The Conversation*, November 21, 2013.

136. GRAIN, "The Global Farmland Grab in 2016: How Big, How Bad?" June 2016.

137. Alliance against Industrial Plantations in West and Central Africa, "Communities in Africa Fight Back against the Land Grab for Palm Oil," September 19, 2019.

138. T. Reardon, C. P. Timmer, C. B. Barrett, J. Berdegué, "The Rise of Supermarkets in Africa, Asia, and Latin America," *American Journal of Agricultural Economics* 85, no. 5 (2003): 1140–46.

139. M. Carlson "Obituary of Earl Butz," *Guardian*, February 7, 2008.

140. B. Popkin, G. Bray, and F. Hu, "The Role of High Sugar Foods and Sugar-sweetened Beverages in Weight Gain and Obesity," *Managing and Preventing Obesity: Behavioral Factors and Dietary Interventions*, ed. T. Gill, (Amsterdam: Elsevier, 2014), 45–57.

141. Food and Water Watch, "The Economic Cost of Food Monopolies," 2012.

142. US Department of Agriculture, Economic Research Service (USDA ERS), Retail Trends, 2017.

143. P. Baker and S. Friel, "Food Systems Transformations, Ultraprocessed Food Markets and the Nutrition Transition in Asia," *Global Health* 12, no. 1 (2016): 80.

144. World Bank, "Commodity Markets Outlook," Washington, DC, 2015.

145. M. Kalkuhl, J. von Braun, M. Torero, "Volatile and Extreme Food Prices, Food Security, and Policy: An Overview," in *Food Price Volatility and Its Implications for Food Security and Policy 2016* (New York: Springer), 3–31.

146. S. Prato, E. Daño, T. Zundel et al., "Policies that Strengthen the Nexus between Food, Health, Ecology, Livelihoods and Identities," Spotlight on Sustainable Development, 2018, 58–76, www.2030spotlight.org.

147. R. Siegel, "As Dollar Stores Move into Cities, Residents See a Steep Downside," *Washington Post*, February 15, 2019.

148. M. Donahue and S. Mitchell, "Dollar Stores Are Targeting Struggling Urban Neighborhoods and Small Towns. One Community Is Showing How to Fight Back," Institute for Local Self-Reliance, December 2018.

149. M. Frazier, "Dollar General Hits a Gold Mine in Rural America," Bloomberg News, October 11, 2017.

150. J. L. Schupp, "Cultivating Better Food Access? The Role of Farmers' Markets in the US Local Food Movement," *Rural Sociology* 82, no. 2 (2017): 318–48; J. Rayner, "The Rise of Social Supermarkets: 'It's Not about Selling Cheap Food, but Building Strong Communities,'" *Guardian*, May 19, 2019; N. Freudenberg, "Healthy-food Procurement: Using the Public Plate to Reduce Food Insecurity and Diet-related Diseases," *The Lancet Diabetes & Endocrinology* 4, no. 5 (2016): 383–84.

151. Jose M. Ordovas, R. Lynnette Ferguson, E. Shyong Tai, John C. Mathers, "Personalised Nutrition and Health," *The BMJ* 361 (2018): bmj.k2173.

152. J. Guthman, *Agrarian Dreams: The Paradox of Organic Farming in California* (Berkeley: University of California Press, 2014).

153. P. Ausick, "Eight Largest Cities without Walmart," 24/7 Wall Street, June 16, 2014.

154. M. Corkery, "Walmart Finally Makes It to the Big Apple," *New York Times*, September 17, 2018, B1.

155. S. Halzack "Walmart Is Ending Its Express Concept and Closing 269 Stores," *Washington Post*, January 15, 2016.

156. J. Dumont, "Walmart to Close 8 Neighborhood Markets," Grocery Dive, March 26, 2019.

157. A. Merrick, "The Walmart-Free City," *The New Yorker*, May 27, 2014.

158. Coalition of Immokalee Workers, "About Us," n.d., https://ciw-online.org/about/.

159. S. Bowen, J. Brenton, E. Sinikka, *Pressure Cooker: Why Cooking Won't Solve Our Problems and What We Can Do about It* (New York: Oxford University Press, 2019), 228.

160. T. Luhby, "Bernie Sanders Unveils Stop Walmart Act," CNN Business, November 15, 2018.

161. World Health Organization, *Guidance on Ending the Inappropriate Promotion of Foods for Infants and Young Children: Implementation Manual* (Geneva: World Health Organization, 2017).

162. Changing Markets Foundation, "Purpose," n.d., https://changingmarkets.org/about/.

163. Changing Markets Foundation, "Milking It: How Milk Formula Companies Are Putting Profits before Science," https://changingmarkets.org/wp-content/uploads/2017/10/Milking-it-Final-report-CM.pdf

164. Changing Markets Foundation, "Busting the Myth of Science-based Formula: An Investigation into Nestlé Infant Milk Products and Claims," 2018.

165. Changing Markets Foundation, "Annual Report 2018," http://changingmarkets.org/wp-content/uploads/2019/04/Changing_Markets_Annual_Report_2018.pdf.

166. J. Lucey, "To Save the Rainforest, We Need to Work with the Palm Oil Industry," *Guardian*, January 15, 2019.

167. Mondelez International, "About Us," n.d., https://www.mondelezinternational.com/about-us.

168. Greenpeace, "Six Greenpeace Activists Arrested on Board a Ship Loaded with Palm Oil Heading to Europe," November 17, 2018, https://www.greenpeace.org/international/press-release/19371/six-greenpeace-activists-arrested-on-board-a-ship-loaded-with-palm-oil-heading-to-europe/.

169. J. Glendary, "Iceland Wriggles Out of Self-imposed Palm Oil Ban by Removing Own Brand Labels," The Drum, January 25, 2019.

170. S. Kadandale, R. Marten, and R. Smith, "The Palm Oil Industry and Noncommunicable Diseases," *Bulletin of the World Health Organization* 97, no. 2 (2019): 118.
171. Friends of the Earth, "Senators Push Financial Firms to Address Global Deforestation," February 6, 2019, https://foe.org/news/senators-push-financial-firms-address-global-deforestation/.
172. C. J. Rhodes, "The Imperative for Regenerative Agriculture," *Science Progress* 100, no. 1 (2017): 80–129.
173. C. Francis, G. Lieblein, S. Gliessman et al., "Agroecology: The Ecology of Food Systems," *Journal of Sustainable Agriculture* 22 (2003): 99–118.
174. A. Wezel, S. Bellon, T. Doré, et al., "Agroecology as a Science, a Movement and a Practice: A Review," *Agronomy for Sustainable Development* 29, no. 4 (2009): 503–15.
175. D. Moss and M. Bittman, "Bringing Farming Back to Nature," *New York Times*, June 26, 2018.
176. K. Hansen-Kuhn, "Bold Farm Plans in Mexico Offer a Ray of Hope in 2019," Institute for Agriculture and Trade Policy, January 15, 2019, https://www.iatp.org/blog/201903/bold-farm-plans-mexico-offer-ray-hope-2019.
177. Agroecology Research Action Collective, "The Need for a Food and Agriculture Platform in the Green New Deal," 2019, https://agroecologyresearchaction.org/green-new-deal/.
178. D. Ortega-Espes, "Agroecology: Innovating for Sustainable Agriculture and Food Systems," Friends of the Earth International, 2018.

CHAPTER 3
1. D. Nasaw, *Schooled to Order: A Social History of Public Schooling in the United States* (New York: Oxford University Press, 1981).
2. J. Bryant and J. Sarakatsannis, "Three More Reasons Why US Education Is Ready for Investment," McKinsey & Company, November 30, 2016.
3. S. Mencimer, "Fox in the Schoolhouse: Rupert Murdoch Wants to Teach Your Kids! News Corp.'s Major Move into the Education Business," *Mother Jones*, September 23, 2011.
4. "Private Education," Special Report, *The Economist*, April 13, 2019, 3–9.
5. M. E. Biery, "These Types of Businesses Have the Highest Returns," *Forbes*, May 5, 2017.
6. L. Lyda Ghanbari, M. D. McCall, "Current Employment Statistics Survey: 100 Years of Employment, Hours, and Earnings," Monthly Labor Review, US Bureau of Labor Statistics, August 2016.
7. L. Uchitelle, "To Add Jobs, Look Past Manufacturing," *New York Times*, May 5, 2019.
8. US Government Spending on Education, https://www.usgovernmentspending.com/spending_chart_1980_2020USb_20s2li011lcn_20t.
9. W. W. Powell, K. Snellman, "The Knowledge Economy," *Annual Review of Sociology* 30 (2004): 199–220.
10. E. S. Savas, E. S. Savas, *Privatization and Public-private Partnerships* (Washington, DC: CQ Press, 2000).
11. D. Hursh, "Neo-liberalism, Markets and Accountability: Transforming Education and Undermining Democracy in the United States and England," *Policy Futures in Education* 3, no. 1 (2005): 3–15.
12. I. W. Martin, *The Permanent Tax Revolt: How the Property Tax Transformed American Politics* (Redwood City, CA: Stanford University Press, 2008), 126.

13. V. Rancaño, "How Proposition 13 Transformed Neighborhood Public Schools throughout California," KQED News, October 25, 2018, https://www.kqed.org/news/11701044/how-proposition-13-transformed-neighborhood-public-schools-throughout-california.

14. M. Fabricant and S. Brier, *Austerity Blues: Fighting for the Soul of Public Higher Education* (Baltimore: Johns Hopkins University Press, 2016), 36.

15. S. Raynes and A. Rutledge, *The Analysis of Structured Securities: Precise Risk Measurement and Capital Allocation* (Oxford University Press on Demand, 2003).

16. A. Fraser, S. Tan, M. Lagarde, N. Mays, "Narratives of Promise, Narratives of Caution: A Review of the Literature on Social Impact Bonds, *Social Policy & Administration* 52 (2018): 4–28.

17. R. W. Lake, "The Subordination of Urban Policy in the Time of Financialization," in *Urban Policy in the Time of Obama*, ed. C. Johnson and J. DeFilippis (Minneapolis: University of Minnesota Press, 2016), 57.

18. A. E. Tse and M. E. Warner, "The Razor's Edge: Social Impact Bonds and the Financialization of Early Childhood Services," *Journal of Urban Affairs* 12 (2018): 1–7.

19. P. Lipman, "Capitalizing on Crisis: Venture Philanthropy's Colonial Project to Remake Urban Education," *Critical Studies in Education* 56, no. 2 (2015): 241–58.

20. B. D. Baker, "Exploring the Consequences of Charter School Expansion in U.S. Cities," Economic Policy Institute, November 30, 2016, https://www.epi.org/files/pdf/109218.pdf.

21. C. Eaton, J. Habinek, A. Goldstein et al., "The Financialization of US Higher Education," *Socio-Economic Review* 14, no. 3 (2016): 507–35.

22. Education Management Corporation (EDMC), 10-K Annual Report," September 2012, https://last10k.com/sec-filings/edmc/0000880059-12-000013.htm.

23. L. Meckler, "Betsy DeVos Reinstates Controversial Gatekeeper of For-profit Colleges," *Washington Post*, November 21, 2018.

24. Project on Predatory Student Lending, " 'Covid College Cons' Series Exposes Predatory For-Profit Colleges Targeting Students during Covid-19 Crisis," April 15, 2020.

25. B. Wakamo, "Instead of Bailing Out For-Profit Colleges, Congress Should Cancel Student Debt," Inequality.org, June 15, 2020.

26. Pearson, "Our Company," no date, https://www.pearson.com/corporate#our-company; J. Reingold, "Everybody Hates Pearson," *Fortune*, January 21, 2015.

27. S. Tanenhaas, "Can Chris Whittle Launch a Truly Global Academy?" Town & Country, July 10, 2018.

28. McKinsey & Company, "Education," n.d., https://www.mckinsey.com/industries/social-sector/how-we-help-clients/education.

29. B. De Smedt, "Applications of (Cognitive) Neuroscience in Educational Research," in *Oxford Handbook of Educational Research*, ed. G. Noblit (New York: Oxford University Press, 2018), 1–23.

30. F. Boninger, A. Molnar, C. M. Saldaña, "Personalized Learning and the Digital Privatization of Curriculum and Teaching," National Educational Policy Center, 2019.

31. J. Pittock and C. Corbin-Thaddies, "Personalized Learning: A Student-Centered Approach for Learning Success," *Medium*, June 26, 2017.

32. J. Spohrer and G. Banavar, "Cognition as a Service: An Industry Perspective," *AI Magazine* 36, no. 4 (2015): 71–86.

33. "The Growing Demand for EdTech during Coronavirus Lockdown," Credit Suisse, April 8, 2020.
34. T. J. McCue, "E Learning Climbing to $325 Billion by 2025," *Forbes*, July 31, 2018.
35. B. Williamson, "Silicon Startup Schools: Technocracy, Algorithmic Imaginaries and Venture Philanthropy in Corporate Education Reform," *Critical Studies in Education* 59, no. 2 (2018): 218–36.
36. K. McClure, "Examining the 'Amenities Arms Race' in Higher Education: Shifting from Rhetoric to Research," *College Student Affairs Journal* 37, no. 2 (2019): 128–42.
37. A. Wolf, *Does Education Matter?: Myths about Education and Economic Growth* (London: Penguin UK), 2002.
38. J. Stein and P. Marley, *More Than They Bargained For: Scott Walker, Unions, and the Fight for Wisconsin* (Madison: University of Wisconsin Press, 2013).
39. E. Schmidt and J. Cohen, *The New Digital Age: Reshaping the Future of People, Nations and Business* (London: John Murray, 2013), 9–10.
40. H. Ryan, "Who Is Behind the Assault on Public Schools?" *Monthly Review* 68, no. 11 (2017): 31–40.
41. S. J. Ball, *Global Education Inc.: New Policy Networks and the Neoliberal Imaginary* (Abingdon, Oxfordshire: Routledge, 2012).
42. D. Ravitch, *The Death and Life of the Great American School System: How Testing and Choice Are Undermining Education* (New York: Basic Books, 2010), 195–222.
43. E. B. Rust Jr., "Higher Standards, Stronger Tests: There's No Turning Back," *Education Week*, January 19, 2000.
44. P. Vogel, "Here Are the Corporations and Right-Wing Funders Backing the Education Reform Movement," Media Matters, April 27, 2016.
45. E. Pilkington, "Revealed: Secret Rightwing Strategy to Discredit Teacher Strikes," *Guardian*, April 12, 2018.
46. J. P. Greene and F. Hess, "Education Reform's Deep Blue Hue," Education Next, March 11, 2019.
47. D. Ravitch, *Slaying Goliath: The Passionate Resistance to Privatization and the Fight to Save America's Schools* (New York: Knopf, 2020), 117.
48. L. M. Anderson, C. Shinn, M. T. Fullilove S. C. Scrimshaw, J. E. Fielding, J. Normand, V. G. Carande-Kulis, and the Task Force on Community Preventive Services, "The Effectiveness of Early Childhood Development Programs: A Systematic Review," *American Journal of Preventive Medicine* 24, no. 3 (2003): 32–46.
49. P. Muennig, D. Robertson, G. Johnson et al., "The Effect of an Early Education Program on Adult Health: The Carolina Abecedarian Project Randomized Controlled Trial," *American Journal of Public Health* 101, no. 3 (2011): 512–16.
50. Ibid.
51. K. A. Magnuson and J. Waldfogel, "Early Childhood Care and Education: Effects on Ethnic and Racial Gaps in School Readiness," *Future Child* 15, no. 1 (2005): 169–96.
52. B. Schulte and A. Durana, "The New America Care Report," New America, September 28, 2016, 1–104.
53. R. Mead, "The Lessons of Mayor Bill de Blasio's Universal Pre-K Initiative," *New Yorker*, September 7, 2017.
54. S. Bishop-Josef, C. Beakey, S. Watson, T. Garrett, *Want to Grow the Economy? Fix the Child Care Crisis* (Washington: Council for Strong America, 2019).

55. E. García and E. Weiss, "Early Education Gaps by Social Class and Race Start US Children Out on Unequal Footing: A Summary of the Major Findings in "Inequalities at the Starting Gate," *Economic Policy Institute*, 2015.

56. See "How Much More Expensive Childcare Is Than Getting a Higher Education," How Much, 2018, https://howmuch.net/articles/child-care-vs-college-costs.

57. R. A. Hahn, W. S. Barnett, J. A. Knopf et al., "Early Childhood Education to Promote Health Equity: A Community Guide Systematic Review," *Journal of Public Health Management and Practice* 22, no. 5 (2016): E1.

58. S. Thomason, L. J. E. Austin, A. Bernhardt et al., "At the Wage Floor: Covering Homecare and Early Care and Education Workers in the New Generation of Minimum Wage Laws," Center for Labor Research and Education, Center for the Study of Child Care Employment, and COWS, May 2018, https://cscce.berkeley.edu/files/2018/05/At-the-Wage-Floor.pdf.

59. Kids Count, "Children under Age 6 with All Available Parents in the Labor Force in the United States," Kids Count Data Center, 2018.

60. Omidyar Network, "Big Ideas, Little Learners: Early Childhood Trends Report 2019," 1–37.

61. National Center for Education Statistics, "2016 National Household Education Survey: Early Childhood Program Participation Survey."

62. L. Schochet and R. Malik, "2 Million Parents Forced to Make Career Sacrifices Due to Problems with Child Care," Center for American Progress, September 13, 2017.

63. P. Neighmond, "Poll: Cost of Child Care Causes Financial Stress for Many Families," *NPR Morning Edition*, NPR, October 26, 2016.

64. Omidyar Network, "Big Ideas, Little Learners," 1–37.

65. D & B Hoover's, "KinderCare Education LLC Profile," 2019.

66. T. Wyatt, "Two Sides of the Private Equity Coin—PE Hub," PE Hub Network, February 26, 2019.

67. M. Strattford, "DeVos Review Identifies 102 Financial Interests with Potential Conflicts," Politico, January 20, 2017.

68. Partners Group, "About Partners Group," n.d., https://www.partnersgroup.com/en/about/.

69. Bloomberg TV, "Partners Group's Path to PE Success," January 9, 2018.

70. T. Mitchenall, "How to Build a 21st Century Returns Factory," Privately Speaking, in Private Equity International, February, 2019, 31–35.

71. T. Wyatt, "Two Sides of the Private Equity Coin," PE Hub, February 26, 2019.

72. KinderCare Education, "KinderCare Education Acquires Rainbow Child Care Center, Expanding to More Than 1,500 Learning Centers, Serving 185,000 Children across the United States," August 27, 2018.

73. "Moody's Says KinderCare's Term Loan Add-on Is Credit Negative; Ratings and Outlook Unchanged," *Moody's*, September 26, 2018.

74. KinderCare, "Leadership: Chief Executive Officer of KinderCare Education— Tom Wyatt," n.d., https://www.kindercare.com/about-us/who-we-are/leadership-and-experts.

75. A. Marum, "KinderCare Uses Big Data to Turn Company Profitable," *The Oregonian*, August 12, 2017.

76. Quotes from "What Are Your Views on the Daycare KinderCare Chain?" Winnie, March 6, 2018, https://winnie.com/post/what-are-your-views-on-18d3efcb.

77. *Eunice Kennedy Shriver* National Institute of Child Health and Human Development, "The NICHD Study of Early Child Care and Youth Development (SECCYD): Findings for Children up to Age 4½ Years (Reference Only)," Washington, DC: US Government Printing Office, 2006.

78. J. Cohn, "The Hell of American Day Care," *The New Republic*, April 15, 2013.

79. US Department of Education, "A Matter of Equity: Preschool in America," 2015.

80. KinderCare Learning Centers, "KinderCare Kids Do Better," n.d., https://www.kindercare.com/about-us/who-we-are/our-approach-to-education.

81. R. Pitzel, The Smart and Easy Choice for Childcare and Preschool: KinderCare Learning Centers," February 7, 2018, http://rachelpitzel.com/2018/02/07/smart-easy-choice-childcare-preschool-kindercare-learning-centers/.

82. Brimhurst Kindercare, Houston Texas, Yelp Review, July 23, 2018, https://www.yelp.com/biz/brimhurst-kindercare-houston.

83. Cohn, "The Hell of American Day Care."

84. J. Wrigley and J. Dreby, "Fatalities and the Organization of Child Care in the United States, 1985–2003," *American Sociological Review* 70, no. 5 (2005): 729–57.

85. New Profit, "Our Impact," n.d., https://oldnp.hiker.co/our-impact/impact-stories/acelero-learning/

86. A. LiBetti, "Leading by Exemplar Data Utilization Practices in Head Start Programs," Bellwether Education Partners, 2019, https://bellwethereducation.org/sites/default/files/Leading percent20by percent20Exemplar percent20Lessons percent20from percent20Head percent20Start percent20Programs_Bellwether.pdf.

87. United States Census Bureau, "School Spending per Pupil Increased by 3.2 Percent, U.S. Census Bureau Reports," May 21, 2018, Release Number CB18-TPS.28.

88. D& B Hoover, "Company Profile, K12 Inc.," 2020.

89. "Attorney General Kamala D. Harris Announces $168.5 Million Settlement with K12 Inc., a For-Profit Online Charter School Operator," Office of the Attorney General of California, July 8, 2016, https://oag.ca.gov/news/press-releases/attorney-general-kamala-d-harris-announces-1685-million-settlement-k12-inc.

90. M. Hensley-Clancy, "Charter School Company Blasts 'Shameless' California Attorney General," Buzz Feed News, July 12, 2016, https://www.buzzfeednews.com/article/mollyhensleyclancy/charter-school-company-blasts-shameless-california-ag.

91. T. Tagami, "Petition for New Online Charter School with K12 Inc. Denied," *Atlanta Journal-Constitution*, August 28, 2019.

92. Forbes, "Forbes 2019 Annual Global 2000 List."

93. A. Kamanetz, "Testing: How Much Is Too Much?" *NPREd*, NPR, November 17, 2014.

94. J. Reingold, "Everybody Hates Pearson," *Fortune*, January 21, 2015.

95. National Commission on Excellence in Education, "A Nation at Risk: The Imperative for Educational Reform," *The Elementary School Journal* 84, no. 2 (1983): 113–30.

96. O. Davis, "No Test Left Behind: How Pearson Made a Killing on the US Testing Craze," TPM (Talking Points Memo), December 19, 2016.

97. V. Strauss, "Report: Big Education Firms Spend Millions Lobbying for Pro-testing Policies," *Washington Post*, March 30, 2015.

98. White House (website), "President Bush Discusses No Child Left Behind," January 8, 2009, https://georgewbush-whitehouse.archives.gov/news/releases/2009/01/20090108-2.html.

99. S. Cavanagh, "Assessing the State of the K-12 Testing Market, as Dynamics Shift," *EdWeek Market Brief*, August 10, 2015.

100. Davis, "No Test Left Behind."

101. G. Spanier, "John Fallon Takes Pearson Helm and Axes Adult Education," *Evening Standard* (London), January 7, 2013.

102. Reingold, "Everybody Hates Pearson."

103. C. R. Pooley, "Pearson Agrees to Sale of US School Textbook Business," *Financial Times*, February 18, 2019.

104. P. Nilsson, "Pearson Chief Executive's £1.5 M Bonus Pushes Up Pay 70 Percent," *Financial Times*, March 25, 2019.

105. S. Cavanagh, "Common-Core Testing Contracts Favor Big Vendors," *Education Week*, September 30, 2014.

106. C. Quintan and R. Nott, "Judge Tosses Challenge to Vendor's Contract for Statewide Student Tests," *The New Mexican*, July 15, 2015.

107. Cavanagh, "Assessing the State of the K-12 Testing Market, as Dynamics Shift."

108. Davis, "No Test Left Behind."

109. V. Strauss, "Pearson Criticized for Finding Test Essay Scorers on Craigslist," *Washington Post*, January 16, 2013.

110. J. Reingold, "Everybody Hates Pearson."

111. J. L. Woodworth, M. E. Raymond, and K. Chirbas et al., "Online Charter School Study, 2015," Credo: Center for Research on Education Outcomes.

112. B. Herold, "Pearson Studies Seek to Shine Light on Cyber Charter Student Mobility," Education Week, July 20, 2018.

113. Open Secrets, "Pearson PLC, Annual Lobbying Contributions, 1998–2019," https://www.opensecrets.org/orgs/lobbying?id=D000068157.

114. S. Simon, "No Profit Left Behind," Politico, February 10, 2015.

115. Davis, "No Test Left Behind."

116. "Glimpse K12 Analysis of School Spending Shows That Two-Thirds of Software License Purchases Go Unused," Glimpse, May 15, 2019, https://www.globenewswire.com/news-release/2019/05/15/1825260/0/en/Glimpse-K12-Analysis-of-School-Spending-Shows-that-Two-Thirds-of-Software-License-Purchases-Go-Unused.html.

117. US Department of Education, "Postsecondary Education," chapter 3 in *Digest of Education Statistics, 2011* (Washington, DC: Department of Education [NCES 2012–001], 2012), 279–412; R. Fry and K. Parker, *Record Shares of Young Adults Have Finished Both High School and College* (Washington, DC: Pew Research Center, 2012); US Department of Education, *Digest of Education Statistics, 2008.* (Washington, DC: Department of Education [NCES 2009–020], 2009), NCES 2009–020.

118. US Department of Education, "*National Postsecondary Student Aid Study* (Washington, DC: Department of Education [NPSAS 96]); and *2015–2016 National Postsecondary Student Aid Study* (Washington, DC: Department of Education [NPSAS:16]).

119. P. Oreopoulos and U. Petronijevic, "Making College Worth It: A Review of Research on the Returns to Higher Education," National Bureau of Economic Research, 2013.

120. National Center for Education Statistics, "Tuition Costs of Colleges and Universities," https://nces.ed.gov/fastfacts/display.asp?id=76.

121. D. Bok, *Universities in the Marketplace: The Commercialization of Higher Education* (Princeton, NJ: Princeton University Press, 2004).

122. S. Goldrick-Rab, *Paying the Price: College Costs, Financial Aid, and the Betrayal of the American Dream* (Chicago: University of Chicago Press, 2016).

123. G. Thrush, "After Scaling Back Student Loan Regulations, Administration Tries to Stop State Efforts," *New York Times*, September 7, 2018.

124. US Government Accountability Office, "Federal Student Loans Actions Needed to Improve Oversight of Schools' Default Rates" (Washington, DC: US Government Accountability Office [GAO–18–163U], 2018).

125. S. Cowley, "California Will be Fourth State to Sue Student Loan Servicer," *New York Times*, June 29, 2018.

126. J. E. Bemel, C. Brower, A. Chischillie, and J. Shepherd, "The Impact of College Student Financial Health on Other Dimensions of Health," *American Journal of Health Promotion* 30, no. 4 (2016): 224–30; K. M. Walsemann, G. C. Gee, and D. Gentile, "Sick of Our loans: Student Borrowing and the Mental Health of Young Adults in the United States," *Social Science and Medicine* 124 (2015): 85–93; J. N. Houle and C. Warner, "Into the Red and Back to the Nest? Student Debt, College Completion, and Returning to the Parental Home among Young Adults," *Sociology of Education* 90, no. 1 (2017): 89–108.

127. Student Debt Crisis, Real Student Debt Stories, https://studentdebtcrisis.org/read-student-debt-stories/.

128. L. Scochet, "The Child Care Crisis Is Keeping Women Out of the Workforce," *Center for American Progress*, March 28, 2019.

129. "New Poll Finds Overwhelming Support for Increasing Investments in Quality, Affordable Child Care," Center for American Progress, September 13, 2018.

130. A. Loewenberg, "Newly Elected Governors Make Early Education a Priority," New America, 2018.

131. B. Covert, "Here's Where Every Democratic Candidate Stands on Child Care and Family Leave," *The Nation*, January 13, 2020.

132. Child Care Providers United, "Caring for California Kids, Raising Up Our Profession," n.d., https://childcareprovidersunited.org/who-we-are/.

133. D. Fernandes, "Child Care Providers Celebrate New Law Allowing Them to Unionize," KCRW, September 30, 2019.

134. C. Veiga, "The Difference a Year Makes: As New York City Expands Pre-K for 3-year-olds, Schools Adapt," Chalkbeat, November 28, 2018.

135. C. Campanile, "State Senator Proposes NYC Payroll Tax to Expand Child Care," *New York Post*, September 16, 2019.

136. Center for Children's Initiatives, Alliance for Quality Education, Citizen Action of New York; Schuyler Center for Analysis and Advocacy, "The State of Early Learning in New York: Too Many Young Learners Still Left Out," January 29, 2019.

137. R. Mead, "The Lessons of Mayor Bill de Blasio's Universal Pre-K Initiative," *New Yorker*, September 7, 2017.

138. E. Stewart, "All of West Virginia's Teachers Have Been on Strike for over a Week," Vox, March 4, 2018.

139. K. Andrias, "Peril and Possibility: Strikes, Rights, and Legal Change in the Age of Trump," *Berkeley Journal of Employment and Labor Law*, 40, no. 1 (2019): 135–49.

140. M. Will, "How Teachers Strikes Are Changing," *Education Week*, March 6, 2019.

141. V. Strauss, "Where Else Teachers Are Primed to Strike in 2019—and Why," *Washington Post*, January 28, 2019.

142. M. Will, "How Teacher Strikes Are Changing," *Education Week*, March 6, 2019.

143. A. Ujifusa, "Buckle Up, Betsy DeVos: Democrats Have Won the House," *Education Week*, November 7, 2018.

144. J. Buterbaugh, "Teachers' Strikes a New Social Movement Researcher Says," Penn State News, May 10, 2019, https://news.psu.edu/story/573753/2019/05/10/research/teachers-strikes-new-social-movement-researcher-says.

145. P. Lipman, The Landscape of Education "Reform" in Chicago: Neoliberalism Meets a Grassroots Movement," *Education Policy Analysis Archives* 25, no. 54 (2017): 54.

146. J. S. Rubin, R. M. Good, and M. Fine, "Parental Action and Neoliberal Education Reform: Crafting a Research Agenda," *Journal of Urban Affairs* 42, no. (2020): 492–510.

147. Associated Press, "New Mexico High School Students Walk Out in Protest of New Standardized Test," *Guardian*, March 2, 2015.

148. UNM Newsroom, "Nava to Lead Learning Alliance New Mexico," October 23, 2017, https://news.unm.edu/news/nava-to-lead-learning-alliance-new-mexico.

149. D. Douglas-Gabriel, "Navient's Student Loan Practices 'Failed Borrowers at Every Stage of Repayment,' Consumer Bureau Says," *Washington Post*, January 18, 2017.

150. "Complaint against Navient Corporation, Navient Solutions, Inc., Pioneer Credit Recovery, Inc., Filed by Consumer Financial Protection Bureau," January 18, 2017.

151. Office of the Inspector General, "Federal Student Aid: Additional Actions Needed to Mitigate the Risk of Servicer Noncompliance with Requirements for Servicing Federally Held Student Loans," Control Number ED-OIG/A05Q0008, United States Department of Education, March 5, 2019, https://www2.ed.gov/about/offices/list/oig/auditreports/fy2019/a05q0008.pdf.

152. US Government Accountability Office, "Federal Student Loans Actions Needed to Improve Oversight of Schools' Default Rates," April 2018, GAO–18–163U.

153. A. Kroll, "The Government's Trillion-dollar Student Loan Office is a Train Wreck," *Rolling Stone*, February 22, 2019.

154. S. Cowley, "Navient Agrees to Settle Teachers' Loan Forgiveness Lawsuit," *New York Times*, May 5, 2020.

155. L. Camera, "Where the 2020 Candidates Stand on Free College and Student Debt," *US News and World Report*, September 12, 2019.

156. "What Is the Debt Collective?" The Debt Collective, n.d., https://debtcollective.org/.

157. A. R. Coleman, "How a Group of Student Debtors Took on Their Banks—and Won," *GQ*, October 8, 2019.

158. S. Peterous, "How Activists Are Moving the Dial on Student Loan Debt, Inequality," Blog of the Institute of Policy Studies, December 21, 2018, https://inequality.org/great-divide/activists-moving-dial-student-loan-debt/.

159. R. Klein, "The NAACP Takes a Major Stand against the Growth of Charter Schools," HuffPost, October 16, 2016.

160. E. Eagan and J. Hauser, "Oversight Targets Abound in Betsy Devos' Education Department," Center for Economic and Policy Research, June 11, 2019.

CHAPTER 4

1. R. L. Siegel, K. D. Miller, and A. Jemal, "Cancer Statistics, 2019," *CA: A Cancer Journal for Clinicians* 69, no. 1 (2019): 7–34.

2. American Cancer Society. Lifetime Risk of Developing or Dying From Cancer, Atlanta, Georgia, 2020.

3. Siegel, Miller, and Jemal, "Cancer Statistics, 2019," 7–34.
4. American Cancer Society, "Facts and Figures," Atlanta, Georgia, 2018.
5. R. L. Siegel, A. Jemal, R. C. Wender, T. Gansler, J. Ma, O. W. Brawley, "An Assessment of Progress in Cancer Control," *CA: A Cancer Journal for Clinicians* 68 (2018): 329–39.
6. Siegel, Miller, and Jemal, "Cancer Statistics, 2019": 7–34.
7. C. Vrinten, L. M. McGregor, M. Heinrich, C. von Wagner, J. Waller, J. Wardle, G. B. Black, "What Do People Fear about Cancer? A Systematic Review and Meta-synthesis of Cancer Fears in the General Population," *Psycho-oncology* 26 (2017): 1070–79.
8. C. Fitzmaurice, T. F. Akinyemiju, F. H. Al Lami et al., "Global, Regional, and National Cancer Incidence, Mortality, Years of Life Lost, Years Lived with Disability, and Disability-adjusted Life-years for 29 Cancer Groups, 1990 to 2016: A Systematic Analysis for the Global Burden of Disease Study," *JAMA Oncology*, 4, no. 11 (November 2018: 1553–68.
9. F. Islami, A. G. Sauer, K. D. Miller et al., "Proportion and Number of Cancer Cases and Deaths Attributable to Potentially Modifiable Factors in the United States in 2014," *CA: A Cancer Journal for Clinicians* 68 (2018): 31–54.
10. E. M. Jaffee, C. Van Dang, D. B. Agus et al., "Future Cancer Research Priorities in the USA: A Lancet Oncology Commission," *The Lancet Oncology* 18, no. 11 (2017): e653–e706.
11. A. Raza, *The First Cell and the Human Costs of Pursuing Cancer to the Last* (New York: Basic Books, 2019), 11.
12. R. L. Siegel, K. D. Miller, A. Jemal, "Cancer Statistics, 2020," *CA: A Cancer Journal for Clinicians* 70, no. 1 (2020: 7–30.
13. S. H. Moolgavkar, T. R. Holford, D. T. Levy et al., "Impact of Reduced Tobacco Smoking on Lung Cancer Mortality in the United States during 1975–2000," *Journal of the National Cancer Institute* 104, no. 7 (2012): 541–48.
14. D. E. Nelson, P. Mowery, K. Asman et al., "Long-term Trends in Adolescent and Young Adult Smoking in the United States: Metapatterns and Implications," *American Journal of Public Health* 98 (2008): 905–15.
15. J. O. DeLancey, M. J. Thun, A. Jemal, and E. M. Ward, "Recent Trends in Black-White Disparities in Cancer Mortality," *Cancer Epidemiology and Prevention Biomarkers* 17, no. 11 (2008): 2908–12.
16. L. C. Richardson, S. J. Henley, J. W. Miller, G. Massetti, C. C. Thomas, "Patterns and Trends in Age-Specific Black-White Differences in Breast Cancer Incidence and Mortality—United States, 1999–2014," Morbidity and Mortality Weekly Report 65 (2016): 1093–98.
17. W. C. Hueper, "Significance of Industrial Cancer in the Problem of Cancer," *Occupational Medicine* 2 (1946): 190–200.
18. M. B. Jakovljevic and O. Milovanovic, "Growing Burden of Non-communicable Diseases in the Emerging Health Markets: The Case of BRICS," *Frontiers in Public Health* 3 (2015): 65.
19. J. Marquart, E. Y. Chen, and V. Prasad, "Estimation of the Percentage of US Patients with Cancer who Benefit from Genome-driven Oncology," *JAMA Oncology* 4 (2018): 1093–98.
20. J. J. Li, *Blockbuster Drugs: The Rise and Fall of the Pharmaceutical Industry* (New York: Oxford University Press, 2014).
21. R. Moynihan, I. Heath, and D. Henry, "Selling Sickness: The Pharmaceutical Industry and Disease Mongering," *BMJ* 324, no. 7342 (2002): 886–91.

22. E. Dolgin, –"Big Pharma Moves from 'Blockbusters' to Niche Busters," *Nature Medicine*, 2010, 16837.
23. Ibid.
24. Community Oncology Alliance, "2018 Community Oncology Practice Impact Report," https://www.communityoncology.org/2018-community-oncology-practice-impact-report/.
25. Community Oncology Alliance, "Cancer Clinic Closings and Consolidation: Ongoing Cuts to Care and Increasing Treatment Costs," June 25, 2013.
26. L. J. Blackhall, P. Read, and G. Stukenborg et al., "CARE Track for Advanced Cancer: Impact and Timing of an Outpatient Palliative Care Clinic," *Journal of Palliative Medicine* 19, no. 1 (2016): 57–63; J. Cohn, J. Corrigan, J. Lynn et al., "Community-based Models of Care Delivery for People with Serious Illness," National Academy of Medicine Perspectives, 2017, 1–13.
27. L. P. Casalino, R. Saiani, S. Bhidya et al., "Private Equity Acquisition of Physician Practices," *Annals of Internal Medicine* 170, no. 2 (2019): 114–15.
28. V. M. Kickirillo, "Oncology on the Rise: Private Equity Investment in Cancer Care," VMG Health, August 13, 2019, https://vmghealth.com/blog/oncology-on-the-rise-private-equity-investment-in-cancer-care/.
29. L. P. Casalino, R. Saiani, S. Bhidya et al., "Private Equity Acquisition of Physician Practices," *Annals of Internal Medicine* 170, no. 2 (2019): 114–15.
30. Buyouts Insider, "Private Equity Fleeing Hospitals," Health Leaders, November 5, 2018, https://www.healthleadersmedia.com/finance/private-equity-fleeing-hospitals.
31. P. K. Modi, L. A. Herrel, S. R. Kaufman et al., "Urologist Practice Structure and Spending for Prostate Cancer Care," *Urology* 130 (2019): 65–71.
32. B. L. Jacobs, Y. Zhang, T. A. Skolarus, B. K. Hollenbeck, "Growth of High-cost Intensity-modulated Radiotherapy for Prostate Cancer Raises Concerns about Overuse," *Health Affairs* 31, no. 4 (2012): 750–59.
33. Gallup Poll, "Healthcare System," https://news.gallup.com/poll/4708/healthcare-system.aspx.
34. L. R. Burns and M. V. Pauly, "Transformation of the Health Care Industry: Curb Your Enthusiasm?" *The Milbank Quarterly* 96, no. 1 (2018): 57–109.
35. IQVIA Institute, "Global Oncology Trends 2018," May 24, 2018.
36. A. M. Gilligan, D. S. Alberts, D. J. Roe, and G. H. Skrepnek, "Death or Debt? National Estimates of Financial Toxicity in Persons with Newly-diagnosed Cancer," *American Journal of Medicine* 131, no. 10 (2018): 1187–99.
37. P. Moore, "The High Cost of Cancer Treatment," *AARP Magazine*, June 1, 2018.
38. K. E. Weaver, J. H. Rowland, K. M. Bellizzi, and N. M. Aziz, "Forgoing Medical Care because of Cost: Assessing Disparities in Healthcare Access among Cancer Survivors Living in the United States," *Cancer* 116, no. 14 (2010): 3493–504.
39. Moore, "The High Cost of Cancer Treatment."
40. A. N. Winn, N. L. Keating, and S. B. Dusetzina, "Factors Associated with Tyrosine Kinase Inhibitor Initiation and Adherence among Medicare Beneficiaries with Chronic Myeloid Leukemia," *Journal of Clinical Oncology* 34, no. 36 (2016): 4323.
41. L. Szabo, "As Drug Costs Soar, People Delay or Skip Cancer Treatments," NPR, March 15, 2017, https://www.npr.org/sections/health-shots/2017/03/15/520110742/as-drug-costs-soar-people-delay-or-skip-cancer-treatments.
42. D. H. Howard, P. B. Bach, E. R. Berndt, R. M. Conti, "Pricing in the Market for Anticancer Drugs," *Journal of Economic Perspectives* 29, no. 1 (2015): 139–62.

43. IQVIA Institute, "Global Oncology Trends 2018."

44. D. Banerjee and J. Sargent, "Therapies Out of Reach: Anticancer Drugs and Global Trade Regimes," *Science, Technology and Society* 23, no. 3 (2018): 371–87.

45. S. Baxi, R. Beall, J. Yang et al., "A Multidisciplinary Review of the Policy, Intellectual Property Rights, and International Trade Environment for Access and Affordability to Essential Cancer Medications," *Globalization and Health* 15, no. 57 (2019).

46. Reuters, "How the North American Trade Deal Will Affect Autos, Digital Trade, Drugs," January 29, 2020.

47. S. Ecks, "Global Pharmaceutical Markets and Corporate Citizenship: The Case of Novartis' Anti-cancer Drug Glivec," *BioSocieties* 3, no. 2 (2008): 165–81.

48. Experts in Chronic Myeloid Leukemia, "The Price of Drugs for Chronic Myeloid Leukemia (CML) Is a Reflection of the Unsustainable Prices of Cancer Drugs: From the Perspective of a Large Group of CML Experts," *Blood* 121, no. 22 (2013): 4439–42.

49. J. Cohen, "The Curious Case of Gleevec Pricing," *Forbes*, September 12, 2018.

50. Banerjee and Sargent, "Therapies Out of Reach," 371–87.

51. K. Stone, "What Are the Top Selling Cancer Drugs?" *The Balance*, December 16, 2018.

52. K. A. McHenry, "Breast Cancer Activism in the United States and the Politics of Genes," *International Journal of Feminist Approaches to Bioethics* 8, no. 1 (2015): 182–200.

53. Association for Molecular Pathology et al. v. Myriad Genetics, Inc., et al. 569 U.S. 576 (2013).

54. D. W. Light and R. Warburton, "Demythologizing the High Costs of Pharmaceutical Research," *BioSocieties* 6, no. 1 (2011): 34–50.

55. Ibid., 47.

56. V. Prasad and S. Mailankody, "Research and Development Spending to Bring a Single Cancer Drug to Market and Revenues after Approval," *JAMA Internal Medicine* 177, no. 11 (2017): 1569–75.

57. Light and Warburton, *Demythologizing the High Costs of Pharmaceutical Research*, 34–50.

58. K. Thomas, "Labor Unions Team Up with Drug Makers to Defeat Drug-Price Proposals," *New York Times*, December 4, 2019.

59. K. Thomas, "Drug Maker Pays $360 Million to Settle Investigation into Charity Kickbacks," *New York Times*, December 6, 2018.

60. S. M. Rothman, V. H. Raveis, A. Friedman, D. J. Rothman, "Health Advocacy Organizations and the Pharmaceutical Industry: An Analysis of Disclosure Practices," *American Journal of Public Health* 101, no. 4 (2011): 602–9.

61. "Amazon in Health Care: The E-Commerce Giant's Strategy for a $3 Trillion Market," CB Insights, 2019.

62. T. Hay, "Google Ventures Leads $130M Round for Big Data Medical Software Company Flatiron Health," *Wall Street Journal*, May 7, 2014.

63. E. B. Peterson, M. J. Shen, J. G. Weber, C. L. Bylund, "Cancer Patients' Use of the Internet for Cancer Information and Support," in *Oxford Textbook of Communication in Oncology and Palliative Care*, 2nd ed., ed. D. W. Kissane, B. D. Bultz, B. W. Butow et al. (Oxford: Oxford University Press 2017), 51–55.

64. A. Pandey, S. Hasan, D. Dubey, S. Sarangi, "Smartphone Apps as a Source of Cancer Information: Changing Trends in Health Information-seeking Behavior," *Journal of Cancer Education* 28, no. 1 (2013: 138–42.

65. F. S. Collins and H. Varmus, "A New Initiative on Precision Medicine," *New England Journal of Medicine* 372, no. 9 (2015): 793–95.

66. K. Monica, "EHR Use, High Administrative Burden Driving Healthcare Spending," *EHR Intelligence*, August 1, 2018, https://ehrintelligence.com/news/ehr-use-high-administrative-burden-driving-healthcare-spending.

67. J. F. Diaz-Garelli, R. Strowd, B. J. Wells et al., "Lost in Translation: Diagnosis Records Show More Inaccuracies after Biopsy in Oncology Care EHRs," AMIA Summits on Translational Science Proceedings, May 5, 2019, 325.

68. R. L. Gardner, E. Cooper, J. Haskell et al., "Physician Stress and Burnout: The Impact of Health Information Technology," *Journal of the American Medical Informatics Association* 26, no. 2 (2018): 106–14.

69. P. Moore, "The High Cost of Cancer Treatment," *AARP Magazine*, June 1, 2018.

70. J. Anderson, "Wall Street Pursues Profit in Bundles of Life Insurance," *New York Times*, September 5, 2009.

71. "Help Save Stephanie from Cancer," https://www.gofundme.com/standing-by-stefanie.

72. J. Snyder and T. Caulfield," Patients' Crowdfunding Campaigns for Alternative Cancer Treatments," *The Lancet Oncology* 20, no. 1 (2019): 28–29.

73. M. Horneber, G. Bueschel, G. Dennert et al., "How Many Cancer Patients Use Complementary and Alternative Medicine: A Systematic Review and Metaanalysis," *Integrative Cancer Therapies* 11, no. 3 (2012): 187–203.

74. S. B. Johnson, H. S. Park, C. P. Gross, and J. B. Yu, "Use of Alternative Medicine for Cancer and Its Impact on Survival," *JNCI: Journal of the National Cancer Institute* 110, no. 1 (2017): 121–24.

75. Snyder and Caulfield, "Patients' Crowdfunding Campaigns for Alternative Cancer Treatments," 28–29.

76. E. Rosenthal, "Time to Rein in Hospital Excesses," *New York Times*, September 25, 2019.

77. Z. Cooper, A. Kowalski, E. Neff Powell, and J. Wu, "Politics, Hospital Behaviour and Health Care Spending" (CEP Discussion Paper No 1523, Centre for Economic Performance, December 2017), http://eprints.lse.ac.uk/86620/1/dp1523.pdf.

78. World Health Organization, "WHO List of Priority Medical Devices for Cancer Management," WHO Medical Device Technical Series, Geneva, 2017.

79. F. Dufour, "Protecting the US Population's Health against Potential Economic Recessions and High Unemployment and the Endemic Inflation of Health Care Costs," available at SSRN 3504249, December 15, 2019, 14.

80. "Medical Devices: Worrying Parallels to Our Nation's Prescription Drug Concerns?" (Altarum Research Brief No. 33, February 2019), https://www.healthcarevaluehub.org/application/files/3915/6391/3206/RB_33_-_Medical_Devices.pdf.

81. G. Donahoe, "Estimates of Medical Device Spending in the United States," AdvaMed, November 2018.

82. D. Grady, "Allergan Breast Implants Linked to a Rare Cancer Face Full F.D.A Recall," *New York Times*, July 25, 2019.

83. S. Chavkin, "Breast Implant Injuries Kept Hidden as New Health Threats Surface," International Consortium of Investigative Journalists, November 26, 2018, https://www.icij.org/investigations/implant-files/breast-implant-injuries-kept-hidden-as-new-health-threats-surface/.

84. "Surveillance, Epidemiology, and End Results Program," Cancer Facts & the War on Cancer, 2002.

85. "Clinton Budget Offers Salvo in War on Cancer," *Toledo Blade*, January 30, 1998.
86. White House (website), "President's Budget Increases Funding for Cancer Research by $629 Million," September 18, 2002, https://georgewbush-whitehouse.archives.gov/news/releases/2002/09/20020918-5.html.
87. A. Rascoe, "Obama Launches Mission to Cure Cancer 'Once and for All,'" Reuters, January 12, 2016.
88. M. P. Coleman, "War on Cancer and the Influence of the Medical-industrial Complex," *Journal of Cancer Policy* 1, nos. 3–4 (2013): e31–34.
89. S. Broder, "Progress and Challenges in the National Cancer Program," in *Origins of Human Cancer: A Comprehensive Review*, ed. J. Brugge, T. Curran, E. Harlow, and F. McCormick (Plainview, NY: Cold Spring Harbor Laboratory Press, 1991), 27–33.
90. "President's Budget Increases Funding for Cancer Research by $629 Million".
91. M. Tindera, "Billionaire Los Angeles Times Owner Patrick Soon-Shiong Accused Of 'Catch-And-Kill' Scheme—With A Cancer Drug," *Forbes*, April 3, 2019.
92. E. Silverman, "A Small Drug Maker Accuses Soon-Shiong of Masterminding a 'Catch-and-kill' Scheme,'" STAT, April 3, 2019, https://www.statnews.com/pharmalot/2019/04/03/soon-shiong-catch-kill-sorrento/.
93. M. Freeman, "Sorrento Therapeutics Get $7 per Share Buyout Offer from Unnamed Suitor; Stock Gains 40 percent," *San Diego Union-Tribune*, January 10, 2020.
94. "Three Questions: Prof. Florian Ederer on 'Killer Acquisitions,'" Yale Insights, April 8, 2019.
95. National Cancer Institute, "Cancer Moonshot Blue Ribbon Panel," Report 2016.
96. H. G. Welch, "Cancer Survivor or Victim of Overdiagnosis?" *New York Times*, November 21, 2012.
97. Coleman, "War on Cancer and the Influence of the Medical-industrial Complex," e31–34.
98. K. Thomas and C. Ornsetin, "Top Sloan Kettering Cancer Doctor Resigns after Failing to Disclose Industry Ties," *New York Times*, September 14, 2018.
99. I. Daalder, "No, We're not at War: The Dangers of How We Talk about the COVID-19 Pandemic," *Bangor Daily News*, May 10, 2020.
100. B. H. Lerner, "Breast Cancer Activism: Past Lessons, Future Directions," *Nature Reviews Cancer* 2, no. 3 (2002): 225.
101. J. R. Osuch, K. Silk, and C. Price et al., "A Historical Perspective on Breast Cancer Activism in the United States: From Education and Support to Partnership in Scientific Research," *Journal of Women's Health* 21, no. 3 (2012): 355–62.
102. S. Chavkin, "Investigative Reporting: Shoe-leather, Data and Empathy," International Consortium of Investigative Journalists, December 10, 2018, https://www.icij.org/blog/2018/12/investigative-reporting-shoe-leather-data-and-empathy/.
103. S. Chavkin, "The Implant Files Sparked Reform around the World. Here's Why We're Still Reporting," International Consortium of Investigative Journalists, February 27, 2019, https://www.icij.org/investigations/implant-files/the-implant-files-sparked-reform-from-around-the-world-heres-why-were-still-reporting/.
104. B. Hoffman, "Health Care Reform and Social Movements in the United States," *American Journal of Public Health* 98, supplement 1 (2008): S69–79.

105. A. J. Davidoff, G. P. Guy Jr., X. Hu et al., "Changes in Health Insurance Coverage Associated with the Affordable Care Act among Adults with and without a Cancer History: Population-based National Estimates," *Medical Care* 56, no. 3 (2018): 220.

106. K. Young and M. Schwartz, "Healthy, Wealthy, and Wise: How Corporate Power Shaped the Affordable Care Act," *New Labor Forum* 23, no. 2 (2014): 30–40.

107. J. Eaton and M. B. Pell, "Lobbyists Swarm Capitol to Influence Health Reform," Center for Public Integrity, February 24, 2010, https://publicintegrity.org/health/lobbyists-swarm-capitol-to-influence-health-reform/.

108. P. Kane, "Lawmakers Reveal Health-Care Investments: Key Players Have Stakes in Industry," *The Washington Post*, June 13, 2009.

109. G. Greenwald, "Obamacare Architect Leaves White House for Pharmaceutical Industry Job," *Guardian*, December 5, 2012.

110. K. Young and M. Schwartz, "Healthy, Wealthy, and Wise: How Corporate Power Shaped the Affordable Care Act," *New Labor Forum* 23, no. 2 (2014): 30–40.

111. Association for Molecular Pathology et al. v. Myriad Genetics, Inc., et al. 569 U.S. 576 (2013).

112. Banerjee and Sargent, "Therapies Out of Reach, 371–87.

113. A. Pollock, "Transforming the Critique of Big Pharma," *BioSocieties* 6, no. 1 (2011): 106–18.

114. S. Wu, S. Powers, W. Zhu, and Y. A. Hannun, "Substantial Contribution of Extrinsic Risk Factors to Cancer Development," *Nature* 529, no. 7584 (2016): 43.

115. M. J. Joyner, N. Paneth, and J. P. Ioannidis, "What Happens When Underperforming Big Ideas in Research Become Entrenched?" *JAMA* 316, no. 13 (2016): 1355–56.

CHAPTER 5

1. "Fordism" describes the system of mass production and mass consumption that was pioneered in the early twentieth century by the Ford Motor Company and the resulting postwar mode of economic growth and its associated political and social order in advanced capitalism. See D. Watson, "Fordism: A Review Essay," *Labor History* 60, no. 2 (2019): 144–59.

2. Keynesian social policies, as described by the economist John Maynard Keynes, proposed that governments should increase consumer demand to boost growth by augmenting government spending on infrastructure, unemployment benefits, and education. See T. Aspromourgos, "The Past and Future of Keynesian Economics: A Review Essay," *History of Economics Review* 72, no. 1 (2019): 59–78.

3. D. Rosner and G. E. Markowitz, eds., *Dying for Work: Workers' Safety and Health in Twentieth-century America* (Bloomington: Indiana University Press, 1987).

4. Centers for Disease Control and Prevention, "Improvements in Workplace Safety—United States, 1900–1999," *MMWR: Morbidity and Mortality Weekly Report*, 48, no. 22 (1999): 461–69.

5. *National Safety Council, Accident Facts, 1998 Edition* (Itasca, IL: National Safety Council, 1998).

6. C. J. Boggs, "Workers' Compensation History: The Great Tradeoff!" *Insurance Journal*, March 19, 2015.

7. C. E. Siqueira, M. Gaydos, C. Monforton et al., "Effects of Social, Economic, and Labor Policies on Occupational Health Disparities," *American Journal of Industrial Medicine* 57, no. 5 (2014): 557–72.

8. A. L. Steege, S. L. Baron, S. M. Marsh, C. C. Menéndez, an J. R. Myers, "Examining Occupational Health and Safety Disparities Using National Data: A Cause for Continuing Concern," *American Journal of Industrial Medicine* 57, no. 5 (2014): 527–38.

9. M. Wilson, "How to Close Down the Department of Labor," The Heritage Foundation, 1995, https://www.heritage.org/node/20681/print-display.

10. S. Barr, "Bureau of Mines Feeling Shafted," *Washington Post*, December 4, 1995.

11. N. Kristof, "Trump's War on Workers," *New York Times*, August 11, 2019.

12. White House (website), "Remarks by President Trump on Deregulation," December 14, 2017, https://www.whitehouse.gov/briefings-statements/remarks-president-trump-deregulation/.

13. J. Hanna, "Unpacking Walmart's Workforce of the Future," *Forbes*, August 2, 2019.

14. Walmart, "Culture Diversity and Inclusion, 2017 Report," https://cdn.corporate.walmart.com/11/0d/f9289df649049a38c14bdeaf2b99/2017-cdi-report-web.pdf.

15. Center for Popular Democracy, "Trapped in Part-Time: Walmart's Phantom Ladder of Opportunity," June 2018.

16. Memorandum from Susan Chambers, Walmart Stores, Inc., to Wal-Mart Stores, Inc. Board of Directors, "Reviewing and Revising Wal-Mart's Benefits Strategy," 2005, cited in "Discounting Rights: Wal-Mart's Violation of US Workers' Right to Freedom of Association," Human Rights Watch, 2007, https://www.hrw.org/report/2007/04/30/discounting-rights/wal-marts-violation-us-workers-right-freedom-association.

17. Center for Popular Democracy, "Trapped in Part-Time."

18. D. Watson, "Fordism: A Review Essay," *Labor History* 6, no. 2 (2019): 144–59.

19. A. Reich and P. Bearman, *Working for Respect: Community and Conflict at Walmart* (New York: Columbia University Press, 2018), Kindle, Locations 2367–2707.

20. J. A. Harrison, review of *Working for Respect: Community and Conflict at Walmart*, by Adam Reich and Peter Bearman, *Social Forces* 97, no. 4 (2019): 1–3.

21. A. Reich and P. Bearman, *Working for Respect*, Location 1603.

22. E. Bonacich and H. Khaleelah, "Wal-Mart and the Logistics Revolution," in *Wal-Mart: The Face of Twenty-First-Century Capitalism*, ed. Nelson Lichtenstein (New York: New Press, 2006), 163–88.

23. Reich and Bearman, *Working for Respect*, Kindle, Location 2317.

24. Ibid., Location 4493.

25. Ibid., Location 242.

26. J. Robinson, *Economic Philosophy* (Chicago: Aldine, 2006), 45.

27. Center for Popular Democracy, "Trapped in Part-Time."

28. S. Greenhouse and M. Barbaro, "Wal-Mart Memo Suggests Ways to Cut Employee Benefit Costs," *New York Times*, October 26, 2005.

29. Reich and Bearman, *Working for Respect*, Location 3818.

30. J. Hanna, "Unpacking Walmart's Workforce of the Future," *Forbes*, August 2, 2019.

31. R. Abrams, "Walmart Is Accused of Punishing Workers for Taking Sick Days," *New York Times*, June 2, 2017.

32. E. Stewart, "Walmart Is Paying $20 Billion to Shareholders. With That Money, It Could Boost Hourly Wages to Over $15," Vox, May 30, 2018.

33. Center for Popular Democracy, "Trapped in Part-Time."

34. A. Bhattarai, "Walmart Store Managers Average $175,000 a Year. Many Employees Still Earn Below the Poverty Line," *Washington Post*, May 9, 2019.
35. Center for Popular Democracy, "Trapped in Part-Time."
36. Reich and Bearman, *Working for Respect*, Location 1995.
37. Ibid, Location 1937.
38. Ibid., Location 1997.
39. N. Lichtenstein, *The Retail Revolution: How Wal-Mart Created a Brave New World of Business* (New York: Metropolitan Books, 2009).
40. Reich and Bearman, *Working for Respect*, Location 3093.
41. Abrams, "Walmart Is Accused of Punishing Workers for Taking Sick Days."
42. Reich and Bearman, *Working for Respect*, Location 2412.
43. A Better Balance, "Pointing Out: How Walmart Unlawfully Punishes Workers for Medical Absences," June 2017.
44. Abrams, "Walmart Is Accused of Punishing Workers for Taking Sick Days."
45. Z. Friedman, "Walmart Expands College for $1 a Day," *Forbes*, June 12, 2019.
46. M. Yglesias, "Walmart's Too-good-to-be-true '$1 a day' College Tuition Plan, Explained," Vox, June 1, 2018.
47. Reuters, "Wal-Mart Settles Lawsuit on Hiring," *New York Times*, February 20, 2009.
48. Center for Popular Democracy, "Trapped in Part-Time."
49. N. Meyerson, "Walmart Discriminated against Pregnant workers, Federal Agency Says," CNN Business News, September 21, 2018.
50. Reich and Bearman, *Working for Respect*, Location 1923.
51. Quoted in S. Greenhouse, *Beaten Down, Worked Up: The Past, Present and Future of American Labor* (New York: Knopf, 2019), 154.
52. A. Zimmerman, "Pro-Union Butchers at Wal-Mart Win a Battle, but Lose the War," *Wall Street Journal*, April 11, 2000.
53. S. Greenhouse, "How Walmart Persuades Its Workers Not to Unionize," *The Atlantic*, June 8, 2015.
54. Reich and Bearman, *Working for Respect*, Location 3492.
55. Ibid., Location 2007.
56. K. Bronfenbrenner, "No Holds Barred—the Intensification of Employer Opposition to Organizing" (Economic Policy Institute Briefing Paper #235, 2009), https://www.epi.org/files/page/-/pdf/bp235.pdf.
57. Reich and Bearman, *Working for Respect*, Location 1954.
58. Center for Popular Democracy, "Trapped in Part-Time."
59. Hoover's, "Kindercare Education LLC Profile," 2019.
60. Partners Group, "About Partners Group," https://www.partnersgroup.com/en/about/.
61. Sources consulted included Indeed, with twenty-nine hundred staff reviews of KinderCare; GlassDoor, with thirteen hundred KinderCare staff ratings; Niche, with twenty-eight reviews; Career Bliss, with twenty-four reviews; and Winnie, with five staff reviews.
62. "KinderCare Learning Centers Salaries in the United States," Indeed, August 2019, https://www.indeed.com/cmp/Kindercare-Learning-Centers/salaries.
63. R. Thomas, "Unions' Win Streak in Legislature Is Broken," *Seattle Times*, March 10, 2008.
64. A. Chen, "Child Care Center Ends Services at USC," *Daily Trojan*, August 12, 2016.
65. Ibid.

66. "KinderCare Learning Centers Salaries in the United States."
67. A. Rosenblat, *Uberland: How Algorithms Are Rewriting the Rules of Work* (Berkeley: University of California Press, 2018), Kindle, Location 537.
68. A. Smith, "Gig Work, Online Selling, and Home Sharing," PEW Research Center, November 17, 2016.
69. Quotes from an interview study with Uber drivers A. Baiyere, N. Islam, and M. Mäntymäki in "Duality of Work in Sharing Economy—Insights from Uber," presented at Twenty-fifth Americas Conference on Information Systems, Cancun, 2019, https://pdfs.semanticscholar.org/2754/548c2bb21d920a84f8f61 76746558efb3189.pdf
70. Ibid.
71. A. Krueger and J. Hall, "An Analysis of the Labor Market for Uber's Driver-partners in the United States" (working paper 587, Princeton University Industrial Relations Section, 2015).
72. D. Farrell and F. Greig, "The Online Platform Economy: Has Growth Peaked?" JP Morgan Chase, November 2016.
73. C. O'Donovan and J. Singer-Vine, "How Much Uber Drivers Actually Make per Hour," BuzzFeed News, June 22, 2016.
74. US Federal Trade Commission, "Uber Agrees to Pay $20 Million to Settle FTC Charges that It Recruited Prospective Drivers with Exaggerated Earnings Claims," January 19, 2017.
75. A. Ravanelle, *Hustle and Gig: Struggling and Surviving in the Gig Economy* (Berkeley: University of California Press, 2019), Kindle, Locations 2013–2016.
76. Rosenblat, *Uberland*, Location 163.
77. Robert Jon Hendricks, cited inibid., Location 176.
78. Ibid., Location 176.
79. Ibid., Location 1648.
80. O. Mehmet, "Race to the Bottom: The Impact of Globalization on Labor Markets—a Review of Empirical and Theoretical Evidence," in *Globalization and the Third World* (London: Palgrave Macmillan, 2006), 148–61.
81. US Securities and Exchange Commission, "Form S-1, Uber Technologies, Inc.," April 11, 2019.
82. "Uber and Lyft Drivers Conduct International Strike," World Socialist Web Site, May 9, 2019, https://www.wsws.org/en/articles/2019/05/09/uber-m09.html.
83. M. Isaac, "Uber's Rocky Ride to Its I.P.O. Ends in Stock Hitting the Skids," *New York Times*, May 11, 2019.
84. Bank for International Settlements, "Global FX Trading Averages $5.1 Trillion a Day in April 2016; Spot Trading Falls While FX Swaps Rise," September 1, 2016, https://www.bis.org/press/p160901a.htm.
85. M. Haiven, "Walmart, Financialization, and the Cultural Politics of Securitization," *Cultural Politics* 9, no. 3 (2013): 239–62.
86. D. L. Barlett and D. B. Steele, "How Special-interest Groups Have Their Way with Congress," *Philadelphia Inquirer*, October 28, 1991.
87. "KinderCare Learning Centers," Indeed, https://www.indeed.com/cmp/ Kindercare-Learning-Centers/reviews?ftopic=mgmt&sort=rating_desc.
88. M. Olsson and J. Tåg, "What Is the Cost of Privatization for Workers?" (working paper 1201, Research Institute of Industrial Economics [IFN],Stockholm, 2018).
89. G. Hodge, *Privatization: An International Review of Performance* (Abingdon, Oxfordshire: Routledge, 2018).

90. M. Abramovitz and J. Zelnick, "Privatization in the Human Services: The Impact on the Front Lines and the Ground Floor," in *Privatization, Vulnerability, and Social Responsibility*, ed. M. A. Fineman, T. Mattsson, and U. Andersson (Abingdon, Oxfordshire: Routledge, 2016), 190–208.

91. J. Manyika et al., *Jobs Lost, Jobs Gained: Workforce Transitions in a Time of Automation* (New York: McKinsey Global Institute, 2017).

92. C. B. Frey and M. A. Osborne, "The Future of Employment: How Susceptible Are Jobs to Computerisation?" *Technological Forecasting and Social Change* 114 (2017): 254–80.

93. K. Taylor, "Fast-food CEO Says He's Investing in Machines because the Government Is Making It Difficult to Afford Employees," Business Insider, March 16, 2016.

94. D. Autor and D. Dorn, "The Growth of Low-skill Service Jobs and the Polarization of the US Labor Market," *American Economic Review* 103, no. 5 (2013): 1553–97.

95. In the Public Interest, "How Privatization Increases Inequality," 2016.

96. G. Rodgers, "Precarious Work in Western Europe: The State of the Debate," *Precarious Jobs in Labour Market Regulation: The Growth of Atypical Employment in Western Europe*, ed. Gerry Rodgers and Janine Rodgers (Brussels: International Institute for Labour Studies, Free University of Brussels, 1989), 3.

97. J. Benach, A. Vives, and M. Amable et al., "Precarious Employment: Understanding an Emerging Social Determinant of Health," *Annual Review of Public Health* 35 (2014): 229–53.

98. G. Standing, "The Precaraiat," *Contexts* 13, no. 4 (2014): 10–12.

99. Bureau of Labor Statistics, "Contingent and Alternative Employment Arrangements—May 2017," US Department of Labor, June 7, 2018.

100. M. Tran and R. K. Sokas, "The Gig Economy and Contingent Work: An Occupational Health Assessment," *Journal of Occupational and Environmental Medicine* 59, no. 4 (2017): e63.

101. A. Bernhardt, R. Batt, S. N. Houseman, an E. Appelbaum, "Domestic Outsourcing in the United States: A Research Agenda to Assess Trends and Effects on Job Quality" (working paper, Upjohn Institute, 2016).

102. A. Aloisi, "Commoditized Workers. Case Study Research on Labour Law Issues Arising from a Set of 'On-Demand/Gig Economy' Platforms," *Comparative Labor Law and Policy Journal* 37 (2016): 38.

103. T. Brown, "The Gig Economy," Daily Beast, January 12, 2009.

104. Rosenblat, *Uberland*, Location 618.

105. M. Ross and N. Bateman, "Meet the Low-wage Workforce," Brookings Institution, November 2019.

106. Center for Law and Social Policy, "The Struggles of Low-Wage Work," 2018.

107. International Labour Office, "Resolution concerning Decent Work and the Informal Economy," General Conference of the International Labour Organization, Meeting in Its 90th Session, 2002 (Geneva: ILO Publications, 2002).

108. D. Smith Nightingale and S. A. Wandner, "Informal and Nonstandard Employment in the United States: Implications for Low-Income Working Families," The Urban Institute, Brief 20, August 2011.

109. M. A. Chen, "Rethinking the Informal Economy: Linkages with the Formal Economy and the Formal Regulatory Environment," *United Nations University, World Institute for Development Economics Research* 10 (2005): 18–27; C. C.

Williams and J. Windebank, "The Growth of Urban Informal Economies," in *Handbook of Urban Studies*, ed. R. Paddison (London: Sage Publications, 2001).

110. A. Valenzuela, N. Theodore, E. Melendez, and A. L. Gonzalez, *On the Corner: Day Labor in the United States* (Los Angeles: Center for the Study of Urban Poverty, University of California, Los Angeles, 2006).

111. L. Medina and F. Schneider, "Shadow Economies around the World: New Results for 143 Countries Over 1996–2014" (discussion Paper, Department of Economics, University of Linz, Linz, Austria, 2017).

112. A. Bracha and M. A. Burke, "Who Counts as Employed? Informal Work, Employment Status, and Labor Market Slack" (working paper 16–29, Federal Reserve Bank of Boston, December 2016).

113. Bureau of Labor Statistics, "Contingent and Alternative Employment Arrangements—May 2017," US Department of Labor, 2018.

114. C. Zillman, "Who Makes Less Than $15 per Hour?" *Fortune*, April 13, 2015.

115. M. Pinto, "Workers in All 50 States Will Need $15 an Hour by 2024 to Afford the Basics," National Employment Law Project, 2017.

116. S. Broder, "Progress and Challenges in the National Cancer Program," in *Origins of Human Cancer: A Comprehensive Review*, ed. J. Brugge, T. Curran, E. Harlow, and F. McCormick (Plainview, NY: Cold Spring Harbor Laboratory Press, 1991), 27–33.

117. T. Gärling, A. Gamble, F. Fors, and M. Hjerm, "Emotional Well-being Related to Time Pressure, Impediment to Goal Progress, and Stress-related Symptoms," *Journal of Happiness Studies* 17, no. 5 (2016): 1789–99.

118. N. Jacobson, "Dignity and Health: A Review," *Social Science & Medicine* 64, no. 2 (2007): 292–302.

119. S. I. Hay, A. A. Abajobir, K. H. Abate et al., "Global, Regional, and National Disability-adjusted Life-years (DALYs) for 333 Diseases and Injuries and Healthy Life Expectancy (HALE) for 195 Countries and Territories, 1990–2016: A Systematic Analysis for the Global Burden of Disease Study 2016," *The Lancet* 390, no. 10100 (2017):1260–344.

120. *Depression and Other Common Mental Disorders: Global Health Estimates* (Geneva: World Health Organization, 2017).

121. World Health Organization, *Preventing Suicide: A Global Imperative* (Geneva: WHO Press, 2014).

122. A. K. Gertner, J. S. Rotter, and P. R. Shafer, "Association between State Minimum Wages and Suicide Rates in the US," *American Journal of Preventive Medicine* 56, no. 5 (2019): 648–54.

123. C. Muntaner, W. W. Eaton, C. Diala, R. C. Kessler, and P. D. Sorlie, "Social Class, Assets, Organizational Control and the Prevalence of Common Groups of Psychiatric Disorders," *Social Science & Medicine* 47, no. 12 (1998): 2043–53.

124. E. O. Wright, *Classes* (Brooklyn, N.Y.: Verso, 1985).

125. S. J. Prins, L. M. Bates, K. M. Keyes, and C. Muntaner, "Anxious? Depressed? You Might Be Suffering from Capitalism: Contradictory Class Locations and the Prevalence of Depression and Anxiety in the USA," *Sociology of Health & Illness* 37, no. 8 (2015): 1352–72.

126. I. Ivandic, A. Freeman, U. Birner, D. Nowak, and C. Sabariego, "A Systematic Review of Brief Mental Health and Well-being Interventions in Organizational Settings," *Scandinavian Journal of Work, Environment & Health*, 43, no. 2 (2017): 99–108.

127. N. L. Sin and S. Lyubomirsky, "Enhancing Well-being and Alleviating Depressive Symptoms with Positive Psychology Interventions: A Practice-friendly Meta-analysis," *Journal of Clinical Psychology* 65, no. 5 (2009): 467–87.

128. S. Vargas, "'It's Not an Easy Conversation': Mental Health in the Workplace. What Role Should Safety Pros Play in Workers' Mental Well-being?" *Safety and Health*, September 23, 2018.

129. M. R. Frone, "Are Work Stressors Related to Employee Substance Use? The Importance of Temporal Context Assessments of Alcohol and Illicit Drug Use," *Journal of Applied Psychology* 93, no. 1 (2008): 199.

130. Ø. Vedaa, E. Krossbakken, I. D. Grimsrud, B. Bjorvatn, B. Sivertsen, N. Magerøy, S. Einarsen, S. Pallesen, "Prospective Study of Predictors and Consequences of Insomnia: Personality, Lifestyle, Mental Health, and Work-related Stressors," *Sleep Medicine* 20 (2016): 51–58.

131. G. Kecklund and J. Axelsson, "Health Consequences of Shift Work and Insufficient Sleep," *The BMJ* 355 (2016): i5210.

132. P. L. Schnall, M. Dobson, and P. Landsbergis, "Globalization, Work, and Cardiovascular Disease," *International Journal of Health Services* 46, no. 4 (2016): 656–92.

133. "The Tokyo Declaration on Prevention and Management of Work-Related Cardiovascular Disorders, Adopted by the Plenary of the Sixth ICOH International Conference on Work Environment and Cardiovascular Diseases under the Auspices of the ICOH Scientific Committee on Cardiology in Occupational Health," Tokyo, Japan, March 30, 2013.

134. Schnall, Dobson, and Landsbergis, "Globalization, Work, and Cardiovascular Disease," 656–92.

135. L. S. Azaroff, L. K. Davis, R. Naparstek et al., "Barriers to Use of Workers' Compensation for Patient Care at Massachusetts Community Health Centers," *Health Services Research* 48 (2013): 1375–92.

136. N. J. Negi, J. Siegel, M. Calderon, E. Thomas, A. Valdez, "'They Dumped Me Like Trash': The Social and Psychological Toll of Victimization on Latino Day Laborers' Lives," *American Journal of Community Psychology* 65, nos. 3–4 (2020): 369–80.

137. L. Topete, L. Forst, J. Zanoni, L. Friedman, "Workers' Compensation and the Working Poor: Occupational Health Experience among Low Wage Workers in Federally Qualified Health Centers," *American Journal of Industrial Medicine* 61, no. 3 (2018): 193.

138. K. H. Kim, E. Kabir, S. A. Jahan, "Exposure to Pesticides and the Associated Human Health Effects," *Science of the Total Environment* 575 (2017): 525–35.

139. M. T. Muñoz-Quezada, B. A. Lucero, V. P. Iglesias et al., "Chronic Exposure to Organophosphate (OP) Pesticides and Neuropsychological Functioning in Farm Workers: A Review," *International Journal of Occupational and Environmental Health* 22, no. 1 (2016): 68–79.

140. C. Hyland and O. Laribi, "Review of Take-home Pesticide Exposure Pathway in Children Living in Agricultural Areas," *Environmental Research* 156 (2017): 559–70.

141. Bureau of Labor Statistics, "Table 5. Employment Status of the Population by Sex, Marital Status, and Presence and Age of Own Children under 18, 2014–2015 Annual Averages," April 22, 2016, http://www.bls.gov/news.release/famee.t05.htm.

142. A. W. Geiger K. Parker, "For Women's History Month, a Look at Gender Gains—and Gaps—in the U.S.," Pew Research Center, March 15, 2018.
143. B. Yeung, *In a Day's Work: The Fight to End Sexual Violence against America's Most Vulnerable Workers* (New York: The New Press, 2020).
144. PL+US: Paid Leave for the United States, "Forging Ahead or Falling Behind? Paid Family Leave at America's Top Companies," 2016, https://actionnetwork.org/user_files/user_files/000/018/893/original/pl_us_corporate_report.pdf.
145. L. Schummers, J. A. Hutcheon, M. R. Hacker et al., "Absolute Risks of Obstetric Outcomes Risks by Maternal Age at First Birth: A Population-based Cohort," *Epidemiology* 29, no. 3 (2018): 379.
146. A. Partanen and T. Corson, "Finland Is Our Capitalist Paradise," *New York Times*, December 8, 2019.
147. S. B. Kamerman and J. Waldfogel, "United States Country Note," in *International Review of Leave Policies and Research 2013*, ed. P. Moss, 147–63, http://leavenetwork.org/lp_and_r_reports/.
148. A. Burtle and S. Bezruchka, "Population Health and Paid Parental Leave: What the United States Can Learn from Two Decades of Research" *MDPI Healthcare* 4, no. 2 (2016): 30–46.
149. A. Case and A. Deaton, "Rising Morbidity and Mortality in Midlife among White Non-Hispanic Americans in the 21st Century." Proceedings of the National Academy of Sciences 112, no. 49 (2015): 15078–83.
150. Trust for America's Health, "Pain in the Nation Update: While Deaths from Alcohol, Drugs, and Suicide Slowed Slightly in 2017, Rates Are Still at Historic Highs," March 2019.
151. Case and Deaton, "Rising Morbidity and Mortality in Midlife among White non-Hispanic Americans in the 21st Century," 15078–83.
152. A. Case and A. Deaton, "Mortality and Morbidity in the 21st Century," *Brookings Papers on Economic Activity* 2017, no. 1 (2017): 397–476.
153. Trust for America's Health, "Pain in the Nation Update."
154. US Centers for Disease Control, "Opioid Overdose," Understanding the Epidemic," 2018, https://www.cdc.gov/drugoverdose/epidemic/index.html.
155. C. E. Siqueira, M. Gaydos, C. Monforton et al., "Effects of Social, Economic, and Labor Policies on Occupational Health Disparities," *American Journal of Industrial Medicine* 57, no. 5 (2014): 557–72.
156. N. Scheiber, "Uber Has a Union. Sort Of . . . ," *New York Times*, May 14, 2017.
157. A. Reich and P. Bearman, *Working for Respect: Community and Conflict at Walmart* (New York: Columbia University Press, 2018), Kindle, Location 3986.
158. D. Schifter, "To those it may concern," Facebook, February 5, 2018, https://www.facebook.com/permalink.php?story_fbid=1888367364808997&id=100009072541151.
159. R. J. Livengood, "Organizing for Structural Change: The Potential and Promise of Workers Centers," *Harvard Civil Rights-Civil Liberties Law Review* 48, (2013): 325.
160. J. R. Fine, *Worker Centers: Organizing Communities at the Edge of the Dream* (Ithaca, NY: Cornell University Press, 2006).
161. D. Gunn, "What Workers Gain at Worker Centers" *Pacific Standard*, April 27, 2018.
162. J. B. Manheim, "The Emerging Role of Worker Centers in Union Organizing: An Update And Supplement," US Chamber of Commerce, Workforce Freedom Initiative, 2017.
163. D. Gunn, "What Workers Gain at Worker Centers?"

164. A. Poo, "Nannies Deserve Rights," *New York Times*, July 15, 2019.
165. C. Frantz and S. Fernandes, "Whose Movement Is It? Strategic Philanthropy and Worker Centers," *Critical Sociology* 44, nos. 4–5 (2018): 645–60.
166. J. Fuld, "Grassroots vs. Grasstops Advocacy," The Campaign Workshop, May 12, 2017, https://www.thecampaignworkshop.com/grassroots-vs-grasstops-advocacy.
167. W. Beaver, "Fast-food Unionization," *Society* 53, no. 5 (2016): 469–73.
168. M. A. Sholar, ed., *Getting Paid While Taking Time: The Women's Movement and the Development of Paid Family Leave Policies in the United States* (Philadelphia: Temple University Press, 2016).
169. United States Department of Labor, Bureau of Labor Statistics, "Table 32. Leave Benefits: Access, Private Industry Workers," National Compensation Survey, March 2018.
170. G. Jones, "Davis to Sign Bill Allowing Paid Family Leave," *Los Angeles Times*, September 23, 2002.
171. National Conference of State Lesgislatures, State Family and Medical Leave Laws. September 21,2020.
172. M. Rossin-Slater, C. Ruhm, and J. Waldfogel, "The Effect of California's Paid Family Leave Program on Mothers' Leave-Taking and Subsequent Labor Market Outcomes," *Journal of Policy Analysis and Management* 32, no. 2 (2013): 224–45.
173. B. Meixell and R. Eisenbrey, "An Epidemic of Wage Theft Is Costing Workers Hundreds of Millions of Dollars a Year," Economic Policy Institute, 2014.
174. K. Conger and N. Scheiber, "California Bill Makes App-Based Companies Treat Workers as Employees," *New York Times*, September 11, 2019.
175. C. Fishman, "The Real Reason for Walmart's Wage Hike. Was It Really the Tax Cut? And Should the Motivation behind Such Good News Even Matter?" Politico, January 12, 2018.
176. N. Meyersohn, "Walmart CEO: America's Minimum Wage Is 'Too Low.'" CNN Business, June 5, 2019.
177. L. Huizar and Y. Lathrop, "Fighting Wage Preemption: How Workers Have Lost Billions in Wages and How We Can Restore Local Democracy," National Employment Law Project, July 2019.

CHAPTER 6

1. R. Pesce, "Death in the 20th Century. The Infographic," April 2, 2013, http://www.medcrunch.net/death-20th-century-infographic/.
2. B. Gardiner, *Choked: Life and Breath in the Age of Air Pollution* (Chicago: University of Chicago Press, 2019).
3. Union of Concerned Scientists, "Car Emissions and Global Warming," n.d., https://www.ucsusa.org/clean-vehicles/car-emissions-and-global-warming.
4. K. T. Jackson, *Crabgrass Frontier: The Suburbanization of the United States* (New York: Oxford University Press, 1987).
5. *Encyclopaedia of Environmental Health*, s.v. "Urban Transportation and Human Health" (Amsterdam: Elsevier, 2011), 578–89.
6. T. Litman, "Evaluating Public Transportation Health Benefits," The American Public Transportation Association, 2010.
7. J. Pucher and R. Buehler, "Walking and Cycling for Healthy Citie," *Built Environment* 36 (2010): 391–414.
8. J. Doyle, *Taken for a Ride: Detroit's Big Three and the Politics of Pollution* (New York: Four Walls Eight Windows, 2000).

9. United States Securities and Exchange Commission, "Form S-1 Registration Statement, Uber Technologies, Inc.," Washington, DC, 2019, 164.
10. Ibid., 10.
11. K. Conger, "Uber's Unsettling Ambitions," *New York Times*, August 8, 2019.
12. E. T. Kim, "How Uber Sees Profit in Public Transit," *New York Times*, June 3, 2019.
13. Conger, "Uber's Unsettling Ambitions."
14. "Brainstorm Tech 2018: Uber's Strategy, Business, Culture, and More," *Fortune*, July 16, 2018, https://www.youtube.com/watch?v=70JgYWOfGYk.
15. L. Bliss, "Uber Was Supposed to Be Our Public Transit," City Lab, April 29, 2019.
16. E. T. Kim, "How Uber Sees Profit in Public Transit," *New York Times*, June 3, 2019.
17. M. McFarland, "Uber Wants to Compete with Public Transit. These Experts Are Horrified," CNN Business, April 25, 2019.
18. R. D. Bullard, "Addressing Urban Transportation Equity in the United States," *Fordham Urban Law Journal* 31 (2003): 1183.
19. R. Chetty, N. Hendren, P. Kline, and E. Saez, "Where Is the Land of Opportunity? The Geography of Intergenerational Mobility in the United States," *The Quarterly Journal of Economics* 129, no. 4 (2014): 1553–623.
20. K. DeGood and A. Schwartz, "Can New Transportation Technologies Improve Equity and Access to Opportunity?" Center for American Progress, April 2016.
21. W. J. Mallett, "Trends in Public Transportation Ridership: Implications for Federal Policy," Congressional Research Services, March 26, 2018.
22. US Department of Transportation, "2015 Status of the Nation's Highways, Bridges, and Transit: Conditions and Performance," Washington, DC, 2017.
23. Kim, "How Uber Sees Profit in Public Transit."
24. D. Sperling, A. Brown, and M. D'Agostino, "How Ride-hailing Could Improve Public Transportation Instead of Undercutting It," *The Conversation*, July 5, 2018.
25. S. Tan, A. Fowers, D. Keating, and L. Tierney, "Amid the Pandemic, Public Transit Is Highlighting Inequalities in Cities," *Washington Post*, May 15, 2020.
26. T. Basu, "Timeline: A History of GM's Ignition Switch Defect," *NPR News*, NPR, March 31, 2014.
27. A. R. Valukas, "Report to Board of Directors of General Motors Company Regarding Ignition Switch Recalls," Jenner and Block, May 29, 2014, https://assets.documentcloud.org/documents/1183508/g-m-internal-investigation-report.pdf.
28. E. D. Lawrence, "GM to Pay $120M in Multistate Defective Ignition Switch Settlement," *Detroit Free Press*, October 19, 2017.
29. M. Daalder, "GM Fulfills Ignition Switch Scandal Terms, Feds Dismiss Case," *Detroit Free Press*, September 20, 2018.
30. G. Colvin, "How CEO Mary Barra Is Using the Ignition-switch Scandal to Change GM's Culture," *Fortune*, September 18, 2015.
31. S. B. Dow and N. S. Ellis, "A New Look at Criminal Liability for Selling Dangerous Vehicles: Lessons from General Motors and Toyota," *Hastings Business Law Journal* 15, no. 1 (2019): 1–53.
32. "Critics Rip GM Deferred Prosecution Agreement in Engine Switch Case," Corporate Crime Reporter, September 17, 2015, https://www.corporatecrimereporter.com/news/200/critics-rip-gm-deferred-prosecution-in-switch-case/ .

33. S. Radu, "Takata Files for Bankruptcy Following Multiyear Air Bag Crisis," *Washington Post*, June 26, 2017.
34. H. Tabuchi, "The Quest to Save a Few Dollars per Airbag Led to a Deadly Crisis," *New York Times*, August 27, 2016.
35. T. Krisher, "Automakers Recall 1.7 Million Cars with Fatal Airbags," Associated Press, February 8, 2019.
36. Ibid.
37. "Takata Airbag Recall: Everything You Need to Know," *Consumer Reports*, March 29, 2019.
38. Radu, "Takata Files for Bankruptcy Following Multiyear Air Bag Crisis."
39. US Environmental Protection Agency, "Notice of Violation of the Clean Air Act to Volkswagen AG, Audi AG, and Volkswagen Group of America, Inc.," September 18, 2015, https://www.epa.gov/sites/production/files/2015-10/documents/vw-nov-caa-09-18-15.pdf.
40. L. Tang, T. Nagashima, K. Hasegawa et al., "Development of Human Health Damage Factors for PM2.5 Based on a Global Chemical Transport Model," *International Journal of Life Cycle Assessment* (2015): 1e11; G. P. Chossiere, R. Malina, A. Ashok et al., "Public Health Impacts of Excess NOx Emissions from Volkswagen Diesel Passenger Vehicles in Germany," *Environmental Research Letters* 12 (2017): 1–9.
41. R. Oldenkamp, R. van Zelm, and M. A. Huijbregts, "Valuing the Human Health Damage Caused by the Fraud of Volkswagen," *Environmental Pollution* 212 (2016): 121–27.
42. M. Sanger-Katz and J. Schwartz, "Assessing the Possible Health Effects from Volkswagen's Diesel Deception," *New York Times*, September 29, 2015.
43. P. Oehmke, "The Three Students Who Uncovered 'Dieselgate.'" *Der Spiegel*, October 23, 2017.
44. D. Fickling, "The Auto Industry Is Overdue a Bout of Mega-Mergers," Bloomberg, April 1, 2019.
45. R. Wright, "Fiat Chrysler Chief Executive Warns Sector of Electric Threat," *Financial Times*, January 11, 2016.
46. J. L. Mashaw and D. L. Harfst, *The Struggle for Auto Safety* (Cambridge, MA: Harvard University Press, 1990), 47–68.
47. J. L. Mashaw and D. L. Harfst, "From Command and Control to Collaboration and Deference: The Transformation of Auto Safety Regulation," *Yale Journal on Regulation* 34 (2017): 167.
48. M. M. Golden, *What Motivates Bureaucrats?: Politics and Administration during the Reagan Years* (New York: Columbia University Press, 2000).
49. K. Laing, "How John Dingell Championed Auto Industry," *The Detroit News*, February 8, 2019.
50. J. Anderson and D. Van Atta, "Detroit's Roadblock on Auto Safety," *Washington Post*, December 5, 1989.
51. Mashaw and Harfst, "From Command and Control to Collaboration and Deference," 182.
52. M. Matthews, "Recalls Rise 13%, Affected Vehicles Fall in 2018," *Automotive Fleet*, April 8, 2019.
53. A. Fuller and A. Roberts, "Car Makers' Struggle with Recalls Leave More Risky Vehicles on the Road," *The Wall Street Journal*, November 1, 2018.
54. K. M. McDonald, "Do Auto Recalls Benefit the Public?" Regulation 32, no. 2 (2009): 12.

55. Mashaw and Harfst, "From Command and Control to Collaboration and Deference," 213.
56. Ibid., 173.
57. A. Taeihagh and H. S. Lim, "Governing Autonomous Vehicles: Emerging Responses for Safety, Liability, Privacy, Cybersecurity, and Industry Risks," *Transport Reviews* 39, no. 1 (2019): 103–28.
58. J. R. Quain, "Autonomous Cars Are Still Learning to See," *New York Times*, September 27, 2019.
59. Society of Automotive Engineers International, Standard "Taxonomy and Definitions for Terms Related to On-road Motor Vehicle Automated Driving Systems, J3016_201401" January 16, 2014, https://www.sae.org/standards/content/j3016_201401/.
60. T. Litman, "Autonomous Vehicle Implementation Predictions Implications for Transport Planning," Victoria Transport Policy Institute, 2019.
61. Strategy Analytics, "Accelerating the Future: The Economic Impact of the Emerging Passenger Economy," June 2017.
62. J. Muller, "Look, Ma, No Steering Wheel or Pedals in GM's Robo-Taxi, Coming In 2019," *Forbes*, January 12, 2018.
63. N. Briscoe, "SSelf-driving Cars: Is the Autonomous Dream Slipping Away from Us?" *Irish Times*, March 13, 2019.
64. World Health Organization, *Global Status Report on Road Safety 2018* (Geneva, World Health Organization, 2018).
65. Litman, "Autonomous Vehicle Implementation Predictions Implications for Transport Planning"; Taeihagh and Lim, "Governing Autonomous Vehicles," 103–28.
66. Litman, ibid.
67. J. B. Greenblatt and S. Shaheen, "Automated Vehicles, On-demand Mobility, and Environmental Impacts," *Current Sustainable/Renewable Energy Reports* 2, no. 3 (2015): 74–81.
68. G. S. Bauer, J. B. Greenblatt, and B. F. Gerke, "Cost, Energy, and Environmental Impact of Automated Electric Taxi Fleets in Manhattan," *Environmental Science & Technology* 52, no. 8 (2018): 4920–28.
69. Litman, "Autonomous Vehicle Implementation Predictions Implications for Transport Planning."
70. I. Austen and D. Wakabayashi, "City of the Future in Toronto? Not Now, Google Sibling Says," *The New York Times*, May 8, 2020.
71. B. W. Smith, "Managing Autonomous Transportation Demand," *Santa Clara Law Review* 52 (2012): 1401.
72. T. Cohen and C. Cavoli, "Automated Vehicles: Exploring Possible Consequences of Government (Non) Intervention for Congestion and Accessibility," *Transport Reviews* 39, no. 1 (2019): 129–51.
73. G. C. Wellman, "Transportation Apartheid: The Role of Transportation Policy in Societal Inequality," *Public Works Management & Policy* 19, no. 4 (2014): 334–39.
74. Ibid.
75. P. M. Smolnicki and J. Sołtys, "Driverless Mobility," *Procedia Engineering* 161 (2016): 2184–90.
76. C. Reinicke, "Autonomous Vehicles Won't Only Kill Jobs. They Will Create Them, Too," CNBC, August 11 2018.
77. A. Balakrishnan, "Self-driving Cars Could Cost America's Professional Drivers Up to 25,000 Jobs a Month, Goldman Sachs Says," CNBC, May 22, 2017.

78. Cohen and Cavoli, *Automated Vehicles*, 129–51; Litman, "Autonomous Vehicle Implementation Predictions Implications for Transport Planning."
79. R. Nader, *Unsafe at Any Speed: The Designed-in Dangers of the American Automobile* (New York: Grossman, 1965); Doyle, *Taken for a Ride*; K. Bradsher, *High and Mighty SUVs: The World's Most Dangerous Vehicles and How They Got That Way* (New York: Public Affairs, 2002).
80. T. Wheeler, "The Tragedy of Tech Companies: Getting the Regulation They Want," Brookings TechTank, March 26, 2019.
81. O. James, "Uber and Lyft Are Lobbying States to Prohibit Local Regulation," Mobility Lab, July 24, 2018.
82. Cohen and Cavoli, "Automated Vehicles," 129–51.
83. J. S. Rothstein, *When Good Jobs Go Bad: Globalization, De-unionization, and Declining Job Quality in the North American Auto Industry* (New Brunswick, NJ: Rutgers University Press, 2016).
84. Mashaw and Harfst, "From Command and Control to Collaboration and Deference," 167.
85. Corporate Europe Observatory, "Two Years after Dieselgate: Car Industry Still Drives Berlin and Brussels," September 18, 2017.
86. S. Miller, "The Dangers of Techno-Optimism," *Berkeley Political Review*, November 16, 2017.
87. P. C. Baker, "Collision Course: Why Are Cars Killing More and More Pedestrians?" *Guardian*, October 3, 2019.
88. Ibid.
89. L. Burns and C. Shulgan, *Autonomy: The Quest to Build the Driverless Car—and How It Will Shape Our World* (New York: HarperCollins, 2018).
90. N. Kitroeff and D. Gelles, "As Boeing Scrutinizes 737 Max, New Safety Risks Come to Light," *New York Times*, January 6, 2020.
91. Centers for Disease Control and Prevention, "CDC Winnable Battles Final Report," US Department of Health and Human Services, 2016.
92. Governor's Highway Safety Association, "Pedestrian Traffic Fatalities by State: 2018 Preliminary Data," 2019.
93. Bradsher, *High and Mighty SUVs*.
94. R. Premack, "America's Obsession with Trucks and SUVs Is Helping Push Car-loan Payments to a 10-year High," Business Insider, March 17, 2019.
95. Baker, "Collision Course."
96. R. Rissanen, H. Y. Berg, and M. Hasselberg, "Quality of Life Following Road Traffic Injury: A Systematic Literature Review," *Accident Analysis & Prevention* 108 (2017): 308–20.
97. A. Arieff, "Cars Are Death Machines. Self-Driving Tech Won't Change That," op-ed, *New York Times*, October 4, 2019.
98. World Health Organization, *WHO Global Status Report on Road Safety 2018* (Geneva: World Health Organization, 2018).
99. Ibid.
100. P. J. Landrigan, R. Fuller, N. J. Acosta et al., "The Lancet Commission on Pollution and Health," *The Lancet* 391, no. 10119 (2018): 462–512.
101. Ibid.
102. United States Environmental Protection Agency, "National Annual Emission Trend, 1970–2018," 2019.
103. United States Environmental Protection Agency, "Fast Facts on Transportation Greenhouse Gas Emissions," 2018.

104. Intergovernmental Panel on Climate Change, "Climate Change and Land: An IPCC Special Report on Climate Change, Desertification, Land Degradation, Sustainable Land Management, Food Security, and Greenhouse Gas Fluxes in Terrestrial Ecosystems," Summary for Policymakers, 2019.
105. Landrigan, Fuller, Acosta et al., "The Lancet Commission on Pollution and Health," 462–512.
106. Arieff, "Cars Are Death Machines."
107. H. Frumkin, "Urban Sprawl and Public Health," *Public Health Reports* 117 (2002): 201–17.
108. P. D. Norton, *Fighting Traffic: The Dawn of the Motor Age in the American City* (Cambridge, MA: MIT Press; 2011), 21–46.
109. Doyle, *Taken for a Ride*, 62.
110. E. Vulliamy, "What Would Jesus Drive? A Disciple Carrier, of Course," *Guardian*, November 24, 2002.
111. Center for Auto Safety, "Center for Auto Safety—What It Is and What It Does, Annual Report 2015."
112. R. McFadden "Clarence M. Ditlow III, Auto Safety Crusader, Dies at 72," *New York Times*, November 12, 2016.
113. Ibid.
114. "Recall Advocates Plan Demonstration at G.M. Meeting," *New York Times*, May 21, 1993.
115. Langer, "Clarence Ditlow, Crusading Consumer Advocate for Auto Safety, Dies at 72," *Washington Post*, November 11, 2016.
116. J. Levine, "Letter to Dara Khosrowshahi," Center for Auto Safety, August 12, 2019.
117. J. Levine, "Counterpoint: Are Self-driving Cars a Good Idea? Think Safety First," *Illinois Business Journal*, October 7, 2019.
118. D. I. Grossman, "Would a Corporate 'Death Penalty' Be Cruel and Unusual Punishment?" *Cornell Journal of Law and Public Policy* 25 (2015): 697.
119. Transportation Alternatives, "We Can Reclaim Our Streets," n.d., https://www.transalt.org/.
120. G. Bellafante, "Crosstown Street, Minus the Cars: A Start," *New York Times*, October 18, 2019.
121. Transportation Alternatives, "A Tactical Urbanist Response to COVID-19," April 8, 2020.
122. Transportation Alternatives, "Families for Safe Streets: About Us," n.d., https://www.transalt.org/getinvolved/familiesforsafestreets/about.
123. M. Conner and E. McDermott, "A City Back in Gear," Medium, May 9, 2019.
124. A. Plitt, "As Traffic Fatalities Rise in NYC, Safe Streets Advocates Demand Action," Curbed NY, May 7, 2019.
125. N. Berman, "Corey Johnson Wants to 'Break the Car Culture' in New York City. What Does That Mean?" *Gotham Gazette*, July 1, 2019.
126. A. Kaswan, "California Climate Policies Serving Climate Justice," *Natural Resources & Environment* 33, no. 4 (2019: 12–16.
127. California Air Resources Board, "California's 2017 Climate Change Scoping Plan," 2017, https://ww3.arb.ca.gov/cc/scopingplan/scopingplan.htm.
128. D. Roberts, "California's Cap-and-trade System May Be Too Weak to Do Its Job," Vox, December 13, 2018.
129. R. Barnes and J. Eilperin, "High Court Faults EPA Inaction on Emissions," *Washington Post*, April 3, 2007.

130. D. Kasler, "In Major Coup against Trump, Gov. Gavin Newsom Strikes Climate Change Deal with Carmakers," *Sacramento Bee*, July 25, 2019.
131. H. Tabuchi, "24 Governors Call for Halt to Emissions Rollback," *New York Times*, July 10, 2019.
132. California Air Resources Board, "California and Major Automakers Reach Groundbreaking Framework Agreement on Clean Emission Standards," July 25, 2019.

CHAPTER 7

1. G. Orwell, *In Front of Your Nose, 1945–1950: The Collected Essays, Journalism and Letters of George Orwell*, ed. S. Orwell and I. Angus, vol. 4, *Essays, Journalism, and Letters* (New York: Harcourt, Harcourt, Brace and World, 1968), 172–73.
2. S. Zuboff, *The Age of Surveillance Capitalism: The Fight for a Human Future at the New Frontier of Power* (London: Profile Books, 2019), 255.
3. N. Klein, *No Is Not Enough* (Chicago: Haymarket Books, 2017), 25–26.
4. "37 Mind Blowing YouTube Facts, Figures and Statistics—2020," MerchDope, February 26, 2020.
5. A. Hawkins, "Sidewalk Labs Wants to Build a City-within-a-City," *Wall Street Journal*, April 26, 2016.
6. E. Schmidt and J. Cohen, *The New Digital Age: Transforming Nations, Businesses, and Our Lives* (New York: Vintage, 2014), 10.
7. N. Reiff, "Top 7 Companies Owned by Amazon," Investopedia, June 25, 2019, https://www.investopedia.com/articles/markets/102115/top-10-companies-owned-amazon.asp.
8. Marist Poll, "NPR/Marist Poll Results June 2018: Digital Economy."
9. F. Frankenfield, "How Amazon Makes Money: Cloud Services, Advertising and Retail Are Growing Fast," Investopedia, June 3, 2019.
10. L. Sumagaysay. "Amazon reaches 1 million workers amid pandemic hiring frenzy," MarketWatch, July 30, 2020 .
11. L. Grossman, "Inside Facebook's Plan to Wire the World," *Time*, December 15, 2015.
12. Statista, "Facebook's Advertising Revenue Worldwide from 2009 to 2019," https://www.statista.com/statistics/271258/facebooks-advertising-revenue-worldwide/.
13. L. Feiner, "Apple's App Store Ads Could Be a $2 Billion Business by 2020," CNBC, October 22, 2018.
14. Statista, "Apple's Global Revenue from 1st Quarter 2005 to 4th Quarter 2019," https://www.statista.com/statistics/263426/apples-global-revenue-since-1st-quarter-2005/.
15. K. Johnson, "GitHub Passes 100 Million Repositories, VentureBeat," November 8, 2018.
16. J. Bort, "Satya Nadella Just Launched Microsoft into a New $ 1.6 Trillion Market," Business Insider, April 15, 2014.
17. S. Nadella, "A Data Culture for Everyone," Official Microsoft Blog, April 15, 2014, https://blogs.microsoft.com/blog/2014/04/15/a-data-culture-for-everyone/.
18. Lekkas, "The Big Five Tech Companies and Their Big Five Acquisitions."
19. M. Phillips, "Giant Stocks Shrug Off Obstacles," *New York Times*, December 11, 2019.
20. N. Singer, "Apple Adds Its Muscle to Medicine," *New York Times*, November 15, 2019.
21. F. Norris, *The Octopus: A Story of California* (New York: Cocimo Classics, 2010 [first published, 1901], 202.

22. Y. T. Wang, V. Mechkova, and F. Andersson, "Does Democracy Enhance Health? New Empirical Evidence 1900–2012," *Political Research Quarterly* 72, no. 3 (2019): 554–69; A. Chandra, C. E. Miller, J. D. Acosta et al., "Drivers of Health as a Shared Value: Mindset, Expectations, Sense of Community, and Civic Engagement," *Health Affairs* 35, no. 11 (2016): 1959–63; National Academies of Sciences, Engineering, and Medicine, *Communities in Action: Pathways to Health Equity* (Washington, DC: National Academies Press, 2017).

23. N. Andalibi, P. Ozturk, and A. Forte, "Sensitive Self-disclosures, Responses, and Social Support on Instagram: The Case of #Depression," in *Proceedings of the 2017 ACM Conference on Computer Supported Cooperative Work and Social Computing*, February 2017, 1485–1500.

24. N. R. Nicolson, "A Review of Social Isolation," *Journal of Primary Prevention* 33, nos. 2–3 (2012): 137–52.

25. M. Pantell, D. Rehkopf, D. Jutte et al., "Social Isolation: A Predictor of Mortality Comparable to Traditional Clinical Risk Factors," *American Journal of Public Health* 103, no 11 (2013): 2056–62.

26. J. S. House, "Social Isolation Kills, but How and Why?" *Psychosomatic Medicine* 63, no. 2 (2001): 273–74.

27. B. DiJulio, L. Hamel, C. Muñana, and M. Brodie, "Loneliness and Social Isolation in the United States, the United Kingdom, and Japan: An International Survey," Kaiser Family Fund, 2018.

28. D. M. Clark, N. J. Loxton, and S. J. Tobin, "Declining Loneliness over Time: Evidence from American Colleges and High Schools," *Personality and Social Psychology Bulletin* 41, no. 1 (2015): 78–89.

29. B. A. Primack, A. Shensa, J. E. Sidani et al., "Social Media Use and Perceived Social Isolation among Young Adults in the US," *American Journal of Preventive Medicine* 53, no. 1 (2017): 1–8.

30. H. B. Shakya and N. A. Christakis, "Association of Facebook Use with Compromised Well-being: A Longitudinal Study," *American Journal of Epidemiology* 185, no. 3 (2017): 203–11.

31. M. Tromholt, "The Facebook Experiment: Quitting Facebook Leads to Higher Levels of Well-being," *Cyberpsychology, Behavior, and Social Networking* 19, no. 11 (2016): 661–66.

32. V. Franchina, M. Vanden Abeele, A. J. Van Rooij, G. Lo Coco, and L. De Marez, "Fear of Missing Out as a Predictor of Problematic Social Media Use and Phubbing Behavior among Flemish Adolescents," *International Journal of Environmental Research and Public Health* 15, no. 10 (2018): 2319.

33. N. Rothchild, "Is Troublesome Facebook Use a Behavioral Addiction?" *American Journal of Medical Research* 5, no. 1 (2018): 73–78.

34. M. E. Duffy, J. M. Twenge, and T. E. Joiner, "Trends in Mood and Anxiety Symptoms and Suicide-related Outcomes among US Undergraduates, 2007–2018: Evidence from Two National Surveys," *Journal of Adolescent Health* 65, no. 5 (2019): 590–98.

35. A. Shensa, C. G. Escobar-Viera, J. E. Sidani et al., "Problematic Social Media Use and Depressive Symptoms among US Young Adults: A Nationally-representative Study," *Social Science & Medicine* 182 (2017): 150–57.

36. B. W. Fisher, J. H. Gardella, and A. R. Teurbe-Tolon, "Peer Cybervictimization among Adolescents and the Associated Internalizing and Externalizing Problems: A Meta-analysis," *Journal of Youth and Adolescence* 45, no. 9 (2016): 1727–43.

37. "The Decade Tech Lost Its Way: An Oral History of the 2010s," *New York Times*, December 15, 2019.

38. M. D. Griffiths, "Adolescent Social Networking: How Do Social Media Operators Facilitate Habitual Use?" *Education and Health* 36, no. 3 (2018): 66–69.

39. Deloitte, "The Deloitte Global Millennial Survey 2019."

40. K. Amadeo, "Personal Consumption Expenditures, Statistics, and Why It's Important: What Do Americans Really Spend Their Money On?" The Balance, June 25, 2019.

41. Statista, "Digital Economy 2019," 132.

42. W. C. Frazier and J. L. Harris, "Trends in Television Food Advertising to Young People: 2017 Update," UConn Rudd Center for Food Policy & Obesity, 2018.

43. Institute of Medicine, *Accelerating Progress in Obesity Prevention: Solving the Weight of the Nation* (Washington, DC: The National Academies Press, 2012); J. L. Harris and F. Fleming-Milici, "Food Marketing to Adolescents and Young Adults: Skeptical but Still under the Influence," in *The Psychology of Food Marketing and Overeating*, ed. F. Folkvord (Abingdon, Oxfordshire: Routledge, 2019), 25–43.

44. UConn Rudd Center for Food Policy & Obesity, "Food Industry Self-regulation after 10 Years: Progress and Opportunities to Improve Food Advertising to Children," 2017.

45. Carol Kruse, cited in "The New Age of Food Marketing: How Companies Are Targeting and Luring Our Kids—and What Advocates Can Do about It," Center for Digital Democracy, Public Health Law and Policy, and Berkeley Media Studies Group, 2011, 10.

46. "The New Age of Food Marketing: How Companies Are Targeting and Luring Our Kids—and What Advocates Can Do about It," Center for Digital Democracy, Public Health Law and Policy, and Berkeley Media Studies Group," 2011.

47. F. Imamura, L. O'Connor, and Z. Ye et al., "Consumption of Sugar Sweetened Beverages, Artificially Sweetened Beverages, and Fruit Juice and Incidence of Type 2 Diabetes: Systematic Review, Meta-analysis, and Estimation of Population Attributable Fraction," *The BMJ* 351 (2015): h3576.

48. "The New Age of Food Marketing: How Companies Are Targeting and Luring Our Kids—and What Advocates Can Do about It."

49. J. Cantrell, O. Ganz, B. Emelle et al., "Mobile Marketing: An Emerging Strategy to Promote Electronic Nicotine Delivery Systems," *Tobacco Control* 26, no. e2 (2017): e1–3.

50. H. Knowles and L. H. Sun, "What We Know about the Mysterious Vaping-linked Illness and Deaths," *The Washington Post*, November 14, 2019.

51. R. K. Jackler, C. Chau, B. D. Getachew et al., "JUUL Advertising over Its First Three Years on the Market," Stanford Research into the Impact of Tobacco Advertising (working paper, Stanford University School of Medicine, January 31, 2019).

52. M. Richtel and S. Kaplan, "Investigators Ask if Vaping Ads Tried to Hook Teenagers for Life," *New York Times*, August 27, 2018.

53. Leonard A. The Story of Stuff," 2009, https://www.youtube.com/watch?reload=9&v=9GorqroigqM&vl=en

54. T. Schlossberg, *Inconspicuous Consumption, the Environmental Impact You Don't Know You Have* (New York: Grand Central Publishing, 2019), 9–63.

55. Statista, "Number of Digital Shoppers in the United States from 2016 to 2021 (in Millions)," https://www.statista.com/statistics/183755/number-of-us-internet-shoppers-since-2009/.

56. S. Kroll, "Retail E-Commerce Sales Rising; Evergage Expands into Europe," Retail Tech News, February 15, 2018.

57. International Air Transport Association, "The Value of Air Cargo, Air Cargo Makes It Happen," IATA, 2018, https://www.iata.org/contentassets/4d3961c878894c8a8725278607d8ad52/air-cargo-brochure.pdf

58. "Boeing Forecasts Air Cargo Traffic Will Double in 20 Years," Boeing, October 16, 2018.

59. T. C. Frankel, "The Cobalt Pipeline," *The Washington Post*, September 30, 2016.

60. P. Whoriskey, "In Your Phone, in Their Air," *The Washington Post*, October 2, 2016.

61. T. C. Frankel and P. Whoriskey, "Tossed Aside in the 'White Gold' Rush," *The Washington Post*, December 19, 2016.

62. J. Bulow, "An Economic Theory of Planned Obsolescence," *The Quarterly Journal of Economics* 101, no. 4 (1986): 729–49.

63. D. Boorstin, *The Americans: The Democratic Experience* (New York: Knopf Doubleday, 1974), 554.

64. "The Decade Tech Lost Its Way."

65. C. P. Baldé, V. Forti, V. Gray, R. Kuehr, and P. Stegmann, *The Global E-waste Monitor 2017* (Bonn/Geneva/Vienna: United Nations University [UNU], International Telecommunication Union [ITU], and International Solid Waste Association, 2017).

66. "Electronics Waste Management in the United States through 2009," United States Environmental Protection Agency, May 2011, EPA 530-R-11-002, https://nepis.epa.gov/Exe/tiff2png.cgi/P100BKLY.PNG?-r+75+-g+7+D%3A%5CZYFILES%5CINDEX%20DATA%5C11THRU15%5CTIFF%5C00000059%5CP100BKLY.TIF

67. N. A. Shah, Y. Rasheed, R. M. Anjum, "Health Effects of E-waste Pollution," in *Electronic Waste Pollution 2019*, ed. M. Z. Hashmi and A. Varma (Cham, Switzerland: Springer), 139–51.

68. K. Grant, F. C. Goldizen, P. D. Sly et al., "Health Consequences of Exposure to E-waste: A Systematic Review," *The Lancet Global Health* 1, no. 6 (2013): e350–61.

69. S. Davies, *Privacy: A Personal Chronicle* (Electronic Privacy Information Center, 2018), Kindle, Location 430.

70. T. Wu, *The Attention Merchants* (New York: Knopf), 342.

71. D. FitzGerald, "5G Race Could Leave Personal Privacy in the Dust," *Wall Street Journal*, November 12, 2019.

72. Ibid.

73. M. Kosinski, D. Stillwell, and T. Graepel, "Private Traits and Attributes Are Predictable from Digital Records of Human Behavior," *Proceedings of the National Academy of Sciences* 110, no. 15 (2013): 5802–5.

74. V. Woollaston, "Facebook Slammed after Advertising Funeral Directors to a Cancer Patient: Promotions Appeared," *Daily Mail*, March 11, 2015.

75. R. Copeland, "Google's 'Project Nightingale' Gathers Personal Health Data on Millions of Americans," *Wall Street Journal*, November 11, 2019.

76. E. Snowden, "Just days left to kill mass surveillance under Section 215 of the Patriot Act," Reddit, May 21, 2015, https://www.reddit.com/r/IAmA/comments/36ru89/just_days_left_to_kill_mass_surveillance_under/crglgh2/.

77. M. Wolff, "Ad Blockers Impair Digital Media," *USA TODAY*, September 13, 2015.

78. Wu, *The Attention Merchants*, 323.

79. Davies, *Privacy*, Location 1421.

80. Ibid., Location 1492.
81. "The Decade Tech Lost Its Way."
82. D. Thompson, "Google's CEO: 'The Laws Are Written by Lobbyists.'" *The Atlantic*, October 1, 2010.
83. Federal Trade Commission, "Facebook Settles FTC Charges That It Deceived Consumers by Failing to Keep Privacy Promises," November 29, 2011, https://www.ftc.gov/news-events/press-releases/2011/11/facebook-settles-ftc-charges-it-deceived-consumers-failing-keep.
84. "The Decade Tech Lost Its Way."
85. A. K. Sen, *Development as Freedom* (New York: Knopf, 1999).
86. M. Wise and P. ainsbury, "Democracy: The Forgotten Determinant of Mental Health," *Health Promotion Journal of Australia* 18, no. 3 (2007): 177–83.
87. A. Deb, S. Donohue, and T. Glaisyer, "Is Social Media a Threat to Democracy?" The Omidyar Group, 2017.
88. "Mark Zuckerberg Stands for Voice and Free Expression," Facebook, October 17, 2019, https://about.fb.com/news/2019/10/mark-zuckerberg-stands-for-voice-and-free-expression/.
89. E. Osnos, "Can Mark Zuckerberg Fix Facebook before It Breaks Democracy?" *The New Yorker*, September 10, 2018.
90. C. Zakrzewski, "The Technology 202: Mark Zuckerberg Says Facebook Is Taking a Long View on Free Speech as Critics Attack Companies' Policies," *The Washington Post*, October 18, 2019.
91. Osnos, "Can Mark Zuckerberg Fix Facebook Before It Breaks Democracy?"
92. "The Decade Tech Lost Its Way."
93. C. Silverman, "This Analysis Shows How Viral Fake Election News Stories Outperformed Real News on Facebook," BuzzFeed, November 16, 2016.
94. C. Kang and M. Isaac, "Zuckerberg Says Facebook Won't Police Political Speech," *New York Times*, October 18, 2019.
95. K. Roose, S. Frenkl, and M. Isaac, "Agonizing at Facebook over Trump," *New York Times*, January 8, 2020.
96. E. Lutz, "George Soros Suggests Facebook Is in Cahoots with Trump," *Vanity Fair*, January 24, 2020.
97. K. Leetaru, "What Is Democracy When Twitter Decides Who Speaks to the President?" *Forbes*, April 25, 2019.
98. B. Lynn, "Google and Facebook Are Strangling the Free Press to Death. Democracy Is the Loser," *Guardian*, July 26, 2018.
99. T. Wu, "The Curse of Bigness: Antitrust in the New Gilded Age," Columbia Global Report, 2018.
100. S. Vaidhyanathan, *Antisocial Media: How Facebook Disconnects Us and Undermines Democracy* (New York: Oxford University Press, 2018).
101. d. boyd, *Why Youth (Heart) Social Network Sites: The Role of Networked Publics in Teenage Social Life*. MacArthur Foundation Series on Digital Learning—Youth, Identity, and Digital Media Volume, ed. David Buckingham (Cambridge, MA: MIT Press, 2007), 3.
102. K. C. Montgomery, "Youth and Surveillance in the Facebook Era: Policy Interventions and Social Implications," *Telecommunications Policy* 39, no. 9 (2015): 774.
103. M. Lynch, "After Egypt: The Limits and Promise of Online Challenges to the Authoritarian Arab State," *Perspectives on Politics* 9, no. 2 (2011): 301–10.
104. A. Semuels, "How Amazon Helped Kill a Seattle Tax on Business," *The Atlantic*, June 13, 2018.

105. S. Shane, "Prime Mover: How Amazon Wove Itself into the Life of an American City," *The New York Times*, November 30, 2019.
106. S. Goldenberg and D. Rubinstein, "With Amazon Deal Dashed, New York's Vast Tax Breaks Called into Question," Politico, February 19, 2019.
107. T. Roosevelt, *A Compilation of the Messages and Speeches of Theodore Roosevelt*, vol. 1, *1901–1905* (London: Arkose Press, 2015), 64.
108. R. Cooper, "The Return of the Trust-busters," *The Week*, January 9, 2018, https://theweek.com/articles/725483/return-trustbusters.
109. E. Kefauver, quoted in Federal Antirtrust Enforcement and Its Impact on Small Business: Hearing Before the Committee on Small Business United States Senate, 98th Cong., (1984) (E. Kefauver) , p. 310. https://www.google.com/books/edition/Federal_Antitrust_Enforcement_and_Its_Im/E-WjtaCDgokC?hl=en&gbpv=0
110. S. Vaheesan, "Accommodating Capital and Policing Labor: Antitrust in the Two Gilded Ages," *Maryland Law Review* 78 (2018): 766.
111. V. Rideout and M. Robb, *The Common Sense Census: Media Use by Tweens and Teens*, 2019 (San Francisco: Common Sense Media, 2019).
112. M. Nestle, "Annals of Marketing: A Sugary Cereal for Toddlers," Food Politics, August 9, 2019.
113. N. Singer and K. Conger, "Google Is Fined $170 Million for Violating Children's Privacy on YouTube," *New York Times*, September 4, 2018.
114. "AG James: Google and YouTube to Pay Record Figure for Illegally Tracking and Collecting Personal Information from Children," September 4, 2019.
115. S. Maheshwari, "YouTube Is Improperly Collecting Children's Data, Consumer Groups Say," *New York Times*, April 9, 2018.
116. Singer and Conger, "Google Is Fined $170 Million for Violating Children's Privacy on YouTube."
117. Campaign for a Commercial-free Childhood, "Tell the FTC: Children Need More Privacy Protection, Not Less," 2019, https://ccfc.salsalabs.org/save_coppa/index.html.
118. Change.org, "SAVE Family-Friendly Content on YouTube," 2019, https://www.change.org/p/youtubers-and-viewers-unite-against-ftc-regulation.
119. "Petition to Sundar Pichai," 2018, https://static01.nyt.com/files/2018/technology/googleletter.pdf.
120. M. Chen, "How Tech Workers Are Fighting Back against Collusion with ICE and the Department of Defense," *The Nation*, June 27, 2018.
121. R. Paulas, "A New Kind of Labor Movement in Silicon Valley," *The Atlantic*, September 4, 2018.
122. B. Menegus, "Amazon's Own Numbers Reveal Staggering Injury Rates at Staten Island Warehouse," Gizmodo, November 25, 2019.
123. L. Fickenscher, "Workers at Amazon's Staten Island Warehouse Hold Rally over High Injury Rates," *New York Post*, November 25, 2019.
124. A. Garcia, "Amazon Workers Walk Out to Protest Climate Change Inaction," CNN Business, September 20, 2019.
125. N. Higgins-Dunn, "Jeff Bezos Is Finally Ending Secrecy over Amazon's Role in Carbon Emissions," CNBC, March 8, 2019.
126. "Coders of the World, Unite: Can Silicon Valley Workers Curb the Power of Big Tech?" *Guardian*, October 31, 2017.
127. A. Glaser and W. Oremus, "A Collective Aghastness," *Slate*, June 28, 2018.
128. Tech Workers Coalition, "Who We Are," n.d., https://techworkerscoalition.org/#learn.

129. Glaser and Oremus, "A Collective Aghastness."
130. Tech Workers Coalition, "Tech Won't Build It Zine," 2018, https://www.slideshare.net/PaigePanter/tech-wont-build-it-zine/1.
131. Silicon Valley Rising, "About Us," n.d., https://siliconvalleyrising.org/about/.
132. D. Streitfeld, "The Amazon Behemoth and Its Would-Be David," *New York Times*, November 26, 2019.
133. Athena, "Tell Amazon: Reinstate Fired Workers Organizing for Health and Safety Protections in Warehouses," n.d., https://actionnetwork.org/petitions/tell-amazon-reinstate-fired-workers-organizing-for-health-and-safety-protections-in-warehouses.
134. T. Wu, "The Curse of Bigness: Antitrust in the New Gilded Age," Columbia Global Report, 2018, 123.
135. "Freedom from Facebook," n.d., https://freedomfromfb.com/.
136. Freedom from Facebook, "Complaint Seeking Investigation, Enforcement, Penalties, and Other Relief as Appropriate against Facebook, Inc.," November 15, 2019, https://www.commondreams.org/newswire/2018/11/15/freedom-facebook-files-legal-complaint-ftc-against-facebook.
137. C. Kang and D. McCabe, "California Sues Facebook for Documents in Privacy Investigation," *New York Times*, November 7, 2019.
138. M. Laslo, "Should Tech CEOs Go to Jail over Data Misuse? Some Senators Say Yes." *Wired*, October 30, 2019.
139. S. Ifill, "Mark Zuckerberg Doesn't Know His Civil Rights History," op-ed, *Washington Post*, October 17, 2018.

CHAPTER 8

1. P. L. Pingali, "Green Revolution: Impacts, Limits, and the Path Ahead," *Proceedings of the National Academy of Sciences* 109, no. 31 (2012): 12302–8.
2. N. Klein, *No Is Not Enough: Resisting Trump's Shock Politics and Winning the World We Need* (Chicago: Haymarket Books, 2017), 237–38.
3. I. X. Kendi, *How to Be an Antiracist* (New York: One World, 2019), 151–65.
4. L. Cox, A. G. Nilsen, "Social Movements Research and the 'Movement of Movements': Studying Resistance to Neoliberal Globalization," *Sociology Compass* 1, no. 2 (2007): 424–42.
5. H. Patomäki and T. Teivainen, "The World Social Forum: An Open Space or a Movement of Movements?" *Theory, Culture & Society* 21, no. 6 (2004): 145–54.
6. A. Lorde, "Learning from the 60s," in *Sister Outsider: Essays and Speeches* (Berkeley, CA: Crossing Press, 2007), 138.
7. J. Stites, "Beyond Hollywood: Domestic Workers Say #MeToo," *In These Times*, February 19, 2018.
8. B. K. Hamilton, *Traveler, There Is No Road . . . : The Way Is Made by Walking* (Iowa City: University of Iowa Press, 2017), 1.
9. O. Balch "Buen Vivir: The Social Philosophy Inspiring Movements in South America," *Guardian*, February 4, 2013.
10. E. Gudynas, "Buen Vivir: Today's Tomorrow," *Development* 54 (2011): 441–47.
11. D. Grandoni, "The Energy 202: Ocasio-Cortez, Markey Unveil Green New Deal with Backing of Four Presidential Candidates," *Washington Post*, February 7, 2019.
12. IPCC, "2018: Summary for Policymakers," in *Global Warming of 1.5°C: An IPCC Special Report*, ed. V. Masson-Delmotte et al., 2019.
13. R. Gunn-Wright and R. Hockett, "The Green New Deal: Mobilizing for a Just, Prosperous, and Sustainable Economy," produced by New Consensus, 2019.

14. "Recognizing the Duty of the Federal Government to Create a Green New Deal," H.R. Res. 109, 116th Cong. (2019–2020).

15. A. Flaccavento, "The Green New Deal—A Compelling Idea that Challenges Both Parties," February 28, 2019, https://www.anthonyflaccavento.com/blog/2019/2/28/the-green-new-deal-a-compelling-idea-that-challenges-both-parties.

16. M. Dickinson, N. Freudenberg, R. Ilieva, "Put Food on the Green New Deal Menu," *City Limits*, July 19, 2019.

17. Sunrise Movement, "About Us," n.d., https://www.sunrisemovement.org/about.

18. "Amazon Employees for Climate Justice," Open Letter to Jeff Bezos and the Amazon Board of Directors, April 10, 2019.

19. J. Greene, "Amazon Threatens to Fire Critics Who Are Outspoken on Its Environmental Policies," *Washington Post*, January 2, 2020.

20. Y. Funes, "The Green New Deal Includes a Powerful Pledge to Indigenous People," Gizmodo, February 15, 2019.

21. J. Rifkin, *The Green New Deal: Why the Fossil Fuel Civilization Will Collapse* (New York: St. Martin's Press, 2019), 233–34.

22. Funes, "The Green New Deal Includes a Powerful Pledge to Indigenous People."

23. A. Flaccavento, "Virginia's Swung Blue, but It Hasn't Trickled Down to the Countryside," Anthony Flaccavento Blog, November 7, 2019, https://www.anthonyflaccavento.com/blog/2019/11/7/virginias-swung-blue-but-it-hasnt-trickled-down-to-the-countryside.

24. Z. Carpenter, "The Political Power of the Green New Deal," *The Nation*, May 17, 2019.

25. A. R. Coleman, "How Black Lives Matter to the Green New Deal," *The Nation*, March 14, 2019.

26. C. Tumber, "Land without Bread: The Green New Deal Forsakes America's Countryside," Common Dreams, September 16, 2019.

27. M. Grunwald, "The Impossible Green Dream of Alexandria Ocasio-Cortez," Politico, February 7, 2019.

28. M. Kelly and T. Howard, *The Making of a Democratic Economy: Building Prosperity for the Many, Not Just the Few* (San Francisco: Berrett-Koehler Publishers, 2019), Kindle, Location 1283.

29. S. Schneider, "Cooperative Home Care Associates: Participation with 1600 Employees," Grassroots Economic Organizing, April 20, 2010, https://geo.coop/node/433.

30. L. Flanders, "How America's Largest Worker Owned Co-op Lifts People Out of Poverty," *Yes!* August 15, 2014.

31. Kelly and Howard, *The Making of a Democratic Economy*, Location 1251.

32. R. Galvin, "Confronting Our Common Enemy: Elite White Male Supremacy," *Medium*, February 14, 2017.

33. J. E. Causey, "In Cleveland, Co-op Model Finds Hope in Employers Rooted in the City," *Milwaukee Journal Sentinel*, April 27, 2017.

34. Evergreen Cooperative, "About Us," n.d., https://www.evgoh.com/about-us/.

35. Causey, "In Cleveland, Co-op Model Finds Hope in Employers Rooted in the City."

36. Ibid.

37. Green City Growers, "Evergreen Cooperative," n.d., http://www.evgoh.com/feature/green-city-growers/.

38. D. J. Guth, "A Bright Future Ahead: Cleveland's Green City Growers Uses LED Lights," *Produce Grower*, January 22, 2019.

39. Evergreen Energy Solutions, ",Your Single Source for Energy-Saving Expertise" n.d., http://www.evgoh.com/e2s/

40. D. J. Hess, *Good Green Jobs in a Global Economy: Making and Keeping New Industries in the United States* (Cambridge, MA: MIT Press, 2012).

41. J. G. Nembhard, "Building a Cooperative Solidarity Commonwealth," The Next System Project, 2016, https://base.socioeco.org/docs/jessicagordonnembhard.pdf

42. M. Peck, "Liberating Our Futures Together: Building the Cooperative Ecosystem in Cincinnati," One Worker One Vote, 2019, http://1worker1vote.org/liberating-futures-together-building-cooperative-ecosystem-cincinnati/.

43. J. Blasi, R. B. Freeman, and D. Kruse, "Evidence: What the US Research Shows about Worker Ownership," in *The Oxford Handbook of Mutual, Co-Operative, and Co-Owned Business*, ed. J. Michie, J. R. Blasi, and C. Borzaga (New York: Oxford University Press, 2017), 211–27.

44. M. Cohen, "Workers—and Consumers—of the World Unite? Opportunities for Hybrid Cooperativism," in *The Oxford Handbook of Co-Operative and Mutual Business*, ed. J. Blasi, D. Borzaga, and J. Michie (Oxford: Oxford University Press, 2015), 374–85.

45. Nembhard, "Building a Cooperative Solidarity Commonwealth," 11.

46. D. Spade, "Solidarity Not Charity," *Social Text* 142, no. 38 (2020): 131–51.

47. J. Tolention, "What Mutual Aid Can Do during a Pandemic," *The New Yorker*, May 18, 2020.

48. E. Cranley, "POLL: 23% of Americans Who Owe a Rent or a Mortgage Payment on Friday Aren't Sure if They'll Have the Money for It," Business Insider, April 30, 2020.

49. T. J. Rosenthal, "It's Time to Cancel the Rent," *The Nation*, May 29, 2020.

50. M. Axel-Lute, "Ilhan Omar Proposes Bill to Cancel Rent, Mortgage Payments During Pandemic", Shelterforce, April 17, 2020.

51. Senator Elizabeth Warren, "Warren, Ocasio-Cortez to Introduce Pandemic Anti-Monopoly Act," Press Release, April 28, 2020.

52. W. J. Barber and J. Kennedy, "The Pandemic Changed Our Definition of 'Essential.' Will We Act on What We Learned?" *The Washington Post*, April 27, 2020.

53. A. Tomer and J. W. Kane, "How to Protect Essential Workers during COVID-19," Brookings, March 31, 2020.

54. *Examining Liability during the COVID-19 Pandemic before the US Senate, Committee on the Judiciary*, 117th Cong. (2020), Rebecca Dixon, National Employment Law Project, https://www.judiciary.senate.gov/imo/media/doc/Dixon%20Testimony.pdf.

55. Saru Jayaraman, "'We're Not Going Back!' The Fight for Unemployed Restaurant Workers," interview with Jon Lovett, *Lovett or Leave It*, Crooked Media, April 10, 2020, https://www.youtube.com/watch?v=Zciney19aww.

CHAPTER 9

1. O. Raimonde, "The Number of Workers on Strike Hits the Highest since the 1980s," CNBC, October 21, 2019.

2. S. Lyford, "A Civic Duty to Improve Access to Generic Pharmaceuticals. Health Affairs Blog," September 26, 2019.

3. W. H. Wiist, "Citizens United, Public Health, and Democracy: The Supreme Court Ruling, Its Implications, and Proposed Action," *American Journal of Public Health* 101, no. 7 (2011): 1172–79.

4. L. Rutkow and S. P. Teret, "Role of State Attorneys General in Health Policy," *JAMA* 304, no. 12 (2010): 1377–78.

5. V. Pickard, "The Strange Life and Death of the Fairness Doctrine: Tracing the Decline of Positive Freedoms in American Policy Discourse," *International Journal of Communication* 12 (2018): 20.

6. P. J. Cooper, *The War against Regulation: From Jimmy Carter to George W. Bush* (Lawrence: University Press of Kansas, 2009).

7. "Tracking Deregulation in the Trump Era," Brookings, 2020.

8. Gallup Poll, "Taxes, Opinions on Fair Share in Federal Taxes, 2005–2019," n.d., https://news.gallup.com/poll/1714/taxes.aspx.

9. "Public Health Awakened: Transforming the Narrative on Taxes," 2018, https://publichealthawakened.com/wp-content/uploads/2018/03/PHA_TaxNarratives_2018.03_fin.pdf.

10. A. Hendrie, "Democrats Want to Repeal Most Important Part of Trump's Tax Cuts," *Washington Examiner*, February 15, 2020.

11. S. Greenhut, "Unions Aiming to Repeal California's Property Tax Caps," *Reason*, September 6, 2019, https://reason.com/2019/09/06/teachers-unions-aiming-to-repeal-californias-property-tax-caps/.

12. E. Saez and G. Zucman, "Progressive Wealth Taxation," Brookings Papers on Economic Activity, 2019.

13. B. Virjee, "Stimulating the Future of Superfund: Why the American Recovery and Reinvestment Act Calls for a Reinstatement of the Superfund Tax to Polluted Sites in Urban Environments," *Sustainable Development Law & Policy* 11, no. 1 (2011): 12.

14. E. Williams and S. Waxman, "States Can Adopt or Expand Earned Income Tax Credits to Build a Stronger Future Economy," Center on Budget and Policy Priorities, 2017.

15. M. A. Eisner, *Regulatory Politics in an Age of Polarization and Drift: Beyond Deregulation* (Abingdon, Oxfordshire: Routledge, 2017).

16. J. L. Pomeranz and M. Pertschuk, "State Preemption: A Significant and Quiet Threat to Public Health in the United States," *American Journal of Public Health* 107, no. 6 (2017): 900–902.

17. C. Roelofs, S. L. Baron, W. Sacoby, and A. Aaron, *Occupational and Environmental Health: Equity and Social Justice.* Occupational and Environmental Health (Oxford: Oxford University Press, 2017), 23–40.

18. United Nations Department of Economic and Social Affairs, 2018 Revision of World Urbanization Prospects, May 16, 2018.

19. J. D. Goodman, "Amazon Scraps New York Campus," *New York Times*, February 15, 2019.

20. D. Geen, "'We Shouldn't Be Inviting Bullies to Our Neighborhood': Alexandria Ocasio-Cortez Defends Her Criticism of Amazon HQ2 in Surprise Queens Appearance," Business Insider, March 20, 2019.

21. B. R. Barber, *If Mayors Ruled the World: Dysfunctional Nations, Rising Cities* (New Haven, CT: Yale University Press, 2013); N. Luangrath and L. S. Wen, "The Role of US Mayors and Health Commissioners in Combatting Health Disparities," *American Journal of Public Health* 108, no. 5 (2018): 588–89; H. P. Aust, "The Shifting Role of Cities in the Global Climate Change Regime: From Paris to Pittsburgh and Back?" *Review of European, Comparative & International Environmental Law (RECIEL)* 28, no. 1 (2019): 57–66.

22. J. Tobias, "Meet the Rising New Housing Movement that Wants to Create Homes for All," *The Nation*, May 24, 2018.

23. J. K. Leon, "Sanctuary Cities in an Age of Resistance," *The Progressive*, February 22, 2017.

24. K. Reynolds and N. Cohen, *Beyond the Kale: Urban Agriculture and Social Justice Activism in New York City* (Athens: University of Georgia Press, 2016).

25. J. Bryant, "'Privatization Is Going to Kill This City': How Progressives are Fighting the Plot to Gut Public Education," AlterNet, April 26, 2019.

26. J. J. L. Candel, "What's on the Menu? A Global Assessment of MUFPP Signatory Cities' Food Strategies," *Agroecology and Sustainable Food Systems* 44, no. 7 (2019): 1–28.

27. C. E. Smith, "Gun Policy: Politics and Pathways of Action," *Violence and Gender* 7, no. 2 (2020): 40–46.

28. The Medicines Patent Pool (MPP) is a United Nations–backed public health organization working to increase access to, and facilitate the development of, life-saving medicines for low- and middle-income countries. See https:// medicinespatentpool.org/.

29. A. Green, "Q&A: James Love on the Biggest Challenges in the Fight for Affordable Drugs," Devex, November 4, 2019.

30. J. H. Marks, *The Perils of Partnership: Industry Influence, Institutional Integrity, and Public Health* (New York: Oxford University Press, 2019).

31. M. A. Rodwin, "Conflicts of Interest in Medicine: Should We Contract, Conserve, or Expand the Traditional Definition and Scope of Regulation," *Journal of Health Care Law and Policy* 21 (2018): 157–87; R. R. Saleh, H. Majeed, A. Tibau, C. M. Booth, and E. Amir, "Undisclosed Financial Conflicts of Interest among Authors of American Society of Clinical Oncology Clinical Practice Guidelines," *Cancer* 125, no. 22 (2019): 4069–75.

32. S. Krimsky, *Conflicts of Interest in Science: How Corporate-funded Academic Research Can Threaten Public Health* (New York: Simon & Schuster, 2019).

33. Charles Perkins Centre, "Engagement with Industry Guidelines," 2016, https://sydney. edu.au/perkins/documents/cpc_engagement_with_industry_guidelines_2016.pdf.

34. D. V. Evans, D. M. Hartung, G. Andeen et al., "One Practice's Experiment in Refusing Detail Rep Visits," *Journal of Family Practice* 60, no. 8 (2011): E1–6.

35. J. Waterson, "Junk Food Ad Ban on London Transport to Take Effect in February," *Guardian*, November 23, 2018.

36. M. Bergen, "YouTube Plans to End Targeted Ads on Videos Aimed at Kids," Bloomberg, August 20, 2019.

37. K. E. Warner, "Selling Health: A Media Campaign against Tobacco," *Journal of Public Health Policy* 7, no. 4 (1986): 434–39.

38. San Diegans for Gun Violence Prevention, "The Activism Marathon," September 23, 2019, https://sd4gvp.org/the-activism-marathon/.

39. G. Mahood, "Tobacco Industry Denormalization: Telling the Truth about the Tobacco Industry's Role in the Tobacco Epidemic," Non-Smokers' Rights Association, 2004, 4–17.

40. J. H. Marks, *The Perils of Partnership: Industry Influence, Institutional Integrity, and Public Health* (New York: Oxford University Press, 2019); I. Hernandez-Aguado and G. A. Zaragoza, "Support of Public-Private Partnerships in Health Promotion and Conflicts of Interest," *BMJ Open* 6, no. 4 (2016): e009342; L. Parker, G Zaragoza, I. Hernández-Aguado I. Promoting population health with public-private partnerships: Where's the evidence?. BMC public health.19(1): 1438, 2019.

41. Ibid.

42. M. Nestle, *Soda Politics: Taking on Big Soda (and Winning)* (New York: Oxford University Press, 2015).

43. K. Buse and A. Waxman, "Public-private Health Partnerships: A Strategy for WHO," *Bulletin of the World Health Organization* 79 (2001): 748–54.

44. K. Lee and J. Smith, "The Role of the Business Sector in Global Health Politics," *The Oxford Handbook of Global Health Politics*, ed. C. McInnes, K. Lee, and J. Youde, 387 (Oxford: Oxford University Press, 2019).

45. J. H. Marks, *The Perils of Partnership: Industry Influence, Institutional Integrity, and Public Health* (New York: Oxford University Press, 2019),. 142.

46. Ibid., 102.

47. S. A. Bialous, "Impact of Implementation of the WHO FCTC on the Tobacco Industry's Behaviour," *Tobacco Control* 28, Supplement 2 (2019): s94–96.

48. S. L. Steele, A. B. Gilmore, M. McKee, and D. Stuckler, "The Role of Public Law-based Litigation in Tobacco Companies' Strategies in High-income, FCTC Ratifying Countries, 2004–14," *Journal of Public Health* 38, no. 3 (2016): 516–21.

49. *Corporations in the Global Food System and Human Rights: Report of the Oslo Conference 11–12 September 2014*, ed. K. Kjæret, A. Eide, W. B. Eide (Oslo: University of Oslo Department of Nutrition and Norwegian Centre for Human Rights), 74, https://www.jus.uio.no/smr/english/research/projects/fohrc/absolute-final-report-from-september-conference_22may2015_korrwbe_26mai-(2).pdf.

50. K. Cullerton, J. Adams, N. Forouhi, O. Francis, and M. White, "What Principles Should Guide Interactions between Population Health Researchers and the Food Industry? Systematic Scoping Review of Peer-reviewed and Grey Literature," *Obesity Reviews* 20, no. 8 (2019): 1073–84; A. Poli, F. Marangoni, C. V. Agostoni et al., "Research Interactions between Academia and Food Companies: How to Improve Transparency and Credibility of an Inevitable Liaison," *European Journal of Nutrition* 57, no. 3 (2018): 1269–73; UK Health Forum, *Public Health and the Food and Drinks Industry: The Governance and Ethics of Interaction. Lessons from Research, Policy and Practice*, 2018.

51. C. S. Brunt, "Physician Characteristics, Industry Transfers, and Pharmaceutical Prescribing: Empirical Evidence from Medicare and the Physician Payment Sunshine Act," *Health Services Research* 54, no. 3 (2019): 636–49.

52. N. Freudenberg, "Public Health Advocacy to Change Corporate Practices: Implications for Health Education Practice and Research," *Health Education & Behavior* 32, no. 3 (2005): 298–319.

53. Fossil Free, "Fossil Fuel Divestment Movement Victory," n.d., https://gofossilfree.org/usa/divest-usa/.

54. A. Lappé, "The Soda Industry's Creepy Youth Campaign," Al Jazeera, August 5, 2015.

55. Corporate Accountability International, "Clowning with Kids' Health: The Case for Ronald McDonald's Retirement," 2017.

56. C. Sittenfeld, "No-Brands-Land," *Fast Company*, August 31, 2000, https://www.fastcompany.com/41238/no-brands-land.

57. Mahood, "Tobacco Industry Denormalization," 4–17.

58. Restaurant Opportunities Center United, "Taking the High Road: A How-to Guide for Successful Restaurant Employers," 2012, https://rocunited.org/publications/taking-the-high-road-a-how-to-guide-for-successful-restaurant-employers-2/.

59. N. Bryner and M. Hankins, "Why California Gets to Write Its Own Auto Emissions Standards: 5 Questions Answered," The Conversation, April 6, 2018.

INDEX

Breast Cancer Advisory Center, 147–48
breastfeeding, 59–60, 62, 324
Breast Implant Illness and Healing, 148
Brecher, Jeremy, 20
Brennan, William, 197
Brier, Stephen, 87
Brigada Ramona Parra, 279f
Bristol-Myers Squibb, 133–34
British Medical Journal, 62
Broad, Eli, 93, 94f
Broder, Samuel, 145, 180–81
Brookings Institution, 178
Brown, Tina, 177
buen vivir, 278–79, 279f
Buffett, Warren, 37–38
bullying on social media, 239–40
Bureau of Mines shutdown (1995), 155
Burger King, 57, 59
Burns, Lawrence, 217
Buse, K., 320
Bush, George H. W., 28
Bush, George W., 28, 67, 106–7,
    143–44, 313
Bush, Vannevar: *Science the Endless
    Frontier*, 32
Business Roundtable Statement on
    Corporate Governance, 22–23
Butz, Earl, 70

California
    drive services organized in, 194–95
    early child care in, 114–15
    education austerity measures
        in, 86–87
    family leave in, 193–94
    Navient sued by, 120
California Air Resources Board (CARB),
    226–29, 306–7, 325
Camp, Garrett, 169
Campaign for a Commercial-Free
    Childhood, 256–57
Canada. *See also* NAFTA; United States-
    Mexico-Canada Agreement
    global food corporations in, 70
    GoFundMe campaigns from cancer
        patients, 141
    patent and intellectual property
        protection in, 33
    ultra-processed food and drink
        consumption in, 46

cancel culture, 317
cancer. *See also specific types*
    activism against corporate care
        for, 147–50
    air pollution and, 127, 180–81, 219
    alternative treatments for, 141–42
    capitalism and, 148–49, 150–52
    control and prevention of, 126–28
    costs of care for, 10, 133–43,
        134f, 151–52
    diet and, 47, 48
    Monsanto's Roundup and, 64
    oncology practices and, 130–32
    palm oil and, 65
    patient advocacy groups, 138
    pesticides and, 186
    precision medicine and, 128–30
    scientific research and, 31
    war on cancer, 151
    "war on" policy approaches to, 143–
        47, 151, 273
CancerCare, 133
Cancer Moonshot Blue Ribbon
    Panel, 145
cap and trade policies, 228
capitalism
    cancer care under, 148–49, 150–52
    corporations' role in, 12–15
    dissatisfaction with, 8–12, 38–39, 299
    education under, 84–104
    financialization and, 21–23
    food sector under, 69–71
    globalization and, 17–20
    ideological influence and, 30,
        35–39, 92
    market concentration and monopoly
        and, 23–25, 53
    mass consumption and, 15–17
    neoliberal agenda and, 25–31, 306–7
    science/technology discoveries
        and, 31–35
    social movements targeting, 269–70,
        275–78, 318–19
    transportation under, 198, 216–17
    types of, 12–13
    well-being undermined by, 15,
        129–30, 278
    work under, 172–75
Caputo-Pearl, Alex, 117–18
carcinogens, 127, 145, 151

labor strategy of, 156–65,
176–77, 188
resistance and alternatives to, 74–76,
160*f*, 190–91
supervision and scheduling at,
161–62, 182–83
training at, 162
work conditions of, 158–59
Walton, Sam, 157
Walton Foundation, 93, 95
Wardynski, Casey, 109
Warren, Elizabeth, 255, 263–64, 294
Waxman, A., 320
Waymo, 211, 236
WeChat, 235
Welch, Gilbert, 146
welfare state, 15–16
well-being. *See also* healthcare;
mental health
capitalism and, 6–8, 276, 296, 297,
304–5, 309
democracy and, 250
education and, 91, 122
global food system and, 43
imagining priorities for,
270–72, 325–26
news media and, 252–53
social connections and, 237–44
social institutions and, 6–8
social movements unified
through, 278–86
transportation and, 215
work and, 153, 154, 180, 182, 184,
196, 286–87
Welle, Ben, 217
WellPoint, 149–50
Wendy's, 58
West Virginia teachers' strike
(2018), 117
WeWork, 291
Whitebook, Marcy, 100
white nationalism and white supremacy,
87, 93, 95, 312–13
Whittle, Chris, 89
Whole Foods, 233, 236
Wiist, William, 29–30
will.i.am, 6
Williamson, Ben, 90–91
Wilmar (food conglomerate), 66,
77, 78–79

Wilson, Bee: *The Way We Eat Now*, 45
Wolff, Michael, 248
women
cancer and, 124, 151–52
child care and, 97, 114
COVID-19 and, 296
gender hierarchies, 274–75,
280, 316–17
leadership development and, 317–18
mass consumption and, 15–16
#MeToo movement and, 275, 304
wage gender gap and, 187
Walmart and, 163–64
work and, 91, 179, 180, 185–86, 187–
88, 194, 287–88
work, 153–96. *See also* independent
contractors
autonomous vehicles and, 214
capitalism's evolution, effect of,
172–75, 180
civil rights movements and, 193–94
contingent labor, 176
deaths of despair and, 188–90
discrimination, 162–64, 181
exposures through, 179,
180–81, 185–87
family conflict with, 174, 181, 187–88
financialization of, 172–74, 176–77
gig economy and, 177–78 (*see also* gig
economy)
grass-roots activism, 193
health inequalities in, 180–81
health risks, exposures to, 127,
179, 180–81
heart diseases and, 184–85
hiring processes, 183
industrialization and, 154, 155
low-wage labor and, 178–81 (*see also*
low-wage labor)
manufacturing, 172–73, 175
mental health and, 181–84, 187
minimum wage, 97, 154–55, 179, 182,
193–96, 261, 295–96, 301
new types of, 175–80
precarious employment, 176
preemption as anti-labor
strategy, 195–96
race and, 155, 185–86, 290
resistance and alternatives in, 190–96,
270, 301

work (*cont.*)
   service sector, 175, 178
   sick leave, 193–94
   stock buybacks and, 158
   surveillance of employees, 157–58,
      161–62, 164
   US policy developments in, 153–56
   wage theft, 194–95
   women employees (*see* women)
   worker centers and independent
      worker organizations, 191–93
   working conditions, effect on
      health, 180–85
worker cooperatives, 286–91, 311
World Bank, 67, 68–69
World Health Assembly, 60
World Health Organization
   on cancer causes, 127
   on chronic conditions, 10
   COVID-19 response of, 20
   on food for infants and toddlers, 76
   on intellectual property rights to
      medicine, 34

   on palm oil, 78
   on traffic deaths, 218–19
World Social Forum, 275
World Trade Organization (WTO), 18,
   20, 33, 134–35, 325
Wu, Tim, 4, 24, 247, 248, 251, 253, 262
Wyatt, Tom, 99
Wyden, Ron, 263–64

X, Malcolm, 272

Yalow, Elanna, 104
Yervoy (cancer drug), 133–34
Yglesias, Matthew, 162
Young, Kevin, 149
YouTube, 232, 255–57
Yum! Brands, 70–71

Zappos, 233
Zoom, 236
Zuboff, Shoshana, 231
Zuckerberg, Mark, 37–38, 234, 251, 252,
   263–64